BENEATH THE WHITE COAT

DOCTORS, THEIR MINDS
AND MENTAL HEALTH

T0172415

BENEATH THE WHITE COAT

DOCTORS, THEIR MINDS AND MENTAL HEALTH

EDITED BY

CLARE GERADA

Medical Director of the Practitioner Health Programme
London, UK

WITH EDITORIAL CONTRIBUTIONS FROM

ZAID AL-NAJJAR

Deputy Medical Director of the Practitioner Health Service
London, UK

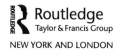

Routledge
Taylor & Francis Group

NEW YORK AND LONDON

First published 2021
by Routledge
52 Vanderbilt Avenue, New York, NY 10017

and by Routledge
2 Park Square, Milton Park, Abingdon, Oxon OX14 4RN

Routledge is an imprint of the Taylor & Francis Group, an informa business

© 2021 Taylor & Francis

Library of Congress Control Number: 2020946034

ISBN: 978-1-138-49981-2 (hbk)
ISBN: 978-1-138-49973-7 (pbk)
ISBN: 978-1-351-01415-1 (ebk)

Typeset in Minion
by Newgen Publishing UK

Contents

Acknowledgements

Writing this book has been a joy, as it has made me reflect on the service that I set up over a decade ago (Practitioner Health). I never intended to be running a mental health service for health practitioners, but I suppose it was inevitable given my background in mental health, medico-legal work and caring for those with addiction. After the interview for the service – which included the biggest interview panel I have ever been at – I really thought I would not get the contract. So sure was I that I had failed in my endeavour that I deleted all references to Practitioner Health Programme (as it was then called) from my computer! I am pleased that my negative prediction did not come true and as such, the first people I must thank are those who trusted me with the formidable task of leading such a service. This includes Rosemary Field and Alastair Scotland. Those first few weeks mobilising the service were frenetic – everything had to be built from scratch and I could not have done it without Lucy Warner – who has stayed with the service ever since and Jane Black. I must also thank all the 200 or so staff who work in the service and have what Jane once named 'It' – the 'It' being a desire to really care for patients, to really put them first and to really hold their needs in mind.

Of course, in writing this book I have drawn on connections I have had with the many thousands of doctors who have attended the service. Thank you all for having the courage and faith to come forward for help. Thank you to the patient group for all your help and guidance, to the members of the Bereavement group for your wisdom – what an amazing group of people you all are, that even in the time of immense grief you reach out to others to help them.

I would like to thank Morris Nitsun for his invaluable support over the years, my sons, Alex and Ben for their patience and love and last, but by no means least, my husband Simon Wessely who has been my rock, my inspiration, my love for nearly 35 years.

Contributors

Mary Doherty, MBChB, FCARCSI
Consultant Anaesthetist
Our Lady's Hospital, Navan
Meath, Ireland

Richard Duggins, MBBS, MRCPsych
Clinical Lead Regional Department of
Psychotherapy, Clinical Lead (North East
and Cumbria)
NHS Practitioner Health
Cumbria, Northumberland, Tyne and Wear
NHS Foundation Trust
Newcastle upon Tyne, UK

Richard Jones, RMN, MSc, BSc, MAREBT
Clinical Director, Mental Health Nurse and
Cognitive Behaviour Therapist
NHS Practitioner Health
Surrey, UK

Sandy Miles, MA, MSc, MBBS, MRCGP
General Practitioner
St Andrew's Surgery
Eastleigh, UK

Isa Ouwehand, BSc, MBBS
Academic Foundation Programme
Trainee
Greater Glasgow and Clyde, UK

Shivanthi Sathanandan, BSc, MBBS, MRCPsych
Consultant Psychiatrist, Addiction Specialist
Camden & Islington Foundation
London, UK

Caroline Walker, MbChB, BSc (MedSci), MRCPsych, PGDip (CBT)
Psychiatrist and Therapist
NHS Practitioner Health
Surrey, UK

Amy Wilson, BMedSci
Medical Student
Sheffield Medical School
Sheffield, UK

Preface

I had to write this book. I needed to try to understand why everywhere one looks, whether in the medical or mainstream press, conference circuit or academic literature, we seem to be in the midst of a crisis of mental illness among the medical profession. Survey after survey has identified that doctors have high levels of burnout, depression and even suicidal behaviour. Many are seeking to leave almost as soon as they have started their career, others are hanging up their stethoscope years before they reach formal retirement age.

Given my role as 'the doctors' doctor' I am in the position, perhaps more than most, to try to make sense of this despair. Since 2008 I have been running a service for doctors with mental illness when I won the contract to deliver the first and only physician health service in the UK NHS. Starting in London, over the years it has expanded to include all doctors across England, meaning that around 180,000 doctors can access my confidential, Practitioner Health Service, and around 3,000 do per year. The catalyst for the service being set up at all was the suicide of a young psychiatrist, Daksha Emson, who killed her three-month-old baby before she killed herself. She, as with other doctors with mental illness, did not have different illnesses from their patients. Most who have come to my service have presented with depression, anxiety and symptoms indistinguishable from post-traumatic stress disorder. Others have problems with substance misuse and a smaller number have, as with Daksha, bipolar disorder or other psychotic illnesses. While the specific proportions may differ, nevertheless, the most common conditions doctors suffer with are those that afflict the general population, namely depression and anxiety disorders.

Where doctors do differ is how, when and why (or more often, why not) they present for care. They often present late or in crisis or following a drink-drive offence. Sadly, for some, especially anaesthetists with substance misuse disorder, the first indication that there is a problem is when they accidently or intentionally kill themselves. The Inquiry following Daksha's and her daughter's death brought to the fore the problems doctors face accessing healthcare, especially for their mental illness. I have seen first-hand the shame many feel just accepting that they might need help. I have seen their fear that if they admit to having a mental illness, this will impact on their career. And I have seen the embarrassment that other doctors have when treating colleagues.

There are other reasons why doctors find it so difficult to accept help. How doctors are trained, in particular how they become socialised in their profession and in doing so accept the unwritten rules of the medical community, especially that they should not become unwell, adds to their risk. This socialisation begins well before doctors reach medical school and resonates with my own personal experience. My life is intertwined with those I write about, well and sick. I share their same foundation, a common ground connecting doctors together, past, present and even into the future. I have a lot invested in medicine and for me, as for many of my colleagues, being a doctor is more than just something I *do*, but something I *am*.

My most memorable moments are tied up with medicine. Getting into University College Hospital, passing finals and being able to use the title 'Dr'; obtaining my GP partnership and winning the contract to provide the sick doctor service. Each day of supporting, treating, diagnosing, being a witness to and just being a doctor has been fulfilling and deeply humbling. I believe that it is this identification with medicine that makes it so difficult for me to become a patient – to literally and metaphorically remove my surgical scrubs and stethoscope and replace them with the patient's gown. Doctors are meant to put others first, to sacrifice their own needs to those of their patient and to make the patient their first concern. Illness is frowned upon and doctors are more likely to go to work when unwell than take time off – presenteeism is more of an issue than absenteeism. This has certainly been my experience. As with my doctor-patients, I have experienced personal, professional and institutional stigma when it comes to accepting that I might be sick. Even when unwell with a broken foot, having just been knocked off my bike, I nevertheless turned up for work, finishing my evening clinic despite the pain, and not for one moment thinking I could ask to go home early. I have shunned help from others and have preferred to suffer in silence than accept I have the same vulnerabilities as my patients, even when, as inevitably happens over the course of one's career, I have suffered from mental health problems. Society puts doctors on a pedestal and the medical culture reinforces this state of elevation. Our bio-medical approach to the doctor–patient relationship takes as a given that the doctor has authority and status of being all-knowing. It is no surprise therefore, that some doctors, me included, view ourselves as invincible and super-human. Hopefully this is now changing as the next generation of doctors have a healthier attitude towards their own weaknesses than previous generations.

Unhappy doctors are not new. In the book I quote from a first-person account given by a Russian doctor at the beginning of the 20th century. He found his work intolerable and talked of the toll of working in the public hospital on his and his colleagues' mental health (with one in ten dying by their own hand). The key emotional drivers for this unhappiness then, as they are now, were shame and stigma associated with disclosing that one might be vulnerable and in need of help.

Given that I am human after all, I have had over the years to move from the authoritative, powerful doctor to the vulnerable patient. This is a giant leap for most doctors to make and I have written about this from a personal as well as professional perspective. I hope that I have made this transition easier by setting up my service, which understands the barriers doctors face when trying to become patients; many of these are self-imposed, though some are put in place by the culture to show no weakness, as well as due to the problems associated with being in a regulated profession. Services that are particularly tailored for doctors are few and far between, but where they do exist, they ensure mentally ill doctors make remarkable recoveries. I compare my service to the more probation-like North American models, giving outcome data along the way.

Even among the medical profession there are some who suffer more than others. I have tried to compare data on different specialities and their risks, though making any meaningful comparisons is a hostage to fortune given the paucity of research and where it does exist, its poor standard, and also give my views based on my experience of now caring for more than 11,000 doctors from different specialities.

I include a chapter looking specifically at the issues facing doctors who undertook their primary medical qualification overseas (International Medical Graduates). These doctors, as with my father, came to seek excitement, a better life and to help their new host country. The vast majority go on to thrive. But we know a significant minority suffer from discrimination and are disproportionately the recipients of regulatory and employment sanctions.

Medical students have always had high rates of mental illness and while this book is about doctors, not including something on the future profession would have left a large gap.

Throughout the years I have also cared for doctors who have transgressed their professional code. There is of course a significant overlap between doctors with mental illness and involvement in regulatory or disciplinary processes. Around 10% of doctors in my service are involved in regulatory procedures, mostly split into two main groups. Those who have had problems relating to drink or drugs – they might have had a drink-drive offence or been caught stealing drugs from work – or they have been involved in behaviour that has drawn them to the attention of the regulator and sought help. I have seen so many doctors become depressed as they progress through a disciplinary process that can take years to complete. Sadly, suicide is a real risk in those doctors who have received a complaint. This is why I have included a section in this book on the basics of the regulatory processes, as it is amazing how few doctors know anything about the workings of the General Medical Council. I also provide some practical advice on how to respond if involved in an investigation.

The vast majority of doctors do not just survive in their job but thrive. This is certainly the case for me over the decades. I have drawn on internal resources, conscious coping and unconscious ego-defence mechanisms. This is probably linked to resilience, which is a complicated area and increasingly used to put the blame on the individual for 'not coping' rather than the system for being unsafe.

This book has been largely written by doctors for doctors. However, I am hoping that the themes I touch on are transferable across the medical profession to any vocational group, such as nurses, social workers, psychological and therapists. Many of the issues are the same – fear of admitting vulnerability, being part of a regulated profession and lack of confidentiality. I hope whichever speciality or area of healthcare you are working in that you enjoy this book.

Royalties for this book are being donated to Doctors in Distress, a registered charity established to support all health professionals and to reduce stigma around mental illness so as to prevent burn-out and suicide of those who care for us.

https://doctors-in-distress.org.uk/about-us/

Charity Registration Numbers: England & Wales (1184953) Scotland (SC049715)

SECTION I

The Making of a Doctor

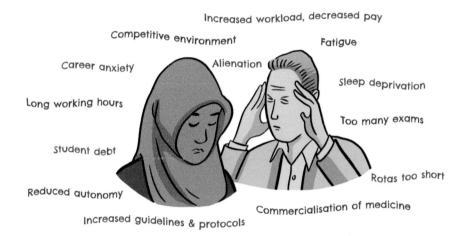

The Making of a Doctor
Medical Self and Group of Belonging

CLARE GERADA

> *Please accept my resignation. I don't want to belong to any club that would accept me as a member.*
>
> **Groucho Marx**

Becoming a doctor involves more than just absorbing the huge volume of information needed to diagnose and treat disease. Doctors have to learn the rules, customs and practices of the profession, evolved over millennia. From the first day at medical school, students have to understand these rules, and in so doing, become part of their chosen group or tribe, 'medicine'. This learning happens not just in the formal lectures, ward rounds or tutorials, but as part of the informal, hidden, uncodified curriculum that happens in the spaces in-between. Individuals are taught to conform to ways of behaving, speaking and dressing; importantly, they also learn and adopt the rules of self-sacrifice. Individuals are largely unaware of this process and how, during it, they take on the persona of 'the doctor'.

'*What do you do?*' is something we ask when introduced to someone for the first time. What we do, by which we mean what *work* do we do, is vital to our identity. For doctors the medical identity is immensely strong, both in terms of the individual as a clinician (doctor) and as a group (medicine). Combined, they create the total professional – **the doctor**. The person and the profession become so intertwined that many doctors, even when retired or unable to work, still use the title 'Dr'. As one of my patients told me, '*a doctor is something you are, not something that you do*'. While this identity helps to ensure they are able to do the job the public expects of them, it also explains the powerful barriers to them seeking and accessing help when needed.

In this chapter, I discuss the formation of doctors' individual and collective identities. Later chapters will unpick various aspects of these concepts and how they are related to the doctor's ability to do their job but also to their vulnerability towards mental illness.

THE MEDICAL SELF

Medicine is still one of the most respected and prestigious professions, with the elevated status of the healer being a common theme cross-culturally and across time. Despite the current difficulties of working as a doctor, places at medical school are still considerably oversubscribed and prospective candidates work hard to show they have the right credentials to obtain entry. Before gaining a place, students have already become inculcated into what it means 'to be a doctor' and this process continues throughout their training. During this time individuals become transformed into the final product, the doctor. The first transformation that occurs is to the individual's sense of self, their core identity. The 'medical self' is a term first used by the North American physician Robert Klitzman in his book *When Doctors Become Patients*[1] and later expanded by Alex Wessely in his work *Why Doctors Make Good Addicts and Bad Patients.*[2] Wessely describes the merging of the professional and personal aspects of the individual doctor to form a single, medical self. The medical self, in fact any 'self', is made up of several identities that change depending on the social situation, and is determined by the world in which we live and by the groups (family, work and wider cultural and social groups) of which we are part.

By way of example, I decided to become a doctor largely because of my late father, who was a general practitioner (GP). Like many doctors in the 1960s, he came as a foreigner to work in the struggling National Health Service. His surgery was our home; what was the living room in the evening became the patient's waiting room by day; the dining room doubled as his consulting room. I learnt to tiptoe upstairs, and I still have vivid memories of peering over the balcony, staring down at the rather plump ladies, all wearing hats and holding screaming babies. Each room in our home was full of the trappings of medicine: textbooks, trade magazines, medical equipment, records and even a full skeleton. Long car journeys were enlivened by my father talking about his experiences in Nigeria when he was posted there as Medical Officer of Health during his long spell working in the Colonial Service. Even when I was young, he would take me on home visits, and from the privileged standpoint of the doctor's daughter I saw poverty and the effects of social deprivation and inequalities. Despite having no medical training, I became the 'embryonic doctor', and friends would seek me out to ask about their health issues. My father stood out as the local GP, priest-like in the reverence he received from patients and the local community. So too did I stand out. The more patients entered my personal space, the more I separated from them. I became and felt different. Unconsciously I defined myself as 'the doctor's daughter'. My personal identity began to incorporate that of other doctors. I answered the phone with authority, abandoning my name and instead giving myself the title of 'Dr Gerada's daughter'. This example gives an illustration of the insidious nature of internalising an identity and particular values, such as being able to maintain confidentiality and being aware of having to behave in an 'appropriate manner' as the daughter of the doctor. Finally, and perhaps most interestingly, learning to make sacrifices, in this instance, personal spaces at home.

Even before arriving at medical school, either implicitly or explicitly, I saw myself as different from others, and I was not alone among my peers in this. Medical school does nothing to disabuse the medical student of this air of 'specialness'. With our longer, more onerous and specific training, our identity is moulded, through the norms and narratives set by relationships with other doctors and patients, into the final product of 'the doctor'. Specialness is reinforced during training as doctors learn a new language, wear new clothes (for me, it was the short white coat as a medical student, moving onto a long white coat post qualification) and carrying the stethoscope (often slung around the neck in a conspicuous way). During medical school, students learn the art of compartmentalising, being able to cognitively partition different aspects of their life. The long training and vast knowledge needed to be assimilated leads to the 'scientising' of the 'self, creating an exclusive cognitive identity, and the finished product (the doctor) as a person embodying knowledge, certainty and authority. Once qualified, the transformation is complete as doctors acquire the new name, 'Dr'. All of these outward symbols register the individual as 'a doctor', but the unseen, internal feelings (power, authority, invincibility) are just as important in creating this identity. The medical self, 'who I am', emerges.

Doctors, like everyone else, have conflicting identities for different times and contexts, being at work or at home, with family or with patients, being a doctor or being a patient. The core 'medical self', however, is particularly strong and pervasive. It is this self that the doctor presents to the outside world and guides them through the 'performances' of their career. Its omnipresence means the work/life balance of a doctor is disrupted: doctors find it hard to leave their working identity at the hospital gate or consulting room door and find it difficult not to adopt an identity other than that of 'the doctor'. This is often evident at social events, where they tend to huddle together, finding each other as if by RADAR among the crowds. Personally, I live and work in the same area and rarely leave the role of 'local GP' even when behind the confines of my own front door, since many of my friends and my children's friends are current or ex-patients and seek me out for advice. While my close contact with patients might be unusual, what is not is the expectation that doctors inhabit their professional role at all times, in all places and can be called upon by friends, family or strangers to offer help. They are, as such, never 'not a doctor'. They are expected to take on the role of the 'good Samaritan'. Over time, therefore, the individual and the doctor become indistinguishable from each other. I can no more take the doctor out of myself than an artist can cast off their creativity; the two are inextricably linked. It is the medical self, which acts, during work, to mask suffering and protects doctors from subjective feelings of guilt, fear and hopelessness.

The 'medical self' acts as a necessary and mature defence mechanism, allowing doctors to cope with close contact with death, despair and disability. However, the 'medical self' can, and often does, get out of hand, especially when not counterbalanced by a healthy working environment or personal support. It can inhibit the development of empathy and limit compassion. This book is scattered with examples where doctors are so intertwined with their caring role that they are unable to pursue any other activity, with negative consequences for their mental health.

One of the best examples of the positive and negative aspects of the medical self is found in the book, *A Fortunate Man: The Story of a Country Doctor*. Written in 1967, the author John Berger gives a portrait of a GP, John Sassall. Sassall worked as a country doctor in the Forest of Dean, and Berger accompanied him on his rounds and in the surgery to produce a fly-on-the-wall account of his life and work. In Berger's book, Sassall emerges as someone who embodies all that is best about the profession. He is described as a saintly individual, 'all-knowing… haggard… and accepted by the villagers and foresters as a man who, in the full sense of the term, lives with them'.[3]

Sassall, like so many doctors, defined himself by his work. When his long-term practice partner died, instead of acquiring a new one, he chose to split the patient list and instead run the practice single-handedly. Berger's book describes how Sassall longed to be woken at night to do house calls. He was incapable of doing nothing and just 'being'. Put simply, Sassall was a workaholic, incapable of taking on any identity other than that of the doctor. His patients of course were the beneficiary of this, in that he was ever-present and available to them. He was the epitome of what many might consider to be the perfect family doctor, but not without consequence. Sassall suffered from regular bouts of depression that affected his ability to do his job properly, and there is no evidence that he sought professional help. Instead, as Berger wrote, 'Sassall needs to work in this way. He cures others to cure himself' (p. 79), becoming the classic 'wounded healer' who plays out his own wounds through his caring role rather than addressing his own psychological needs. As the 'total doctor', Sassall could not protect his patients from the impossible task of curing the incurable, a failure Sassall took personally and felt deeply. Sadly, after the death of his wife, things became too much for him and he took his own life.

THE GROUP OF BELONGING (THE COLLECTIVE SELF)

Becoming a doctor involves an increasingly narrowing network of relationships, with and within the medical establishment. Not surprisingly therefore, the second transformation that occurs during training is to doctors' collective identity.

Nina arrived just in time for the lecture. The theatre was full. Almost everyone there was a doctor and they waited in anticipation for the start of a keynote speech given by a distinguished professor who had won a prestigious prize; this was his valedictory lecture. Just before delivering his oration, he was told that among the audience of around 500 was Nina, who had just found out that she had quali-fied as a doctor. Though this was his day, his glory, he shared it with the young woman, announcing her achievement to all. The audience all stood and cheered and clapped her. She had joined their group.

In the vignette, Nina had passed through the required rite of passage by qualifying as a doctor and had joined the 'tribe' that is medicine.[4] Such rituals connect with the changes in the individual's life cycle to their attendant change in the social hierarchy, thus uniting the physical and social aspects of their biography. Rites of passage have three stages. Rituals of separation, between the medical and non-medical student, rituals of transition, that of absorbing biomedical knowledge, skills, attitudes, values and so on, and a ritual of incorporation through the swearing of the Hippocratic oath, label of 'Dr' and distinctive uniform.

Again, as with the 'medical self' this process happens gradually, reinforced as medical students and later doctors spend many hours in the bounded space of their 'total institution', where they live, work, suffer, play, learn and even love together (as many form lifelong partnerships with other doctors). Total institutions, as defined by the Canadian sociologist Erving Goffman, are places where people work and live, cut off from their wider community for considerable lengths of time, leading an enclosed life.[5] Typical examples are the old mental health institutions, prisons and boarding schools. The physically enclosed spaces of these institutions lead to divisions between 'them' and 'us' (nurses and patients, prisoners and prison officers, teachers and pupils), with other features reinforcing the differences such as admission rituals, clothing, language and so on. Medical schools are less physically confined in terms of the space created by bricks and mortar, rather more, as the anthropologist, Simon Sinclair suggests, in terms of time spent within the conceptually and cognitively limited organisation of the profession itself.[6] They therefore share many of the core features of Goffman's total institution: the student is seen as just one of a 'crowd' and training of individuals is conducted in the proximity of others. Furthermore, routines are imposed from top-down regimes and enforced by formal/informal rules and bodies of officials (bureaucracy), irrespective of whether this is best for either student or the profession.

Sinclair undertook a year-long study observing medical students and newly qualified doctors at University College London (UCL) Medical School (where I studied), writing his findings in *Making Doctors: An Institutional Apprenticeship*. For Sinclair,

> the unceasing need for medical students to work for never-ending examinations ultimately results in professional cognitive membership of the institution, of which they are an inmate (that is, the profession of medicine), a passage and a membership that may exclude the lay world just as surely as the asylum walls.

I would rather consider a more benevolent, but no less total, description of medicine's total institution, as the 'group of belonging'.

During medical school, and later when working, I became unconsciously enmeshed within my group of belonging, which has contained me ever since. I learnt about the rules of my group, even as a teenager helping my father; how, for example, never to tell what I saw or heard; how to behave in public; and how to appear confident. I held secrets concerning others, including my close friends and their families. This group linked me to the past, present and even to a future community of doctors and gave me a pre-established notion of what it meant to be a doctor. Medical school therefore creates a finished product of an individual who embodies the tremendous power that a medical education brings, manifest in how the doctor speaks, acts, writes and interacts. This has positive connotations, allowing doctors to do the job that patients demand of them, but also places extreme pressures on the doctor and their families. For many doctors, work literally and metaphorically replaces their family. The final product of 'the doctor' is immersed in their 'group of belonging' (medicine), a group strengthened by a profession that has strict hierarchies, behaviours (in and out of work), professional solidarity, cultures, norms and values built up over time. The 'group' of course is not a single entity, but a matrix of different interconnecting groups that change over time, including for myself: my dissection group, my hospital firms, my hospital ward teams, my medical trade union, my professional body, my GP partnership and so on. However, the common medical thread links each group, reinforced by trappings such as group rules, clothing (surgical scrubs, robes, chains of office) and rituals, all of which serve to strengthen group cohesion.

DOCTORS AND WORK

Given the transformations that occur during the training of a doctor, it is hardly surprising that work becomes central to their identity.

> *Richard was a senior consultant surgeon in a large teaching hospital. The hospital was in special measures, failing to meet waiting list targets and running into serious financial deficit. The hospital was run almost entirely by locums. Richard, as head of his department felt guilty that he could not meet the needs of his patients. He addressed this by taking on the workload of absent colleagues, giving patients direct access to him via his private mobile number and arriving earlier (6am) and staying longer in the department (10pm). The working hours were made worse by his hour drive to and from work each day. He became irritable, anxious and found he was drinking to help him fall asleep at night. As the workload increased, his mood deteriorated.*

Richard's attendance at my service was precipitated by a suicide attempt, designed to mimic an accident. He had crashed his car into the central reservation on the way to work. Fortunately, his airbag had saved his life and other than a few cuts and bruises he was none the worse for wear. He admitted to his partner what he had planned to do, and then made contact with my service. As with John Sassall, the protagonist of *A Fortunate Man*, Richard felt (and acted) as if it was his duty to solve the failures of his hospital single handedly and to deal personally with the problems within it. In his first appointment at the service, Richard said, 'the more I worked the more I deluded myself that I was OK'.

It is hardly surprising, given that doctors' identity is so emmeshed in their work, that presenteeism, that is, coming into work when unwell, is more of a problem among doctors than absenteeism. Presenteeism can be seen as the visible manifestation of how central work is to a doctor's identity. Doctors, as

Richard did, will work when impaired, and attempt to fulfil their responsibilities, in part driven by the shame associated with not working as well as the desire not to let their colleagues down if they are absent from work. This means that sick doctors who work harder become more entrenched within their group and 'medical self', as they take on extra hours and see more patients. This reaction becomes akin to magical thinking or manic defence, as one doctor-patient makes clear: 'I thought that if I work harder, I can't be ill, so I got in earlier and earlier to work, saw more and more patients. But in the end, it all fell apart when I crashed the car on the way to work'. It is not just doctors who work when unwell, so do teachers, police officers and these professions share many of the features discussed in this chapter.

Absence from work, especially for prolonged periods, produces a negative effect on physical and mental health, as well as professional and financial stability. Not working, especially if enforced, can lead to substantial demoralisation, depression and even suicide. Unemployed and suspended doctors are among the most isolated members of the profession, with increased risk of developing serious mental health problems. Self-stigmatisation among doctors who are not working is also common, with doctors describing themselves as failures and internalising the negative views of others. Feelings of alienation from their 'total institution' undoubtedly develop, creating a loss of identity and questioning of their sense of self and worthiness. There is a paradox. Goffman's model suggests that it is being in the total institution and the processes of institutionalising that ultimately produces loss of individuality, alienation, lack of future orientation and learned helplessness. For doctors it is being excluded from the 'institution of medicine' that produces these personal experiences, and this speaks to the depth of internalisation of the identity of being a doctor.

One doctor, Belinda Brewer, writing about her own depressive illness, tells us that,

> Being a doctor and not being able to work robs you of more than just your health. This is not just a job, being a doctor is fundamentally integrated into everything we are.[7]

For doctors, working harder means that they can hide behind the mask of legitimacy that their medical self offers. Insight into their own health condition is obscured by this mask, which protects them from the full force of what their life has become. As one patient said,

> I held onto it [being a doctor] desperately. For about three months I was only happy when I was at work. I was pulling extra shifts, staying late. I felt like I had purpose and had a meaning. Work was my crutch; I thought 'I must be alright because I'm still working'.

Amy Wilson, when still a medical student, examined doctors' narratives written when they were unwell.[8] In some, doctors talk about the struggle to find a balance between having expert scientific knowledge and the sudden influx of emotions and adversity that comes with personal illness. In other words, they find it difficult to become patients. Recurring themes are denial, self-stigmatisation, shame and concerns about their professional reputation and competence. These themes are common and will be addressed later in this book and in Chapter 2 Mental illness in doctors: a historical context. Amy Wilson's research and that in the academic literature tells us that there is an informal contract that means doctors work through illness, ignoring symptoms of distress, and expecting colleagues to do the same, summed up by one GP: 'Unless you're unable to get out of bed you'll crawl in and work'.

This lack of acceptance of personal illness results in continued denial of vulnerability, poor health-seeking behaviour, concealment of ill health and an attempt to give the illusion of an outwardly highly functioning individual. Doctors will often 'keep going' at work, even after their marriages break up, their friends disappear and their interests dwindle. They hold onto their professional role, seeing it as the *one* domain in their life in which they can exert the most influence and control and receive the validation they may perceive to be lacking elsewhere. Where these doctors run into difficulty is when the sole source of their validation as a doctor (and in their view as a human being) is threatened.

The psychiatrist Max Henderson and his colleagues interviewed doctors who were on long-term sick leave due to physical and mental health issues.[9] The main themes that emerged from their interviews was the importance of their working identity and feelings of emptiness when not at work. Being on sick leave was associated with a fundamental change in this identity, one which they perceived as 'humiliating, shameful and isolating'. When unwell and unable to work, doctors tend to blame themselves. This in turn can further worsen self-esteem and create a vicious cycle where the doctor needs work to improve their self-esteem but cannot work. Viewing themselves as a failure becomes the new identity, exacerbated by perceived negative views from colleagues. Once unwell, sick doctors feel excluded from their group of belonging (medicine). Self-stigma describes the phenomenon whereby people adopt and internalise external social stigma, experiencing loss of self-esteem and self-efficacy.[10-12] Overall, feelings of failure becomes a generalised self-perception rather than specific to the loss of the work role, and the experience of being a doctor away from work culminates in an internalised, altered sense of self. Of course, not all doctors behave in this manner. Some accept the sick role when needed, seek and adhere to the advice of others and are model patients. Sadly, though, in my experience of now overseeing the care of more than 10,000 mentally ill doctors, most find it difficult to accept they are unwell and leave it until they are in crisis before seeking help.

CONCLUSION

I hope this opening chapter begins to explain why doctors find it so difficult to accept the sick role, that the problem goes beyond the practical aspects of merely making an appointment but to the core of what it means to be a doctor. A doctor's deep-rooted attachment to their medical identity and the rules of 'belonging' to 'medicine' preclude them showing vulnerability. I will pick up many of themes as the book progresses.

REFERENCES

1 Klitzman R. *When Doctors Become Patients*. Oxford University Press, 2008.

2 Wessely A, Gerada C. When doctors need treatment: an anthropological approach to why doctors make bad patients. *BMJ* 2013;**347**:f6644. Available from: www.bmj.com/content/347/bmj.f6644

3 Berger J, Mohr J. *A Fortunate Man*. New York: Vintage, 1995.

4 Van Gennep A. *The Rites of Passage*. London: Routledge and Kegan Paul, 1960.

5 Goffman E. *Asylums; Essays on the Social Situation of Mental Patients and Other Inmates*. Garden City: Anchor Books, 1961.

6 Sinclair S. *Making Doctors*. Oxford: Berg, 1997.

7 Brewer B. Depression has many faces. In: Jones P. *Doctors as Patients*. Oxford: Radcliffe Publishing, 2005, pp. 11–13.

8 Wilson A. The art of medicine. Physician narratives of illness. *Lancet* 2019;**394**:20–21.

9 Henderson M, Brooks SK, del Busso L, *et al*. Shame! Self-stigmatisation as an obstacle to sick doctors returning to work: a qualitative study. *BMJ Open* 2012;**2**:e001776. doi:10.1136/bmjopen-2012-001776.

10 Watson A, Corrigan P, Larson J, Sells M. Self-stigma in people with mental illness. *Schizophr Bull* 2006;**33**(6):1312–18.

11 Ritsher J, Otilingam P, Grajales M. Internalized stigma of mental illness: psycho-metric properties of a new measure. *Psychiatry Research* 2003;**121**(1):31–49.

12 Schomerus G, Matschinger H, Angermeyer M. The stigma of psychiatric treatment and help-seeking intentions for depression. *Eur Arch Psychiatry Clin Neurosci* 2009;**259**(5):298–306.

2

Mental Illness in Doctors
An Historical Context

AMY WILSON

THE HEROIC PHYSICIAN IN THE NEW CENTURY

The challenges of modern medicine (long hours, the responsibility to patients and an unforgiving medical culture) are not new.[1] While contexts and societies have changed, insights into the mental health and illness of doctors can be found throughout history. During the nineteenth and early twentieth centuries, medicine existed in a different landscape: as a predominantly male and low-income profession, witnessing the rise of science and technology within a society that deeply stigmatised mental illness.[2] Much of the stoic nature of medicine was established during this time, with the Victorian stiff-upper-lip enforcing emotional repression and the ability to face adversity unscathed. Yet, dissatisfaction and disillusionment can be dated as far back as 1869. A physician lamented that: 'Medicine has ever been and is now, the most despised of all the professions which liberally-educated men are expected to enter' and advised undergraduates: 'don't study medicine.'[3]

The doctor Vikenty Veresaeff shared his struggles with medicine in his memoir, *Confessions of a Physician*.[4] Although well-received by the press and the public, *Confessions* was met with a storm of indignation from medical peers. They were unimpressed by his 'self-exploitation' to the 'lay-man'.[3] As the swift rejection would suggest, Veresaeff was in the minority of doctors in the early 1900s. For many, the medical memoir was about celebrating one's achievements and demonstrating heroism. But even in these texts, an implicit conflict appears to slip through the cracks. A sense of nervous tension, burnout and an unrelenting workload is mirrored in Francis Galton's 1908 memoir, *Memories of My Life*.[5] Galton, most well-known for his work in eugenics, also studied medicine at Cambridge. In one short paragraph, he discusses the time off he took for his health:

It was during my third year I broke down entirely in health and had to lose a term and go home. I suffered from intermittent pulse and a variety of brain symptoms of an alarming kind. A mill seemed to be working inside my head; I could not banish obsessing ideas; at times I could hardly read a book... it would have been madness to continue the kind of studious life that I had been leading... I had been too much zealous, had worked too irregularly and in too many directions, and done myself serious harm.[6]

The experience is intense and emotive, but only fleetingly discussed. Galton emphasises that the workload was simply too much, resulting in 'brain symptoms' and 'obsessing ideas', that 'a mill seemed to be working inside [his] head'. The imagery is clear, and demonstrates the significance of such a memory, contradicting the brevity if its presentation.

Providing greater insight into the pressures of medicine, it was during this era the conflict between medical professionals and their work was first examined. The earliest texts on medical sociology were published in 1894, 1902 and 1909.[6–8] McIntire states that

The labors of the physicians... would furnish a history abounding in scenes of greater self-sacrifice and permeated with more unassuming bravery than the recital of all our wars would afford.[7]

Warbasse elaborates on such sacrifice and bravery, reflecting that the medical profession fails to look beyond its peers as a whole, where the individual is but an isolated, often imperfect, human expression.[8] These are among the first discussions to critique the medical profession for an unmatched devotion and perfectionism that may lead to a sense of isolation. Further to this, we see the earliest reports on physician suicide rates. A one-page editorial published in 1897 claimed a high degree of unhappiness in the profession[9] (coincidentally the same year that Durkheim published his ground-breaking book, *Suicide*[10]).

The editorial, entitled *Suicide among physicians*, suggests that:

there [are] special reasons for discontent which apply with exaggerated force to the physician... the practice of medicine affords little in return for the demands which it makes, including no compensation of short hours and holidays... [and] many ethical and moral burdens to bear without loyal support.[9]

Despite the recognition of the demands of medicine, the exposure of 'discontent' within the profession was, once again, met by contemporary doctors with objection. Such dismissal of the challenges doctors faced at the turn of the century, and the decline of medical sociology in the subsequent decades, hints at how the vulnerability of medical professionals would be approached in the years to come.

INCREASING STATUS, INCREASING CONFLICT

Between 1903 and 1947 very few articles considering physician well-being were published.[11-14] Over this period, both medicine and society underwent significant changes. The biomedical model became fully integrated into medical practice, the NHS would be established in the UK in 1948 and healthcare would become privatised in the USA. The medical profession was gaining political and scientific prestige, providing a platform on which the heroic physician could flourish. The developing theories of Sigmund Freud introduced the idea that mental illness could exist among the general population. Suicidology shifted in light of this, now focusing on the individual, and mental health care was beginning to take shape in the form of psychiatry and psychoanalysis.

The issue of physician suicide became somewhat problematic. How could the profession protect its success and its newly earned image? In other words, if suicide was due to individual factors, how could a suicidal doctor meet the demands of the profession? In the *New York Medical Journal*, Knopf reports that medicine has 'the greatest number of suicides of all the professional classes', yet these rates are 'pathetic' – that 'one could not expect deviant colleagues who self-destructed' to be successful in medicine.[14]

The first in-depth analysis of the psychiatric well-being of physicians was conducted by Anchersen in 1947. His paper, *On the Prognosis of Narcomania*, exposed the high prevalence of drug addiction in physicians in the USA and UK.[15] Physician suicide arose again as an issue that required solution. DeSole, Singer and Aronson published a list of the reported suicide rates in physicians at this time:

> In 1950, the age-adjusted rate of physician-suicide compared to all other white males between the ages of 25–59 in America was 1.11:1;
> The rate of suicide among physicians in Great Britain is approximately two-and-a-quarter times the rate for all males.[16]

The authors discuss the cause for these high rates, suggesting that the statistics 'do not reflect a true reaction to the new social relations established as a result of socialised health services'.[16] While it may be possible that the context of these physicians contributed towards suicide risk, this explanation attributes 'social transition and stress' as the cause of suicidality. They go on to outline factors for physician suicide likened to those in the early century: an overwhelming stress, workload and role strain. Yet, their explanation wanders into the realm of individual blame, suggesting that some individuals just could not cope with the stress. Another paper published in the *BMJ* attributed the cause to 'harsh working conditions' and 'intellectual types who work under some degree of pressure'.[17] Again, there is an assumption that doctors lacked resilience. While these papers begin to address physician suicide (and the associated issues of workload and stress), the necessity of doctors to be strong and resilient overshadowed this.

Excerpts of personal experience provide a closer look into the dissatisfaction and stressors of the wider medical society in the 1950s. A doctor, writing in the medical journal the *Lancet*, in 1950, wrote, 'In a profession, one of whose chief glories was what the Minister called "in-breeding", fathers are now discouraging their sons from following in their footsteps'.[18] Pinner's *When Doctors are Patients*, published in 1952, is the first collection of illness narratives written by doctors. Here, the experience of anxiety is illuminating. On seeing black marks on people's foreheads, a surgeon writes,

> I was terribly afraid to ask someone. The secret would be out, and I'd be labelled a psychotic. I decided that I had to gamble. I tried to be casual…He answered, unaware of my inner panic, 'Today is Ash Wednesday.[19]

He also recalls seeing a medical student being treated for depression:

> Among these charts I stumbled on one belonging to a medical student whose name I knew… Here he was, hidden away, gradually recovering from severe emotional depression… I recalled his normal appearance, my vague discomfort and apprehension came on again… My mouth felt dry, and I was sweaty all over.[19]

These narratives reveal that mental illness occurred in physicians just as it did in the general population. They show a progression from the personal torment of the individual to the deep shame felt by the wider profession. In the *Bulletin of Suicidology*, a physician's wife, whose husband took his own life, describes the complete lack of support from colleagues:

> [his colleagues] were unable to believe that the person I knew at home was the person they knew as a doctor. I begged for help for the last two years to have him admitted to a hospital to keep him from killing himself, but no one could believe me.[20]

These texts begin to outline some themes common to illness experience in doctors even today – an innate fear of mental illness, a sense that mental ill-health would be the end of their career, difficulty seeking help and the cover-up of doctors who experience mental illness or are receiving treatment.[21]

THE UNSTABLE, PATHOLOGICAL AND UNWELCOME DOCTOR

In the 1950s, mental illness, suicide rates and dissatisfaction in medicine were slowly beginning to be linked. From 1960 to 1975, we see a surge in the literature and research of physician mental health. Individual accountability and a lack of support penetrates through to these later decades, as literature over this period considered doctors with mental illness as pathological and unsuitable for medicine. It was also determined that doctors 'were more likely to have relatively poor marriages, to use drugs and alcohol heavily and to obtain psychotherapy'.[22] Researchers from this time state that only the physicians with the least stable childhoods and adolescent adjustments appeared vulnerable to the occupational hazards and stress of medicine.[22] Many studies ostracised psychiatrists, who apparently went into the field 'seeking solutions to their own unconscious problems', learnt the success of suicide from patients and whose own suicide showed a failing of knowledge for his own specialty. As women began to enter the profession, they also faced scrutiny – described as compulsive, competitive and preoccupied with marriage.[23] Although the high pressure and anxiety-provoking nature of the work was highlighted, the cause of psychiatric illness was ultimately placed down to failing self-respect and personality traits.[24]

By 1972, drug addiction and suicide occurring in physicians were noted. It was also during this year a doctor who had schizophrenia killed three children in a UK hospital; interest was rising in the field, but this event dramatically increased professional and public interest in psychiatric illness in physicians.[25] Reviews emerged in multiple psychiatry journals and the *Lancet*. In terms of assessment two proposals were recommended by the General Medical Council (GMC) and British Medical Association (BMA): to establish mental health panels and a committee with the powers to suspend mentally ill doctors, and for medical school deans to assess the mental state of their students (and if deemed acceptable, issue a certificate of fitness to practise).[25] In 1973, the American Medical Association (AMA) published an article that defended the commitment of medicine to competent patient care, while also emphasising the scope of psychiatric illness in physicians.[26] It listed the programs arising in some states, and offered recommendations underlining 'physicians' ethical responsibility in reporting affected colleagues and how to notify the state disciplinary board.[23]

The mentally ill physician as intrinsically hopeless, pathological and unwelcome in the profession may be shocking to a modern reader. Stigma and individual blame were deep-rooted in the ideals of the medical profession, and its growing status and power were protected at any cost. While doctors may have wanted to support their colleagues with mental illness, the consequences of raising concern about another doctor placed them in a difficult position. In many cases, the idea was reiterated that 'doctors don't report problem doctors because they don't want to destroy the other doctor's career'.[27] Simultaneously, research was reinforcing the idea that these individuals didn't deserve help; they weren't fit for medicine, they were a lost cause.

Doctors with mental illness seemingly had nowhere to turn. This was recognised by those who were ill, as illustrated in the narratives from this time (which became increasingly outspoken and explicit).[21] This had detrimental consequences on the individuals most in need of support. Many did not feel able to seek help and continued practising medicine until the point of breakdown. In some cases, this resulted in investigation into these individuals. It is a tragic but common theme that many who were under investigation died by suicide:

> He was reported to the local medical society and was investigated by the impaired physician's committee. Finally, during one of his depressive episodes, he killed himself.[27]

For those who did manage to seek help, a sense of isolation and self-stigma is tangible. Taken from a narrative of addiction, one doctor described:

> Finally, the therapist asked how I was doing, and through the tears, I spilled out in guilt and despair. I'm a doctor, and I'm in a hospital for drug addiction. Would you send your mother or wife or sister to a doctor like me? I'm a medical doctor; I should know better![28]

Examples of personality problems are also evident:

> I was the only chemically dependent person in this hospital, and the psychiatrists had no idea how to treat me. They said I had a character disorder, that I was too tense, that I had to learn to take life easier.[27]
>
> My psychiatric colleagues... say that in alcoholism there is 10% depression, 90% inadequate personality. I cannot accept this contention.[29]

These quotations highlight the consequences of perceptions towards mentally ill physicians in the 1970s. Treatments were becoming available, but they often showed the same stigma and blame as outlined in the literature. Nonetheless, it was support from unsuspecting colleagues, and even other ill or addicted doctors, that seemed most significant to those who were ill:

> These two men were remarkably knowledgeable about alcoholism because they were also recovering from the disease...They showed me true love, compassion and understanding, and made me believe in my self-worth and led me to recovery.[28]

RECONSIDERING THE CHALLENGES OF MEDICINE

In the last quarter of the century, the profession began to demand a change in the ideals of medicine. Throughout the 1980s, junior doctors were consistently working more than 100 hours a week, with on-call weekends starting on Friday morning and ending on Monday afternoon. In the form of articles relating to physician lifestyle and stress, research began to consider the other factors involved in physician mental health. Much as in the early 20th century, the stresses of medical school and practice became a central part of the discourse. By this point, it was believed that the culture of the medical profession created imperfect personality traits and poor coping behaviours, where 'lack of sleep, competitive one-upmanship, marriages strained or broken by a perpetual 24-hour-a-day medical commitment – these stresses join forces to impose anxiety and insecurity'.[30]

The predisposing personality factors noted in physician mental illness and suicide were instead recognised as risk factors that could serve as a targets for intervention, rather than qualities of professional exclusion.[31] Unlike earlier in the century, dissatisfaction among doctors was becoming openly acknowledged and discussed. By 1981, in a survey of doctors in British Columbia, one-half said they would not recommend medicine as highly as they would have a decade earlier.[32]

Although the unrealistic ideals of the heroic physician were beginning to be broken down, a direct solution to dissatisfaction and mental illness in medical professionals remained unfound. In 1989, Pilowski and O'Sullivan published an article in the *BMJ*, in response to yet another health study, stating many of both sexes and all ages regret becoming doctors, and offer a review of the existing research.[33] They consider the counselling programmes available for ill physicians:

> Although this service is to be valued, it will probably not be sufficient. Other measures, including real career reforms, will be necessary.[33]

This marks a significant change in the literature, analysing the effectiveness of programmes available and demanding a re-evaluation of working culture. The subsequent need for prevention and management was undeniably essential, and the first major reforms for the well-being of ill doctors emerged throughout the 1990s in the UK and the USA, including recommendations for counselling for medical students and guidelines on improving the health of the NHS workforce.[34,35]

Simultaneously, it was in the 1990s that research began into the 'hidden curriculum' of medical education, exploring the learned rules and customs of medicine and its institutions.[36] This exposed some of the more challenging cultural issues of medicine: establishment of hierarchy, humiliation and competition with peers.[36,37] Ultimately, medical students are required to adopt the deep-rooted characteristic of stoicism, to detach emotionally and accept disrespect and humiliation as a part of hierarchy. Further studies of medical culture arose, examining that of doctors in general and doctors with illness. An interesting study by Thompson *et al.* looked at GPs' culture towards their own health, offered insightful results. They noted denial, viewing personal psychiatric illness as weakness, concerns about confidentiality, reluctance to accept treatment and an explanation that in medical school and hospital, 'illness was not really tolerated and you were expected to do the job'.[38]

Such a culture can be seen in the narratives of doctors from all specialities. Self-stigma persists into modern narratives of mental illness – echoing those of the 1980s, and even the 1950s. Taken from Petre Jones' 2007 *Doctors as Patients*, one doctor describes:

> Mental illnesses are very common, and doctors are just as vulnerable as anyone else. But there are vulnerable taboos against 'admitting' to having one (as if that were a crime)… Would patients and colleagues ever trust me? Would I ever trust myself? So, doctors keep quiet about their problems and the system colludes with them, often with tragic results.[39]

Despite a steady shift across the century towards challenging the ideals of the profession, the common difficulties of medical culture are unwavering throughout. Although the modern narratives of mentally ill doctors begin to challenge stigma and show a greater reflection upon their vulnerabilities and the taboos surrounding them, the innate issues appear to remain. The above quotation begins to separate two distinct subjects, asking '*Would patients and colleagues ever trust me? Would*

I ever trust myself?' Attitudes towards the self, compared to attitudes from the wider profession, are arguably the two major aspects of mental illness in doctors throughout the century. Although it is hard to determine the aetiology of mental illness, at the very least we can say that there is a persistent strain on medical professionals, between their individual identity, values and beliefs, and the environment in which they are working.

Denial, stigma, a sense of failure; these are seen across the century in the illness narratives of doctors and discussed as themes in this book. In the majority of cases, harmful beliefs about the self are reinforced by the wider profession, as a reflex reaction of medical culture's historical caricature of heroism. Quite simply, I use a quotation from Pamela Wible's 2016 *Physician Suicide Letters Answered* to demonstrate this:

> How cruel we physicians are to each other. How can we be so cruel?[40]

Even in modern narratives, so many feel unable to seek help. So many who seek help are provided with little support from colleagues and managers. Many mentally ill doctors discuss ongoing stigma from others, where they are seen as incompetent, considered a liability and unfit for the profession.[21]

CONCLUSION

Today, there is a greater acknowledgement of mental illness and suicide in physicians than ever before. While it is hard to say whether statistics of mental illness and suicide are increasing, it is clear that our doctors are struggling. The profession is facing recruitment and retention problems, as more young doctors refuse the pressures of medicine and older doctors are retiring as early as possible.[41] Some have been lucky to find support in their colleagues. Taken from her 2015 memoir of depression, psychiatrist Linda Gask describes a turning point in the path to her recovery:

> 'What do you do when you think you probably feel worse than some of your patients?'
>
> 'Get some help.'
>
> 'Where from?'
>
> 'Leave it to me', she said, 'I'll organise something.'[42]

The offering of help is profound, and the words unsaid are perhaps the kindest offerings of understanding.

It is tempting to look for blame, for a cause, in the case of mental illness in physicians. It is even the tendency of doctors to search for the cause of illness – the tumour, the virus or the parasite – and remove it. Over the 20th century, the potential reasons for mental ill health oscillate between the individual and the environment. In truth, we are all accountable for how we treat each other. Although the root causes of mental illness in physicians are complex and create areas of vulnerability, perhaps the greatest shortcoming of the medical profession is in its struggle to embrace this.

ACKNOWLEDGEMENTS

This research was conducted under the supervision of Chris Millard and Ian Sabroe. I wish to acknowledge their role in the creation of this work. Both always engaged with my writing and offered intellectual insight, while trusting me with freedom over its direction.

REFERENCES

1 Kinman G, Teoh K. What could make a difference to the mental health of UK doctors? A review of the research evidence [Internet]. 2018. Available from: http://eprints.bbk.ac.uk/24540.
2 Porter R. *Blood and Guts: A Short History of Medicine*. London: Penguin Books, 2002.
3 Beauchamp DE, Starr P. The social transformation of American medicine: the rise of a sovereign profession and the making of a vast industry. *Polit Sci Q* 1983;**98**.
4 Veresaeff V. *Confessions of a Physician*, 1st edn. London: Grant Richards, 1904.
5 Galton F. *Memories of My Life*. London: Methuen & Co, 1908.
6 Blackwell E. *Essays in Medical Sociology*. London: E Bell, 1902.
7 McIntire C. The importance of the study of medical sociology. Bull Am Acad Med 1894;**19**:425–34.
8 Warbasse J. *Medical Sociology*. New York: Appleton & Co, 1909.
9 Suicide among physicians. *Med Surg Report* 1897;**76**:271–3.
10 Durkheim E. *Suicide: a Study in Sociology*. New York: The Free Press, 1897 [1951].
11 JAMA. Suicide of physicians and the reasons. *JAMA* 1903;**41**(4):263–4.
12 Emerson H, Hughes H. Death rates of male white physicians in the United States, by age and cause. *Am J Public Health* 1926;**16**:1088–93.
13 Dublin L, Spiegelman M. The longevity and mortality of American physicians. *JAMA* 1947;**134**:1211–5.
14 Knopf A. Suicide among American physicians – its causes and suggestions for prevention. *New York Med J* 1923;**118**:84–7.
15 Anchersen P. On the prognosis of narcomania (euphomania) (to clarify some problems of narcomania). *Acta Psychiatr Scand* 1947;**22**:153–93.
16 DeSole DE, Singer P, Aronson S. Suicide and role strain among physicians. *Int J Soc Psychiatry* 1969;**15**(4):294–301.
17 Sponar J, Pivec L, Sormova Z. Suicide among doctors. *BMJ* 1964;**1**(5386):789–90.
18 Batten L. Letter to Lancet. *Lancet* 1950;780.
19 Pinner M. *When Doctors are Patients*, 1st edn. New York: WW Norton & Co, 1952.

20 Blachly P, Dishner B, Roduner G. Suicide by physicians. *Bull Suicidol* 1968;**4**:1–18.

21 Wilson A, Millard C, Sabroe I. Physician narratives of illness. *Lancet* 2019;**394**(10192):20–1.

22 Vaillant GE, Sobowale NC, McArthur N. Some psychologic vulnerabilities of physicians. *N Engl J Med* 1972;**287**(8):372–5.

23 Legha RK. A history of physician suicide in America. *J Med Humanit* 2012;**33**(4):219–44.

24 A'Brook MF, Hailstone JD, McLaughlan I. Psychiatric illness in the medical profession. *Br J Psychiatry* 1967;**113**(502):1013–23.

25 Murray R. Psychiatric illness in doctors. *Lancet* 1974;**1**(7868):1211–3.

26 Council of Mental Health. The sick physician: impairment by psychiatric disorders, including alcoholism and drug dependence. *JAMA* 1973; **223**(6):684–8.

27 Pekkanen J. *Doctors Talk About Themselves*. New York: Dell Pub Co, 1988.

28 Gehring WR. *Rx for Addiction*. Michigan: Zondervan Publishing House, 1985.

29 Spiro H, Mandell H. *When Doctors get Sick*. New York: Plenum Publishing Corporation, 1987.

30 Preven D. Physician suicide. *Hillside J Psychiatry* 1981;**1**(1):61–70.

31 AMA Council on Scientific Affairs. Physician mortality and suicide: results and implications of the AMA-APA Pilot Study. *Conn Med* 1986;**50**(1):37–43.

32 Zuger A. Dissatisfaction with medical practice. *New Engl J Med* 2004;**350**(1):69–75. Available from: www.uft-a.com/PDF/NEJMPhysician Dissatisfaction1-03.pdf.

33 Pilowski L, O'Sullivan G. Mental illness in doctors. *BMJ* 1989;**298**(6669):269–70.

34 Hays L, Cheever T, Patel P. Medical student suicide, 1989–1994. *Am J Psychiatry* 1996;**153**(4):553–5.

35 Williams S, Michie S, Pattani S. *Improving the Health of the NHS Workforce*. London: Nuffield Trust, 1998.

36 Lempp H. Papers. The hidden curriculum in undergraduate medical education: qualitative study of medical students' perceptions of teaching. *BMJ* 2004;**329**:770.

37 Sinclair S. *Making Doctors. An Institutional Apprenticeship*. Oxford: Berg Publishers, 1997.

38 Thompson WT, Cupples ME, Sibbett CH, Skan DI, Bradley T. Challenge of culture, conscience, and contract to general practitioners' care of their own health: a qualitative study. *BMJ* 2001;**323**(7315):728–31.

39 Jones P (ed). *Doctors as Patients*, 1st edn. Oxon: Radcliffe Publishing Ltd, 2005.

40 Wible P. *Physician Suicide Letters Answered*. Pamela Wible; 2016.

41 Read C. Driving retention by supporting doctors [Internet]. *HSJ* March 2019. Available from: www.hsj.co.uk/workforce/driving-retention-by-supporting-doctors/7024583.article.

42 Gask L. *The Other Side of Silence: A Psychiatrist's Memoir of Depression*. Chichester: Summersdale Publishers, 2015.

3

What Makes Medicine Such a Difficult Task Master and Doctors at Higher Risk of Mental Illness?

CLARE GERADA

While mental illness in doctors is not new, levels of unhappiness and disillusion are reaching worrying levels. It is hard for those not working in medicine to understand why doctors are so unhappy, and even though I work with mentally ill doctors, it still surprises me that they do become so unwell, and at such high rates. Of course, I know on one level that having a medical degree does not confer immunity from mental illness nor protect against experiencing traumatic life events. Yet given that doctors have a host of protective factors (rewarding career, good social networks, high status, financial stability and flexibility in their working lives) it would be expected that their rates of mental illness should be considerably lower, not as research suggests, higher than in the general population.

The reasons why doctors are so unhappy are complex: some contributing factors are associated with the job itself (especially the emotional toil of working close to suffering); others stem from the common characteristics of those who choose to become doctors; and some are due to wider, socio-political factors that relate to the changing place doctors have in society. Perhaps the best narrative I have read about doctors' causes of distress is by the American, Abigail Zuger.[1] Her article is written from a USA perspective and as such mentions stressors that might not currently be so relevant in the UK, such as managed care and the malpractice crisis. Others, such as the inability to care for patients in the way one was trained to do due to lack of time and the increasing burden of observation and scrutiny, are common across the world.

THE EMOTIONAL WORK OF MEDICINE

Perhaps the best place to start in understanding why doctors are so distressed is by looking at the job itself. A previous editor of the *BMJ*, Richard Smith, wrote an opinion piece titled *Why are doctors so unhappy?*, and concluded that doctors are overworked and under-supported.[2] Smith is right. It seems obvious, but the most important risk factor is **the job**. Medicine is a hard taskmaster, and is intellectually, physically and emotionally demanding.

It is not just the unsocial hours or long shifts that make it so (though they add to the stress). Nor is medicine difficult simply due to the vast amount of knowledge we need to remember (after all, lawyers have to learn the equivalent of several telephone directories to do their work well). What makes medicine difficult is having to deal with human suffering and all its attendant emotions.

The sociologists Harold Lief and Renée Fox *wrote that medicine is about:*

exploring, examining, and cutting into the human body; dealing with fears, anger, sense of helplessness, and despair of patients; meeting emergency situations; accepting the limitations of medical science in dealing with chronic or incurable disease; being confronted with death itself.[3]

All of these are difficult. However, it is more than the visible manifestations of disease that we have to deal with (and one can argue it is nurses who carry much of this burden) but the hidden, emotional aspects that are perhaps even harder to deal with.

Working with people is complicated and deeply satisfying but can also be psychologically painful. Patients bring their unique histories, expectations, beliefs and desires into the consultation room. They bring their emotions – joy, sadness, shock, fear, aggression, worries and everything else wrapped up in being mortal. For those brief moments we become guests in their lives as they share with us their most intimate concerns and using all our senses, we become attuned to their needs. We must create a space, if only for a few minutes, that is entirely theirs, uncluttered by our own needs. Forty years on, I am still in awe how, within seconds of a stranger meeting me, they are willing to disclose the most personal parts of their minds and bodies, parts that are forbidden in all other human encounters, even to those nearest and closest to them.

Patients rarely come with fully formed diagnoses and rather present with undifferentiated symptoms ('pain all over', 'feeling odd', 'out of sorts'), which, detective-like, we need to gently piece together into a coherent diagnosis. They do not follow textbook descriptions of illness. I remember a patient who presented with 'watering eyes', only when he passed a certain street. It turned out to be tears of grief for a long dead friend, resurrected each time he passed by the house. Patients make personal choices that might be out of kilter with our medical training. Georgina refused all conventional treatment for her cancer and I had to watch for years as her health deteriorated and the only 'treatment' she accepted was that recommended by her herbalist. My role was to be present and ready when and if she changed her mind; she never did and died prematurely. One cannot see patients, day in day out for years, without being profoundly affected by this experience and the struggles we witness. Even now, as I write this chapter, I see the faces of my patients and hear their words, some long deceased. I see their ghosts as I walk my dog, shop in the supermarket or walk past their old homes. Many of my patients still live in my mind.

It is not only the patient's emotions that enter the consulting room. Our emotions are there as well. Patients often stir up powerful feelings in us, which, in the main, have to be understood rather than responded to. These feelings, not always generated directly from the patients, but indirectly, are brought to life through the encounter with the patient, due to a doctor's past painful experiences. For example, a doctor who lost their mother at an early age might overidentify with someone who has recently been bereaved following a death of a parent, or with a female patient who stirs up memories of their mother. This is commonly referred to in the psychoanalytic literature as transference and countertransference. Both can occur with any doctor–patient interaction, though more frequently where there are intense and close therapeutic relationships, such as during psychotherapy. Without safe spaces to think about why a patient makes one feel or act in a certain way, these emotions can 'stick' to the doctor who is left to carry them unsupported.

Patients also create powerful negative emotions in us, not because they 'remind' us of past experiences, but just because they can be dislikeable, difficult or rude. They may be drunk, violent, demanding or engage in activities that we as doctors have deemed unacceptable. We may feel guilty if we harbour these negative feelings and are loath to admit to them, except in the safety of staff support groups or individual supervision.

There are very few jobs that require individuals to be constantly attuned to the needs of others, yet, at the end of the day, literally and metaphorically leave them behind in the consulting room or hospital ward. Irrespective of how we feel or how tough a time we've had, or the traumas we have endured or sorrows waiting for us in our personal life, in the consulting room we must always be engaged with our patient, attentive to their needs, objective and professional. The day my mother died I had to finish a busy clinic. It was too late to delegate the session to someone else (though I imagine this says more about my failure in accepting vulnerability than management's response if I had cancelled). Despite my grief, I had to focus on my patients, I had to make them my first concern. This is what I understand to be the 'emotional labour' of our work, a term first used by the American sociologist Arlie Hochschild.[4] It is about managing or supressing our personal feelings so that they do not interfere with the act of caring or giving to others. It is the emotional labour that accompanies the work of doctors that places them at particular risk of mental illness. The trope of the smiling waitress asking, 'have you had a nice day?' when she is having a terrible one is similar to the doctor maintaining their composure when confronted with patients or situations that make them recoil in fear or revulsion. On a surface level, emotional labour means that the professional controls or changes their emotional reaction so that the observer (in this case the patient) is not able to recognise what he/she really feels. The mismatch between what one expresses and what one feels can lead to cognitive dissonance – and if the gap is too large, it can cause guilt, anxiety, depression and burnout.[5]

Understanding how one modulates emotional interactions with patients, how to manage the dissonance between acting and reality, is hard, and especially so when one does not have time to stop and reflect with peers or teams.

Our job is essentially about managing human expectations and dealing with the suffering our patients bring. Patients try unconsciously to 'offload' their fears by 'giving them' (in the psychoanalytic term, projecting) onto doctors. These projections find fertile ground and, given doctors' desire to care, easily become accepted by the medical profession. Patients see doctors at their most vulnerable moments. They come wanting to be given hope and for us to contain their fear of death. Some even want us to prevent it happening at all, even when impossible. I see this fantasy of doctors and healthcare expected to have magical powers in my working life. For example, when terminally ill patients reach the end of their life, their relatives call 999 at the last moment, demanding their loved one is taken from their bed to hospital in the hope that medicine can give them 'one last chance', only for them to die a few hours later on an A&E trolley. In the case of Charlie Gard, a baby with a severe, rare and untreatable genetic disorder, his parents took the hospital to High Court, demanding they should be allowed to take the child abroad to receive experimental interventions only ever tested on mice. Even the Pope and Donald Trump got involved, buying into the delusional belief that death, even in those with life ending diseases, can be put off for ever. Of course, death cannot be prevented and even though not spoken about, it is the shadow of all healthcare, and while services are generally geared to saving and prolonging life, the spectre of death is never far away.[6] There is a reason why most hospitals have morgues onsite. I believe it is this mismatch between the expectations of medicine and its reality that fuels the development of burnout in doctors, and our hopelessness in the face of suffering that leads to depression. Denial of death is widespread.

The psychoanalyst Isabel Menzies-Lyth, who conducted studies on student nurses in the 1950s talked about how society defends itself from problems it finds too difficult to deal with by locating, and then disavowing, associated anxieties into institutions such as hospitals, nursing homes and prisons.[7] Once split off from normal consciousness, the left-over anxiety is acted out through either idealising or denigrating those who have taken the unpalatable tasks away. It is no surprise to me therefore, that my speciality, general practice is increasingly portrayed as both the scapegoat and the saviour of the NHS, as health leaders locate their fear of the very survival of the health service onto us. This might also explain why paediatricians, until now the darlings of the health system, are increasingly the recipients of verbal abuse, litigation and complaints. As medicine is keeping alive children with chronic and complex diseases, parents project onto paediatricians their emotions of having an unwell child and paediatricians accept and have to deal with these painful projections. Holding these emotions for others is psychologically difficult, yet largely unspoken about. So is confronting the shadow side of our work, day in, day out, learning to cope with the knowledge that we will always fail our patients and that failure is a quintessential part of medicine. These are hard lessons to learn, needing support, supervision and spaces to explore our feelings, which are sadly lacking in modern healthcare systems.

SOCIO-POLITICAL FACTORS

I was brought up to believe that medicine is an art underpinned by science. Sound clinical judgements are the result of personal relationships as well as scientific knowledge and textbooks can never prepare us for the uniqueness of every patient we encounter. Learning to strike the right balance between the science and art of medical practice isn't easy, and failure to do so creates anxiety.

Across the world, we are facing something of a crisis in healthcare, with doctors made to focus on the disease rather than on the patient, on the science rather than the caring. This was something that Francis Peabody, professor at Harvard, identified as early as in 1927:

> The most common criticism made at present by older practitioners is that young graduates have been taught a great deal about the mechanism of disease, but very little about the practice of medicine – or to put it more bluntly, they are too 'scientific' and do not know how to take care of patients.[8]

Nearly a century later the art of caring is under even more pressure, as medicine becomes a numbers game of measurement, monitoring and productivity. Doctors now have less opportunity to practise their craft, uncluttered by the market or external forces such as inspection or monitoring. These act to negate the individuality of the patient and the creativity of the doctor. Writing about general practitioners, the geriatrician Steve Illife talks of the dissonance created as the role of medicine changes from:

> a craft concerned with the uniqueness of each encounter with an ill person to a mass manufacturing industry preoccupied with the throughput of the sick.[9]

Iona Heath, a former President of the Royal College of General Practitioners reminisced that when she embarked on her career in 1974, to be a public servant meant doing something good. With the shift towards a market economy and through a painful and demoralising process, this pursuit of a career in medicine has changed to something 'somehow despicable'.[10] What these individuals are articulating, which I am not completely in agreement with, is the loss of their professional ideal, of the doctor having a unique and personal relationship with their patient. It is becoming harder to deliver personalised care, but I think it is the struggle to do so, at all odds, that is making doctors unhappy. Doctors are as altruistic, caring and committed as in Iliffe's and Heath's day, just that today these doctors need to work harder to achieve their desired aims.

The practise of medicine is also becoming increasingly difficult as many of the protective factors within organisations, which would have acted as a counter to work-related mental distress, have been lost. Harold Ellis, a surgeon who qualified in 1948 (and who taught me as a medical student) recalls his time working as a positive experience. Despite never being off-call, he has fond memories: 'we all knew each other… the firm was a happy band of brothers'.[11] When one reads first person accounts written by doctors of his generation, they talk about their teams (firms) and how well supported they felt. This was my experience too. These interactions between colleagues were invaluable, offering not just access to education but support and a sense of belonging. My hospital had a doctors' mess and even a doctors' dining room where we could eat our meals and share our stories without the fear of being overheard by patients. I felt I belonged not just to my firm, but to the hospital. Today, there is a general lack of connection between individuals, and between individuals and institutions.

How doctors have been treated has also changed over the decades. Ellis woke each morning with breakfast delivered to his room by a porter; his shoes had been polished overnight; other doctors were given free accommodation, all meals, laundry and a maid service in the doctors' mess.[11] Now doctors barely even have a hook to hang their coats on, let alone hot meals and a room to rest. Poorly designed rotas, staffing gaps and increasing shift work – with the consequent loss of continuity of care – also negate a sense of belonging to, and being cared for by their employer, leading to feeling more like itinerant workers than resident doctors. Training has now become atomised and rather than coming together doctors are at risk of becoming singletons, only capable of defending their own psychological skin.

The unconscious hierarchy between patients and doctors is rapidly disappearing as patients are living longer with chronic illnesses, and doctors' exclusive access to medical knowledge is being eroded with the proliferation of 'Dr Google' and online communities. In *The Changing Face of Medicine* (2017), the British Medical Association (BMA) with contributors from across the world focused on factors impacting on physician well-being and morale, and how the traditional role of doctors and their status in society is changing and contributing to the profession's mental health crisis.[12] The themes were all familiar: the inability to deliver continuity of care; the harmful effects of bringing the market to healthcare; the changing nature of professionalism; and the intensity of workload. Another major cause of distress in the NHS, but also across many other health systems, is endless reorganisations.

It is not just doctors who are unhappy today. Many other professions, including law and teaching, have become constrained by corporate structures, resulting in loss of autonomy, status and respect. In 1982 the sociologist Paul Starr wrote that, for most of the 20th century, medicine was 'the heroic exception that sustained the waning tradition of independent professionalism… But the exception may now be brought into line with the governing rule'.[13] His ground-breaking book talks about the growth of medical authority (surpassing that of religious authority), brought about in part by the increasing body of knowledge held by doctors. Authority signifies the possession of special status and power, which doctors have largely been the recipients of until the more recent technological revolution, where knowledge is now more equally shared.

INDIVIDUAL FACTORS

Aside from socio-political factors and the realities of the profession, doctors, as individuals carry our own risk of mental illness.[14] The process for deciding which individuals enter medical school is highly selective. We have to meet difficult entrance requirements, involving excellent examination results and challenging interviews. Aspiring applicants need to show determination, intelligence, ability to work hard under pressure; they must be good communicators and demonstrate a desire to care. The University Clinical Aptitude Test (UCAT) is an admissions test used by many medical schools in the UK to assess students' suitability to study medicine. It assesses potential students against attributes such as verbal, quantitative and abstract reasoning, decision making and situational judgment. Nowadays, unlike when I gained a place at medical school, prospective doctors must also have flawless school reports. Those who get over these hurdles are likely to share a set of attributes that are deemed to foster the makings of a good doctor. These include being patient, unselfish, responsible and highly ethical. When stressed, and in the face of demands, individuals must not show weakness or indecision and must put others first. These formidable attributes can become exaggerated, leading to doctors becoming less tolerant of errors in themselves or their colleagues, striving for perfection and never feeling 'good enough'. The academic Jenny Firth-Cozens in her research on doctors suggests that the difficult and emotionally demanding job of a doctor leads to them being overly self-critical when stressed.[15] Some practitioners can have maladaptive coping strategies – emotional distancing, for example, rather than actively dealing with stressors – which may add to psychological distress.[16] Other common psychological vulnerabilities include an excessive sense of responsibility, desire to please everyone, guilt for things outside of one's own control, self-doubt and obsessive–compulsive traits.[17]

Perfectionism is one of the most pervasive personality traits found in doctors. Perfectionists strive for flawlessness and set extremely high standards for themselves and others, which can lead to individuals becoming increasingly self-critical.[18,19] As the practise of medicine becomes less tolerant of mistakes, having perfectionists on the team is seen as positive and desirable and as such the wish for 'the perfect doctor' is a collective collusion between the doctor, the patient and the health system. This collusion is evidenced by the current 'zero suicide' initiatives, the quest for endlessly improving quality and the elimination of so-called 'never events' (which are, as they say, events that are deemed to be such catastrophic errors that they must never happen, such as amputating the wrong limb during an operation). Across the industrialised world, young people now face tougher social and economic conditions than their parents and the increasing pressure to achieve is pervasive throughout their lives.[20] Today's students are under constant scrutiny, and they know it. Every attachment is graded, and these grades contribute to final scores, influencing the young doctor's ability to obtain training posts, research grants and other positions. Striving for perfection has become the new norm.[21]

Behaviour that encourages perfectionism (increased engagement, working longer hours and being more motivated) is negatively counterbalanced by the increased risk of burnout, depression and anxiety, which have serious consequences beyond just the workplace. Far from producing better outcomes, research has shown that perfectionism leads to more detrimental work and non-work outcomes, as well as higher levels of mental illness.[22]

Charlotte, an accomplished 27-year-old medical trainee, was always the best at school, not just academically, but also in sports and music. When things got tough, which they did when her younger brother died suddenly, she focused on her schoolwork to avoid thinking about her loss. She sailed through medical school, winning prizes. She was critical of her colleagues for not working as hard as she did. Once in training she found herself becoming increasingly anxious and fearful of making errors. She was always checking her work, even coming in on her days off to make sure her clinical decisions had not caused any harm to her patients. One day, while on call, a patient died unexpectedly. She blamed herself, even though her colleagues and the case review exonerated her. After this her fear of getting things wrong intensified. She arrived at work two hours early for each shift. She split up with her partner as she felt she had to remain focused on her work. Unable to bear things any longer, Charlotte took an overdose of tablets and was found by her flatmate.

We have hundreds of Charlottes in my service. She, as with other doctors, have internalised the need to be 'perfect'. This need was primed even before starting medical school and then reinforced during training, modelled by other doctors she encounters and by the culture of medical practice in which she works, where individuals who make errors are punished. At medical school, studying hard predictably translates into achievements, but there is no guarantee that this will achieve similar outcomes once qualified. Perfection, which doctors demand of themselves, is impossible in the real world of medical care, and can be harmful.[22]

In *The House of God*, the satirical description of a young doctor's journey through his internship in an American hospital, Samuel Shen describes an inter-action between a more senior doctor (called Fat Man) and a junior intern. Fat Man gives the junior important lessons on how to cope with no sleep and endless patient admissions during the night:

Key concept, said the Fat Man, to think that you're doing a shitty job. If you resign yourself to doing a shitty job, you go ahead and get the job done, and since we're all in the ninety-ninth percentile of interns, at one of the best internships in the world, what you do turns out to be a terrific job, a superlative job.[23]

Fat Man is teaching the intern an important coping mechanism, that is *not* to strive for perfection and accept that good enough is good. Maybe this is a lesson we all need reminding of. Understanding the limits of our capabilities is perhaps one of the most important antidotes to dealing with a lifetime in medicine.

The decision to study medicine, as with all choices, is influenced by conscious and unconscious motivations. Consciously, the most obvious reason might be the individual is good at science, and wants an interesting career helping others. It may be parental pressure that pushes someone into applying for medical school in the hope of fulfilling their own failed ambitions. Problems arise of course when the child finds themselves in the wrong career. Unconscious components are important as well, especially as they might predict why some individuals are more at risk of developing mental illness. While the unconscious motivations are often speculative, there is some evidence to suggest that a desire to make reparation for traumatic childhood experiences is an important factor.[24–26] This might have been at the root of my desire to become a doctor. I chose medicine due to my admiration for my father, a GP. Fostering a love of medicine and all that went with it meant I had a 'legitimate' reason to spend more time with him, important as he left the family home when I was still very young. Through my interest in medicine I could visit him in his surgery, go on home visits with him and spend time with him talking about being a doctor. My attachment to him – and, I am sure, his to me – grew, and I felt 'special'. It is no surprise therefore that I became a doctor and then went on to be a GP.

A medical career might give individuals the information and skills to resolve previous conflicts and to give to others the care and attention they would have wished for themselves. These are not bad motives for wanting to study medicine, though there is evidence that these students might be more likely to present with mental health problems when particular clinical experiences resonate with their earlier conflicts.[27] The unconscious desire to heal a loved one and the guilt associated with failing to do so can become channelled into a relentless drive to care more, be more altruistic and work harder. These are the actions of the wounded healer. If unchecked this will not lead to reparation or healing; instead, it risks repeating the failure to cure the incurable, which further feeds the associated emotional drive to apply oneself to an impossible task. This does not mean that these individuals should not become doctors. I have flourished in my career and I hope I have been a good (enough) doctor to my patients. Having experience of personal trauma might predispose individuals to a real gift and capacity for empathy and caring, especially if their childhood conflicts have been acknowledged and the vulnerability held in awareness.[28] This is partially supported by the work of Firth-Cozens.[29] She found that those students who were more depressed both as students and as junior doctors tended to be more empathetic, more self-critical and then their peers, all of which would appear to be desirable attributes for a doctor to possess.

CONCLUSION

I have discussed in this chapter how the emotional work of medicine together with what the individual brings (especially perfectionism) and wider socio-political factors make doctors at risk of mental illness, and increasingly so. Addressing these factors is not easy, as some of them have been hard wired into doctors and society for millennia. Given the difficulties discussed, it is important to remember that most doctors thrive in their work. Working with people and having a career in which one can make such a difference to others is itself rewarding and self-fulfilling. The joy, personal satisfaction and sense of achievement at the end of a day's work, replenishes one's psychological batteries and makes it possible to face another day, refreshed and with enthusiasm.

REFERENCES

1 Zuger A. Dissatisfaction with medical practice. *N Engl J Med* 2004;**350**:1.

2 Smith R. Why are doctors so unhappy? *BMJ* 2001;**322**:1073–4.

3 Lief HI, Fox RC. Training for 'detached concern' in medical students. In: HI Lief, VI Lief, NR Lief (eds). *The Psychological Basis of Medical Practice*. New York: Harper & Row, 1963, p. 13.

4 Hochschild AR. *The Managed Heart: Commercialization of Human Feeling*. Berkeley: University of California Press, 1983.

5 Schwenk T, Gold K. Physician burnout – a serious symptom, but of what? *JAMA* 2018;**320**(11):1109.

6 Nitsun M. *Beyond the Antigroup: Survival and Transformation*. London: Routledge, 2015.

7 Menzies Lyth I. *Containing Anxiety in Institutions*. London: Free Assoc. Books, 1992, p. 209.

8 Peabody FW. *The Care of the Patient*. 1927;**88**:877–82.

9 Illife S (2008). *From General Practice to Primary Care. The Industrialisation of Family Medicine*. Oxford: Oxford University Press, 2008, pp. 2–3.

10 Heath I. *Love's Labours Lost: Why Society is Straitjacketing its Professionals and How We Might Release Them*. Presentation at The Royal Society of Edinburgh Michael Shea Memorial Lecture; organised in partnership with the International Futures Forum, 2012.

11 White C. Feature, Junior Doctors Was there ever a golden age for junior doctors? *BMJ* 2016;**354**:i3662. https://doi.org/10.1136/bmj.i3662 (published 6 July 2016).

12 British Medical Association. *The Changing Face of Medicine and the Role of Doctors in the Future*. Presidential project, 2017.

13 Starr P. *The Social Transformation of American Medicine: The Rise of a Sovereign Profession and the Making of a Vast Industry*. USA: BasicBooks, a division of HarperCollins Publishers, 1982.

14 Brooks S, Gerada C, Chalder T. The specific needs of doctors with mental health problems: qualitative analysis of doctor-patients' experiences with the Practitioner Health Programme. *J Mental Health* 2017;**26**(2):161–6. DOI: 10.1080/09638237.2016.1244712.

15 Firth-Cozens J. Predicting stress in general practitioners: 10 year follow up postal survey. *BMJ* 1997;**315**:34–5.

16 Tattersall AJ, Bennett P, Pugh S. Stress and coping in hospital doctors. *Stress Medicine* 1999;**15**: 109–13.

17 Vaillant GE, Sobowale NC, McArthur C. Some psychological vulnerabilities of physicians. *N Engl J Med* 1972;**287**:372–5.

18 McManus IC, Keeling A, Paice E. Stress, burnout and doctors' attitudes to work are determined by personality and learning style: a twelve-year longitudinal study of UK medical graduates. *BMC Med* 2004;**2**:29.

19 Brewin CR, Firth C. Dependency and self-criticism as predictors of depression in young doctors. *J Occup Health Psychol* 1997;**2**:242–6.

20 MORI. Global Trends Survey [Internet]. 2014. Available from: www.ipsos.com/sites/default/files/publication/1970-01/ipsos-mori-global-trends-2014.pdf.

21 Curran T, Hill A. Perfectionism is increasing over time: A meta-analysis of birth cohort differences from 1989 to 2016. *Psychol Bull* 2019;**145**(4):410–29.

22 Swider B, Breidenthal A, Bujold Steed L. *The Pros and Cons of Perfectionism, According to Research* [Internet]. Harvard Business Review. 2018 [cited 28 September 2019]. Available from: https://hbr.org/2018/12/the-pros-and-cons-of-perfectionism-according-to-research.

23 Shen S. *The House of God*. London: Black Swan, 1985, p. 75.

24 Johnson WDK. Predispositon to emotional distress and psychiatric illness amongst doctors: The role of unconscious and experiential factors. *Br J Med Psychol* 1991;**64**:317–29.

25 King E, Steenson C, Shannon C, Mulholland C. Prevalence rates of childhood trauma in medical students: a systematic review. *BMC Med Educ* 2017;**17**(1):159.

26 Bowlby J. The making and breaking of affectional bonds. *Br J Psychiatry* 1977;**130**(3):201–10.

27 Sacks MH, Frosch WA, Kesselman M, Parker L. Psychiatric problems in third year medical students. *Am J Psychiatry* 1980;**137**:822–5.

28 Zigmond D. Physician heal thyself: the paradox of the wounded healer. *Br J Holistic Med* 1984;**1**:63–71.

29 Firth-Cozens J. Emotional distress in junior house officers. *BMJ* 1987;**295**:1177–80.

4

Rising Levels of Mental Illness
Fact or Fiction?

CLARE GERADA

The current focus on mental illness in doctors tends to imply that this is a new phenomenon and that mental illness did not exist in the past. It did exist, as Amy Wilson illustrates in Chapter 2, with examples of narratives of doctors through the ages describing their experience of mental illness. These include that of the Russian doctor Vikenty Vikentyevich Veresaeff, who gave a first-hand account of the misery of being a doctor in his memoir *Confessions of a Physician*.[1] Amy Wilson mentioned it is worth looking at this book in greater detail as many of the issues written in it as are pertinent today as they were when it was published in 1904. Veresaeff began to write his book as he entered medical school training and for a decade or so after qualifying, and his confessions referred to in the title are those concerning the hypocrisy of the 'powers' of medicine and the faith the public has in the medical profession. The book is a pretty sorry account of his experience training and later working as a doctor. As with many students today, he started out excited but very soon became demoralised and dejected by what he was experiencing. He wrote 'learning the truth, the lay-person may lose his or her confidence in medicine and its exponents'. In fact, Veresaeff lost confidence in his own ability to help his patients, describing medicine as consisting of 'moments of terrible nervous tension... a sudden turn for the worse in a recovering patient, an incurable who cries for relief, the impending death of a patient, the ever-present possibility of an untoward accident or mistake'.

He discusses the horror, when only a first-year clinical student of 'studying the suffering of living men'. He complained about the stress of his job, his disillusionment working as a doctor and of the high rates of depression and suicide among his colleagues, with 10% of them to die by their own hands. He blamed the problems he and his colleagues faced on the unrealistic expectations of patients as to 'the scope of the powers vested in the physician'; the pay and conditions; the culture of complaints and litigation; and the unrelenting workload. He even made reference to 'the cheap newspapers, which constantly run the doctors down'. So, it appears nothing much has changed in the intervening century. Though he doesn't use the term 'burnout' (it took another 70 or so more years before this was described), he certainly exhibited many features of it and gave what must be the first description of its symptoms in the published literature:

> there are times... when you are seized with such depression that only one thought remains – to turn your back on all and flee far from the madding crowd and feel, if only for a time, free and at peace.[2]

The woes of doctors at the turn of the 20th century were ignored and denied. A review in the *BMJ*, for example, concluded 'we find a Russian physician washing his dirty linen in public with every sensational accompaniment that is calculated to attract attention to the nasty business'. And went on to say: 'The proper place for Veresaeff "Confessions" is not the drawing-room table, but the dustbin'.[3]

I qualified in 1983, and while I was aware that some doctors struggled, this was never talked about (certainly not openly). Doctors disappeared, left training rotations or consultant posts. It was only in whispers that people mentioned that they had become depressed, or even killed themselves. In 1986 I wrote in the *Maudsley Gazette* (the in-house magazine for the Maudsley hospital) about my experience of working as a junior doctor. The article I wrote, which I did not stumble across until 20 years later was called *Lest We Forget*, and in the centre of it was a photo of four junior doctors, myself and three others. The article described my experience of performing a six-month obstetric job. I wrote of the unremitting nights on call, and their devastating impact on myself and my friends. We couldn't sleep. We couldn't concentrate. We found little to enjoy in life. And, like many of my peers at the time, I blamed myself for not being able to cope. I wrote:

> for the first time I understood the process where junior doctors could become so depressed as to take their own lives, sometimes performing the act in their own on-call room.

Very few doctors talked about their mental distress, though they did talk about their fatigue, their anger at the hours worked, the lack of support, their fear of making errors and of complaints. A doctor writing a personal account of her own mental illness asked the reader to consider:

> what profession would allow some of its members to go without food or drink, two basic human necessities, on a such a regular basis. I felt I was being emotionally and physically tortured.[4]

IS MENTAL ILLNESS RISING?

In recent years there has been increasing concern over the seemingly relentless increase in mental illness among the medical profession. However, good research is largely lacking to make an objective analysis of whether rates are rising, falling or staying the same. There are few studies that use the same methodology with similar cohorts across different time periods, and the best studies are now more than 30 years old.[5,6] Nevertheless, if one were to judge solely by reports in newspapers, radio or television programmes, social media or on the conference circuit, one would conclude that we are in the midst of a crisis of 'mental illness'. It appears to be in most other professional groups as well, such as social workers, teachers, journalists and police officers, not to mention students and school children. Indeed, all groups seem to be 'in crisis'. However, we need to be somewhat careful, because none of this may actually indicate a rise at all. Before we assume the worst, we need to consider a range of alternative explanations. It might be due to better case finding; of addressing unmet need, through improved training of health professionals to identify mental health problems in their patients; it could be related to greater willingness to talk about mental illness and to come forward for help. Saying this, while today's doctors might have a healthier attitude towards mental illness, I think we have a long way to go before we make it as easy to disclose depression as it might be to disclose dyspepsia.

A perception of rising levels of mental illness might be due to the tendency to categorise normal 'distress' or experiences such as failing exams, shyness or loneliness, as a mental illness. There is some evidence for this as we are seeing increasing numbers of (mainly younger) doctors who, having exhibited any sign of distress in the work place (such as being tearful after the death of a patient) are encouraged to attend counselling services for help rather than seek support through friends and colleagues.

> *Arvind was completing the end of his paediatric accident and emergency job. This was the fourth failed resuscitation of a child in as many months. He felt gutted, a failure, and very down. He knew that for each there was nothing he could have done, the children were all too sick to have survived. This didn't stop him feeling so sad and he started to cry. The clinical director (CD) asked him what the matter was, and he told him how the deaths had left him feeling. The CD told him to report to occupational health the next day and to take time off until his 'mental health was better'.*

Arvind was experiencing a normal (acute adjustment) response to an abnormal situation. Yet this has now become pathologised with the referral to occupational health and the label of mental illness. A gentle (metaphorical) arm around him, an offer of a chat from a senior to a junior, might be a far better, more adaptive response.

Other factors that might skew the results, could include bias related to how we 'measure' mental distress, and also *who* asks the questions. Occupation-specific surveys can suffer from systematic bias.[7] For example, one review compared studies focusing on single occupational groups only (for example, teachers, doctors, social workers, police) with larger, randomly sampled population-based studies. This study concluded that people are less likely to report symptoms of common mental disorders in the context of a population-based study rather than in a study of the identified work group to which they belong. This means we risk overestimating the levels of distress when members of samples identify as belonging to particular professional groups (such as doctor, nurse, teacher). Responses in occupational studies may be further biased with the emphasis on work-related questions potentially leading to individuals expressing overall dissatisfaction through the medium of questionnaires. Only once we have eliminated these biases can we perhaps conclude that there is indeed a true rise in the rate of mental illness among doctors.

RISING CONCERN AND REAL NUMBERS

Where research does exist, it gives conflicting results. One longitudinal study found no significant increase in the prevalence of psychiatric morbidity over a three-year period,[8] while another found a significant increase over an eight-year period.[9] The Firth-Cozens longitudinal studies found the proportion of doctors showing above threshold levels of stress stayed remarkably constant at around 28%.[10,11] Finally, a more recent meta-analysis, involving 54 studies published between 1963 and 2015 suggests the prevalence of depression has increased by an average of 0.5% per year,[12] though this might reflect the general increase in mental illness in the general population (particularly among young women).

Each year an increasing number of doctors come to my service for care, as sick as those attending any outpatient mental health service.[13] Given the results of numerous recent surveys it does not appear there is any respite in the rising levels of distress I am seeing in my clinic. Whether there has been a true increase in the rate of mental illness among doctors or not, there is rightly an escalation in the concern from bodies such as the NHS,[14–16] Health Education England[17] (who oversee all training of doctors in England), General Medical Council (GMC)[18] (who regulate doctors in UK), British Medical Association (BMA),[19,20] (the UK medical trade union) and the World,[21] Canadian[22] and American Medical Associations.[23] Concerns are related not just to the numbers presenting to mental health services such as my own, but also due to the rise in proxy measures of discontent, such as the number of doctors leaving medicine prematurely (some even only two years after qualifying), numbers choosing to work part time and increasing levels of sickness. Problems with mental illness are at both ends of one's career. One percent of medical students are excluded for health reasons and one-half of these result from mental health problems. The same pattern continues later in life – 40% of early retirement is due to psychiatric problems.[24]

All doctors are suffering, though it appears that general practitioners are experiencing particularly high rates of mental distress. The GMC's annual report (State of Medical Education, 2019)[25] found that while doctors are struggling to cope with their workload, it is especially problematic among GPs; when asked, one-sixth of GPs reported feeling unable to cope with workload on a daily basis. This is more than twice the proportion reported by specialists, four times non-consultant grade doctors and more than five times doctors in training. GPs also had the highest risk of burnout compared with other doctors. Given their position at the 'front door' of the health system, GPs are probably bearing a disproportionate burden of workload against diminishing resources. It is hardly surprising therefore that studies from across the world have found that GPs have some of the highest rates of mental distress and burnout compared to other doctors,[26–29] with variability across the world largely related to workload (volume and complexity).[30] The University of Manchester has been surveying the wellbeing of GPs for a number of years, with the latest report published in 2018.[31] The survey focuses upon GPs' experiences of their working lives, asking questions about: satisfaction with various aspects of their work, sources of pressure at work (including resource pressures, demands from a variety of sources and workload); overall experience of their work and future working intentions (including intentions to increase or decrease working hours and intentions to quit practice). While there has been little change in the satisfaction and stressor results from the 2015 survey to the most recent one, low levels of satisfaction and high levels of pressure have remained. A more recent survey conducted by the General Medical Council found that 90% of GPs and 75% of specialists felt they were struggling with high workloads and high demand in their working lives.[18]

It is not just GPs who are experiencing higher levels of mental illness. Hospital doctors are also suffering under the strain of increased intensity of their working day. As general practice becomes unable to meet the demands of their patients, patients attend accident and emergency departments instead. Bed shortages compound the problem as hospital doctors rush around many wards over a large hospital site looking after their seriously ill patients. Whereas in the past hospital doctors could expect some down time during their on-call shift, perhaps to share tea and toast with the ward nursing staff, everyone is now working flat out, with no time even for basic human needs. The *Adapting, Coping, Compromising* research carried out in 2018[32] reported how rising pressure caused by workforce shortages are leading doctors to becoming stressed and unwell. Other staff surveys of those working in the NHS find that over one-third of doctors working in hospital settings have indicated that they have been unwell as a result of work-related stress,[33–35] 10% in the last year. The GMC report found level of sickness due to stress was rising, and 18% of doctors in training reported taken leave due to stress in the previous year, 11% of doctors overall.[32] In 2018 the Canadian Medical Association conducted a survey of mental illness among their doctors. While nearly 60% of respondents reported that their mental health was flourishing, the survey also revealed areas of concern, such as high rates of burnout, depression and lifetime suicidal ideation, especially among women doctors.[22]

CONCLUSION

It feels as if there is a real crisis, whether backed by numbers or not. While rates of mental illness might not be rising as fast or as far as the background dialogue would suggest, nevertheless there is a sense of a change in the mood of the profession, towards that of depression, burnout and despondency. It is essential that we address the causes of this discontent. Dinesh Bhugra, past president of the BMA, after his report showing that 25% of doctors were suffering from mental health problems was published, said:[36,37]

This report shines an important light on the alarming mental health crisis currently burdening the medical workforce as the link between the current pressures on doctors and poor mental health can no longer be ignored.

I would echo this. A system that fails to support and protect its own staff will flounder.

REFERENCES

1 Veresaeff V. Simeon Linden (translator). *The Confessions of a Physician.* London: Grant Richards, 1904, p. ix.
2 Veresaeff V. Simeon Linden (translator). *The Confessions of a Physician.* London: Grant Richards, 1904, p. 176.
3 Lichterman B. *Memoirs of a Physician. BMJ* 2007;**335**(7614):307.2–307.
4 Paiba N. Running on empty. In: Jones P (ed). *Doctors as Patients.* Oxford: Radcliffe Publishing, 2005, p. 31.
5 Scheurer D, McKean S, Miller J, Wetterneck T. US physician satisfaction: a systematic review. *J. Hosp Med* 2009;**9**:560–8.
6 Murray A, Montgomery J, Chang H, Rogers W, Inui T, Safran D. Doctor discontent. A comparison of physician satisfaction in different delivery system settings, 1986 and 1997. *J Gen Intern Med* 2001;**16**(7):452–9.
7 Goodwin L, Ben-zion I, Fear NT, Hotopf M, Stansfeld SA, Wessely S. Are reports of psychological stress higher in occupational studies? A systematic review across occupational and population-based studies. *Plos One* 2013;**8**(11). doi: 10.1371/journal.pone.0078693.
8 McManus I, Winder B, Gordon D. The causal links between stress and burnout in a longitudinal study of UK doctors. *Lancet* 2002;**359**:2089–90.
9 Taylor C, Graham J, Potts H, Richards M, Ramirez A. Changes in mental health of UK hospital consultants since the mid-1990s. *Lancet* 2005;**366**:742–4.
10 Firth-Cozens J. The psychological problems of doctors. In: Firth-Cozens J, Payne R (eds). *Stress in Health Professionals: Psychological and Organizational Causes and Interventions.* London: Wiley, 1999.
11 Wall T, Bolden R, Borrill C, *et al.* Minor psychiatric disorder in NHS trust staff: Occupational and gender differences. *Br J Psychiatry* 1997;**171**(6): 519–23.
12 Mata DA, Ramos MA, Bansal N, *et al.* Prevalence of depression and depressive symptoms among resident physicians: a systematic review and meta-analysis. *JAMA* 2015;**314**(22): 2373–83.
13 Gerada C, Ashworth M, Warner L, Willis J, Keen J. Mental health outcomes for doctors treated at UK Practitioner Health Service: a pilot study. *Res Adv Psychiatry* 2019;**6**(1):7–14.
14 NHS England. National NHS Staff Survey 2018 [Survey]. Data accessed 30 October 2019. Available from: www.england.nhs.uk/statistics/2019/02/26/2018-national-nhs-staff-survey-in-england. Additional analysis conducted on data provided by NHS England.

15 2015 HSC staff survey regional report | Department of Health [Internet]. Health Available from: www.health-ni.gov.uk/publications/2015-hsc-staff-survey-regional-report.

16 NHS Wales. NHS Wales Staff Survey 2018: National report [Internet]. 2018. Available from: www.wales.nhs.uk/sitesplus/documents/866/4.3b%20 National%20Staff%20Survey%20Report.pdf. Additional analysis conducted on data provided by NHS Wales.

17 NHS Health Education England. NHS Staff and Learners' Mental Wellbeing Commission [Internet]. 2019. Available from: www.hee.nhs.uk/sites/default/files/documents/NHS%20%28HEE%29%20-%20Mental%20Wellbeing%20Commission%20Report.pdf.

18 ComRes (2019) *What it means to be a doctor*. Available from: www.gmc-uk.org/-/media/documents/what-it-means-to-be-a-doctor-report_pdf-79704293.pdf (accessed 1 November 2019).

19 British Medical Association. The changing face of medicine and the role of doctors in the future [Internet]. 2017. Available from: www.bma.org.uk/collective-voice/policy-and-research/education-training-and-workforce/changing-face-of-medicine.

20 British Medical Association. Caring for the mental health of the medical workforce [Internet]. 2019. Available from: www.bma.org.uk/collective-voice/policy-and-research/education-training-and-workforce/supporting-the-mental-health-of-doctors-in-the-workforce#report1.

21 World Medical Association. WMA statement on physicians wellbeing. Available from: www.wma.net/policies-post/wma-statement-on-physicians-well-being.

22 Canadian Medical Association. CMA National physician health survey. Available from: www.cma.ca/sites/default/files/2018-11/nph-survey-e.pdf.

23 IHS Markitt Ltd. The Complexities of Physician Supply and Demand: Projections from 2017 to 2032 [Internet]. Washington D.C.: Association of American Medical Colleges; 2019. Available from: www.aamc.org/system/files/c/2/31-2019_update_-_the_complexities_of_physician_supply_and_demand_-_projections_from_2017-2032.pdf.

24 Pattani S, Constantinovici N, Williams S. Who retires early from the NHS because of ill health and what does it cost? A national cross-sectional study. *BMJ* 2001;**322**:208–9.

25 General Medical Council. The state of medical education and practice in the UK: the workforce report. 2019. Available from: www.gmc-uk.org/about/what-we-do-and-why/data-and-research/the-state-of-medical-education-and-practice-in-the-uk/workforce-report-2019.

26 McCain R, McKinley N, Dempster M, Campbell W, Kirk S. A study of the relationship between resilience, burnout and coping strategies in doctors. *Postgrad Med J* 2017;**94**(1107):43–7.

27 Imo U. Burnout and psychiatric morbidity among doctors in the UK: a systematic literature review of prevalence and associated factors. *B J Psych Bull* 2017;**41**(4):197–204.

28 Halliday L, Walker A, Vig S, Hines J, Brecknell J. Grit and burnout in UK doctors: a cross-sectional study across specialties and stages of training. *Postgrad Med J* 2016;**93**(1101):389–94.

29 Orton P, Orton C, Pereira Gray D. Depersonalised doctors: a cross-sectional study of 564 doctors, 760 consultations and 1876 patient reports in UK general practice. *BMJ Open* 2012; **2**:e000274.

30 Baird B, Charles A, Honeyman M, Maguire D, Das P. Understanding pressures in general practice [Internet]. The King's Fund; 2016. Available from: www.kingsfund.org.uk/sites/default/files/field/field_publication_file/Understanding-GP-pressures-Kings-Fund-May-2016.pdf.

31 Gibson J, Sutton M, Spooner S, Checkland K. Ninth National GP Worklife Survey [Internet]. University of Manchester: Policy Research Unit in Commissioning and the Health Care System; 2018. Available from: www.research.manchester.ac.uk/portal/en/publications/ninth-national-gp-worklife-survey(4192e8f5-b256-45db-ad90-45274acda242).html.

32 Community Research (2019) *Adapting, Coping, Compromising*. Available from: www.gmc-uk.org/about/what-we-do-and-why/data-and-research/research-and-insight-archive/adapting-coping-compromising-research-exploring-the-tactics-and-decisions-doctors-are-applying (accessed 12 November 2019).

33 NHS Wales. NHS Wales Staff Survey 2018: National report [Internet]. 2018. Available from: www.wales.nhs.uk/sitesplus/documents/866/4.3b%20National%20Sta %20Survey%20Report.pdf. Additional analysis conducted on data provided by NHS Wales.

34 2015 HSC staff survey regional report. Department of Health [Internet]. Available from: www.health-ni.gov.uk/publications/2015-hsc-sta-survey-regional-report.

35 NHS England. National NHS Staff Survey 2018 [Survey]. (accessed 30 October 2019). Additional analysis conducted on data provided by NHS England.

36 Independent. One in four NHS doctors suffering from mental health issues, report warns. Available from: www.independent.co.uk/life-style/nhs-doctors-mental-health-stress-british-medical-association-a8881936.html.

37 British Medical Association. Serious mental health crisis among doctors and medical students revealed in BMA report [Internet]. 2019. Available from: www.bma.org.uk/news/media-centre/press-releases/2019/may/serious-mental-health-crisis-among-doctors-and-medical-students-revealed-in-bma-report.

5

Surviving and Thriving in Medicine

CLARE GERADA

Just as doctors don physical protection when dealing with patients, such as surgical gloves, face mask and theatre scrubs, so to must we use psychological protection to protect from emotional spillages. Given the day-to-day nature of medicine, the interesting issue is not why do so many doctors become unwell, but why do so few? Anxiety provoking events begin early in medical school with the first sight of the cadaver in the dissecting room (even today that sickly-sweet smell of preservative has still not left me), then continue as for me, needing to get over the repulsion of the sight of blood and the unnatural act of putting a needle into human flesh. We then have to continue to learn to deal with our errors and omissions (hard when you are chosen for your per-fectionistic, obsessional, compassionate traits). If we are not just to survive but thrive in our career, we have to learn to use a suite of cognitive, psychological and behavioural approaches to deal with the anxiety of working so close to death, despair, disability and failure. As the psychoanalysts Robert Hale and Liam Hudson wrote, doctors:

> are required to transform the shocking into the mundane; and, in doing so, to contain the unacknowledged anxieties their patients project into them. In coping, we each rely on defensive structures, institutional and individual, which for the most part serve us well.[1]

These mechanisms are made up of conscious **coping mechanisms** and uncon-scious **ego defences**. They are what prevents doctors collapsing into a psycho-logical heap every time they have to break bad news or deal with a severely injured patient. They allow us to move from one intensely traumatic event, such as the death of a child, to a more mundane one, seemingly effortlessly. The work environment can provide extra psychological protection through compassionate working practices, which foster team cohesion, predictable routines and fairness.

Learning different coping strategies are done frontstage, during the formal ward rounds, lectures and tutorials, and backstage, informally, through modelling on one's peers and trial and error. They are as important in the day-to-day practise of medicine as knowing how to take the blood pressure of a patient. They give us the skills and psychological armour to do the work expected of us. Over time doctors become desensitised to human emotion and this is normal. We all need to find the sweet point that Harold Lief and Renee Fox called 'detached concern'.[2] Lief and Fox were referring to the process whereby medical students learn through objectifying and intellectualising their experiences to distance themselves from their initial emotions of anxiety and fear. Doctors must learn to keep these emotional boundaries in place and the use of distancing, or detachment, when balanced with the appropriate amount of concern for the patient, has long been considered a recipe for a healthy patient–physician relationship. As they note: 'The empathic physician is sufficiently detached or objective in his attitude toward the patient to exercise sound medical judgment and keep his equanimity, yet he also has enough concern for the patient to give him sensitive, understanding care'.[2]

Detached concern is a hard balance to achieve and even harder to maintain. A balance needs to be found, as with too little armour we risk becoming broken by our patients' pain, too much and we can become hardened and unempathetic. Even with all the methods we use to protect ourselves, sometimes contact with our patients affects us deeply, and spills over into our private lives. This is where supervision and team working become so important, as they provide the safe space where we can show our emotional fault lines without fear of sanction.

This chapter on coping and Chapter 6 on resilience will explore how we do this. I distinguish in this chapter between coping (which I believe to be largely under conscious control) and unconscious ego-defences.

What students must learn at medical school to help cope with their job
How to understand and deal with transference and countertransference arising from the doctor–patient interaction
How to stay emotionally present without becoming emotionally labile
How to prevent overidentification with patients
How to 'forget'
How to not project one's own feelings onto patients
How to remain patient-centred
How to recognise and deal with compassion fatigue
How to maintain professional boundaries
How to break bad news

COPING STRATEGIES

Coping is a broad concept covering a range of thoughts and actions (cognitive, as in thinking, and behavioural, as in doing) that we use to make a situation more tolerable. In other words, using techniques to prevent or diminish threat, harm and loss or to reduce associated distress. Coping in itself does not imply **success**, but **effort**. All of us use coping mechanisms to deal with anxiety and to deal with difficult situations. I have used different strategies over the course of my career. For the stress of everyday general practice and more recently caring for sick doctors, I have relied heavily on talking, either to my peers or outside professionals. I have been part of a weekly reflective practitioner group for more than a decade and having a confidential space and the time to talk about patients who get under my skin has been invaluable. Less formal peer support has been through weekly multidisciplinary team meetings, which have been the bedrock of my clinical practice for over 30 years. For trickier and more personal issues, I have sought help on a one-to-one basis with outside professionals, over the years seeing a clinical supervisor, mentor, occupational psychologist, cognitive behaviour therapist and when, under immense pressure and felt things were becoming more difficult, a psychotherapist, who helped locate difficulties into a more personally historical context. I trained as a group therapist; joining and running therapy groups has helped me cope with dysfunctional groups I have encountered during my career. I have used running, and perhaps my favourite way of de-stressing at the end of a difficult day, watching back to back episodes of the TV programme 'Come Dine with Me'. I have also 'coped' by avoiding the stressor, walking away and hoping it will go away. It rarely does.

The literature classifies coping methods into **problem focused**, and **emotion focused**.

Problem-focused coping strategies act to minimise distress by reducing or eliminating the stressor, as well diminishing its impact. These are used where the individual has the power to change things. Techniques might include altering working patterns or working longer hours to get through a difficult period such as preparing for an examination. In the main, this helps deal with a (hopefully) temporary period of additional stress. Emotion-focused coping refers to strategies that regulate emotions and minimise the pain triggered by stressors. These include seeking out emotional support, meditation and using exercise or other relaxation methods.

There appears to be gender differences in what might be used. A study of Canadian physicians found females reported seeking out more social support when stressed than their male counterparts.[3] There is even some evidence that doctors in different specialities might prefer different ways of coping. For example, psychiatrists have been found to prefer relaxation techniques, organisational problem solving, staff support groups, confidential counselling and staff sensitivity sessions.[4] Doctors working in hospice and palliative medicine commonly reported using 'making time for oneself', meditation and reflection.[5] A survey of American doctors found nearly one-half used exercise to cope with burnout and one-third by eating junk food and one-quarter used alcohol.[6] In the short term, these of course can help. Who hasn't filled themselves up with stodge (after all it's called comfort food) or had a large gin and tonic to cope with a stressful day?

This brings me to the third category of coping. This is based on **avoidance** or **disengagement**, either through action (physically removing oneself from a situation or using drugs or alcohol to gain mental disengagement) or thinking (using denial or wishful thinking). While avoidance may temporarily be beneficial in distancing an individual from the stressor, the longer it is used, the more intractable problems can become, nor does it address the underlying issue. Prolonged use of avoidance can lead to an increase in intrusive thoughts about the stressor and as such more anxiety and/or further problems; for example, developing substance misuse. The most common avoidance technique I find in the doctors I treat is that they try and work themselves out of the problem. They work harder, stay longer hours and 'burn the candle at both ends'.

Elizabeth Cotton, psychoanalyst and author of *Surviving Work*, describes unhealthy coping mechanisms used by those struggling at work.[7] Among them is the unhelpful use of anger and blaming others. This might mean directing their frustration about lack of resources towards hospital managers, or even blaming the patient for their own illness. Similarly, an individual already struggling at work is an easy recipient for other people's projections and it is not uncommon for them to be scapegoated for problems in the workplace.

In 2019, the UK regulator, the General Medical Council (GMC) commissioned research on the tactics and decisions doctors use to survive in a system under pressure.[8] What they found was that doctors used different overlapping and interlinking methods that could be broadly be thought of as belonging in three areas:

- **Compromising**: looking for ways to reduce workload such as prioritising patients and their problems or what the service can offer; delegating tasks, encouraging patients to take more responsibility for their own health.
- **Adapting**: trying to change the way of working, such as improving effective team working, working longer and harder; spreading the workload with colleagues, using telephone or technology to save time; developing more effective triage systems and reducing administration.
- **Coping:** learning how to live with the pressure, having micro-breaks during the day; keeping their role varied, looking after their emotional wellbeing, such as using meditation, exercise and spending time with family or friends.

Specific coping mechanisms

Mapped onto the broad classification of coping are examples of different interventions that can be used. They can be what the **individual** does alone, or what can be done with **others**, either as one-to-one (mentoring, supervision, coaching) or in a group.

INDIVIDUAL

Setting boundaries

Setting boundaries, whether in a single consultation or across one's working life is a skill doctors must learn. Boundary setting starts in the consultation, especially important in general practice where it is not uncommon for patients to present with many (seemingly) unrelated problems, wishing to discuss them all in a 10–15-minute consultation. Even if time were not the issue, I express my concern to the patient that I am unable to focus on so many different matters at the same time. This is not about me denying their needs, but accepting that I have needs as well, and the most important one is to remain focused (and reasonably keep to time). Dealing with many different problems ranging from the psychological, social, physical and practical at a single time is not possible. This technique requires skill and experience – and it is important not to dismiss the 'oh by the way doctor' as the patient heads out of the room. The 'oh by the way' problem is often the most serious.

Boundary setting is also about learning to leave the patient behind at the end of the working day. Ruminating on difficult consultations or operations serves no purpose other than to increase anxiety. The blurring of boundaries between home and work is increasingly commonplace as we are encouraged to log in remotely into work computers, complete our paperwork at home or answer emails out of hours. Home should be a place where we recharge our psychological batteries and recover from the day's workload, not a surrogate consulting room. Setting boundaries also means being realistic as to what can be achieved and accepting of oneself if we cannot do everything. Setting limits requires practice as it is all too easy to say 'yes' rather than 'I can't'. This is even more important since COVID-19 where home working has become the norm. Doing that extra shift or staying longer in a crisis is fine, but when it is required, day in day out, then the doctor has to learn to say 'no'. Standing up for oneself should be part of the medical curriculum. For non-patient work, I have learnt deadlines are largely man-made and usually can be extended. Maintaining a clear boundary between work and home life is very important, as is taking all one's annual leave allowance. Boundary setting also happens between consultations, building in small amounts of time between difficult consultations to gather one's psychological equilibrium, asking oneself between time, 'am I in good condition for the next patient?' This is called 'housekeeping'.[9]

Dike Drummond, a charismatic American physician, who is also an expert on burnout has written his advice (based on an 800-pound, silverback gorilla) on maintaining personal work–life boundaries. It is well worth reading.[10]

Cognitive techniques

'Thinking' one's way out of psychological distress is efficacious. One of the most constructive coping mechanisms is called '**cognitive reframing**'. Much of the anxiety we feel in stressful situations is linked to how we interpret the threat we face. For example, if we haven't obtained the necessary blood result needed for the ward round, our automatic thoughts might be something along the lines, 'I am terrible, I am a bad doctor, I am never going to get passed as competent'.

These thoughts are more than likely then to induce feelings of anxiety. Identifying and challenging these negative and largely irrational thoughts and replacing them with more realistic ones is the essence of cognitive reframing. It is the technique that underpins cognitive behavioural therapy (CBT). Many doctors fret about failing exams. Failure for them equates with imperfection and thoughts of being useless and undeserving. Reframing this cognitive distortion by perhaps thinking, 'well, it was a very difficult exam' or 'others have failed exams before and gone on to have really good careers', can help. I talk more about these techniques in Chapter 23.

WITH OTHERS

If there was a single intervention that would enhance doctors' ability to cope (other than the obvious one of reducing workload) it would be to create the spaces where they can come together to talk about their work, in a psychoanalytical, reflective manner rather than focusing on the bio-medical aspects of our interactions with patients. Working with others, either in a one-to-one as in clinical supervision or in groups, provides for a sense of community, 'we're in this together' and reduces isolation and emotional disconnection from others. They also give us a reality check – normalising our experiences in the context of others. Working with others involves effective team working, multidisciplinary team meetings or more formal reflective group activities.

Team working

Belonging to a supportive team is probably the most effective way of dealing with workplace stressors. Teams that meet regularly, value each other's skills and support each other provide better preparation for individuals to cope with their work. It is the need to be connected to, cared for and caring of others, and to feel valued and respected that is most helpful. Teams help share the burden of complex cases and decrease professional isolation.[11] At my general practice, with sandwiches provided (I always feel teams bond best over food), we have a weekly team meeting where we discuss all safeguarding issues (child and adults), any new diagnosis of cancer and all deaths. These meetings are protected in the working week and everyone is expected to attend. This simple team event is now a rarity (especially so in general practice). The current arrangement of practising medicine has resulted in the loss of opportunities in which teams can be formed or sustained. The removal of the traditional 'firm', increased shift working, working across multiple wards, complex rotas, reliance on locums and frequent moves in training means that doctors have less opportunity to belong to a team. Now, no-one seems to notice the presence or absence of an individual, except how it relates to their function on the rota. This was the finding by the psychologist Michael West when asked to conduct an independent review on the increasing levels of mental illness among doctors.[12] Paradoxically, while working in teams contributes to high levels of job satisfaction, they can also be a source of stress as a poorly functioning team can expose role ambiguity and opposing values and leads to interpersonal conflict. Well-functioning teams need time and space to iron out their difficulties and resolve conflicts. This requires channels of communication, trust and spaces to bring people together. Sadly, as team members become more separated, through increasing part time working, reduced hours and shift working, these opportunities become scarcer.

Mentors and external support

Time with family and friends creates a refuge of stability and understanding,[13] provides a buffer for work-related stress[14] and a vital source of emotional support.[15] Mentors also assist stress reduction and adaptation to change.[16,17]

Clinical supervision

I want to focus a little on clinical supervision as I think it is a vital missing ingredient in the lives of most health professionals. Supervision, if provided to all staff (either on a one-to-one or as a group activity) would go a long way to improving the quality of care patients receive and increase professional resilience and more reflective ethical decision making.[18] Our psychotherapist colleagues seem to be one of the only professional groups that prioritise and see the value of this essential discipline. Clinical supervision is a safe and contained meeting with a colleague, which takes place on a regular basis (typically monthly) where the effect of working with patients can be explored, analysed and understood. The supervisee sets the agenda and brings what they wish to discuss and explore. The supervisor may offer guidance, seek clarification, and even challenge the supervisee. Within this meeting, the thoughts, feelings and actions of the supervisee are the focus. This is a rare space within medicine where the patient is not the focus. It's this very aspect that doctors often find very hard to grasp. The people we interact with on a daily basis will knowingly or unknowingly 'push our buttons' to some degree. These 'buttons' are *our* buttons, and with practice, experience and learning we can influence the degree to which those around us get to press them and if they do, how deeply they get pressed (if at all).

Supervision is not about performance monitoring or being pulled up on things not being quite right. When explaining what clinical supervision is, I often use the following visualisation. Imagine you and your patient are both wearing Velcro suits, yours is over your white coat. Most things that these suits come into contact with will stick. The patient arrives laden down with pain, distress or anger. This is too much for them to bear, so they understandably try and throw some at you, their clinician (this is largely done unconsciously). Our desire to help and heal means that if we are not careful, our metaphorical white coats become covered with these negative feelings and experiences thrown at us. They can weigh us down, and actually make us feel the same as our patients. Psychologists sometimes call this **emotional contagion**. This emotion is not yours, but the patient's and supervision can help untangle what belongs where. Once aware that the 'mood' does not belong to you, the doctor, it can be removed, examined, and disposed of, without I hasten to add, needing to throw it back to the person who gave it to you in the first place.

Supervision can occur in one-to-one or in groups, face-to-face or online, informally or formally, and between peers or in a more hierarchical relationship. The boundaries between coaching, supervision and mentoring are sometimes unclear, though I am not sure strict differences or definitions really add much. What is important is that any discussion about the individual's performance is kept separate.[19]

The GP John Launer, who has written about and practiced narrative-based supervision for a number of years, is careful to state that supervision is not therapy, though there is no clear dividing line where our need for supportive supervision ends and our need for psychotherapy begins.[20] As a supervisee I have been helped with my struggles dealing with complaints, errors, and how seriously ill relatives impact on my working day. Equally, as a supervisor, I would not ask my supervisee to leave their real-life issues at the door of the consulting room.

Reflective practice groups

During my GP training, I read the psychoanalyst Michael Balint's book *The Doctor, his Patient and the Illness*, which was published in the 1950s.[21] This ground-breaking book was the first time in my training I was introduced to the concept that the interaction between the patient and the doctor could be influenced by more than the medical condition the patient presented with. Michael was a Hungarian immigrant who, together with his wife Enid, started holding psychological training seminars for GPs. There were no lectures or directive 'teaching'. Instead, the work focussed on small group discussions (later called Balint Groups) using a psychodynamic rather than traditional clinical approach to understanding the doctor–patient relationship and dynamics of the consultation. Balint groups help doctors comprehend the interpersonal aspects of their work. They allow clinicians to reach a deeper understanding of their patient's feelings, exploring how one's own experience might interfere with the therapeutic relationship. In addition to Balint groups,[22] participation in practice-based groups,[23] Schwartz rounds,[24,25] and protected learning schemes all help doctors cope with their work.[26-29] These all enhance the connections between team members. They also improve the care patients receive as well as providing doctors with the space to talk about the emotional impact of their work.[30,31] Groups play an important function in giving us a space to remember our patients (for better or worse) and where needed to mourn their loss.

This case gives a practical example of different techniques that can be used:

Philip, a consultant surgeon was at the end of his tether. Workload pressures, which included a job split on two sites and a day a week in private practice, meant that he was always on the go. He constantly felt guilty that he was not spending enough time with his young family and was becoming grumpy with his wife as soon as he walked through the door. All he wanted was to have a double gin and tonic before speaking to anyone. Given an ultimatum by his wife, 'do something or I'll leave you' he decided to act.

Actions Philip took:

Problem focused (largely behavioural) Aim was to create more time for his family and not be so frazzled at the end of the day	Reduced his private practice by one session per week. Reduced his management session in his main work Cycled to work instead of driving to provide space for exercise Delegated work to his junior
Emotion focused (largely cognitive) Aim was not to be so tense and angry	Took up mindfulness Asked for a mentor at work
Avoidance (behavioural and cognitive) Aim was to get a bit of respite in his workload and prioritise his clinical work	Stopped doing discharge letters

Mentors, coaches and therapists can all help relieve the difficulties we face and help us survive into the future. An analyst once remarked to me that for those in the caring professions, it should be considered as normal to see a therapist, to keep our mind healthy, as it might be to go to the gym, to keep our body fit.

DEFENCE MECHANISMS

I will now move to those unconscious coping mechanisms, so-called **psychological ego defences**. First described by Sigmund Freud, psychological defences are techniques brought into play by the unconscious mind to manipulate, deny or distort reality to protect oneself against feelings of anxiety, unacceptable impulses or potentially harmful stimuli.[32] To be without psychological defences would be akin to going out in cold weather without a coat or in the rain without an umbrella. Defences allow for the maintenance of a healthy emotional distance between 'us', the carer, and 'them', our patients, such that we are able to leave our patients in the consulting room (so to speak) at the end of a day's work. They all act to reduce the intensity of the emotional arousal inherent in our work and help us achieve the ideal balance of detached concern discussed earlier in this chapter.

The psychologist George Vaillant explained the features of ego-defences[33] as the following:

- They mitigate the distressing effects of both emotion and cognitive dissonance.
- They are unconscious and involuntary.
- They are discrete from one another.
- They can be adaptive, even creative, as well as pathological.

Psychological defences start to be formed in early infancy, are refined during adulthood and used throughout life. They are learnt through modelling and attachments to family and peer groups.[34] The so-called **mature defence** mechanisms are often the most constructive and helpful. Most defence mechanisms are fairly unconscious – in other words, the individual does not know they are being used in the moment. They provide temporary relief to make a situation more manageable. If overused, and if the individual is not given the time, space and support to process their feelings, then problems can arise. Defensive styles can become entrenched as psychological walls build up and feelings of vulnerability and sadness become more deeply buried.

DEFENCE MECHANISMS USED BY DOCTORS

INTELLECTUALISATION

Intellectualisation is a mature defence mechanism enhanced during medical school training. When a person intellectualises, (s)he shuts down their emotions and approaches a situation solely from a rational standpoint. It helps deal with anxiety caused by real patients with real suffering. It allows us to think about events in a dispassionate, clinical way to avoid engaging with the emotional aspects of it. I remember the first time I saw cancer, really saw, this monstrous, fungating, malodourous mass, filling the entire side of a patient's face, and I nearly fainted. That evening, I spent time comparing his pathological features with those in the textbook. I learnt how to lose myself in the scientific and technical details of this man's suffering and, in so doing, avoid overidentification with him. I had learnt the defence of intellectualisation. Over the next few days, as I visited him after his heroic operation, I was able to blend professional detachment with human attachment – a vital skill for any doctor.

DENIAL

Denial is one of the most primitive of the defence mechanisms, as it is one of the first to occur developmentally. Denial is essentially the refusal to accept reality or fact and instead act as if a painful event, thought or feeling did not exist. It provides the capacity to detach from disturbing emotional states. It is perhaps one of the most commonly used defence mechanisms, used in everyday life. The culture of medicine encourages denial, as it emphasises the need for self-sacrifice and denial of personal needs over others, as epitomised in the first line of the GMC's *Duties of a doctor*, namely, *Make the care of your patient your first concern.* Doctors also use a classic defence triad to avoid admitting they are unwell, which is also often seen in addiction. These are denial (*I can't have an alcohol problem because I don't get withdrawal effects*), minimalisation (*I drink the same amount as my spouse*) and rationalisation (*I only drink in the evenings to relax, and I can stop at any time*).

Perhaps the worst example of denial I have seen was a patient, having been the subject of a serious complaint, put all his mail into bin-liners. In hiding the letters, he hoped to convince himself that there was no problem; if he didn't open the letters the problem would disappear. However, unlike a problem that is merely avoided or postponed, a denied problem does not go away, it just grows and grows. Individuals require immense psychological work to control their anxiety in the face of mounting evidence (in his case, full bin bags).

DEPERSONALISATION

Depersonalisation allows us to detach from a disturbing emotional situation, and to get on with the task in hand. For example, the emergency department doctor might only be able to perform well by seeing the patient as a series of biometric values, rather than the critically ill, young mother fighting for her life. Depersonalisation could be considered an adaptive response to intolerable situations and a protection against becoming overly involved with suffering (certainly in the short term when exposed to traumatic situations) as it helps to shut down emotions.

HUMOUR

Humour, when used as a defence mechanism, is the re-directing of unacceptable impulses or thoughts into a light-hearted story or joke. Like other defences, it reduces the intensity of a situation, and places a cushion of laughter between the person and the impulses. It is considered to be a mature defence mechanism and is often used by doctors to convert an intolerable situation into something more manageable. The thoughts retain a portion of their innate distress, but they are 'skirted around' by witticism, for example self-deprecation.

> They met behind the curtain, emergency department doctors and nurses desperately trying to save the life of a young man with serious head trauma and crush injuries to his chest. He was bleeding to death. They worked efficiently for 50 minutes, but even they could not reverse what a lorry had done to him that morning as it turned left, oblivious to the young man continuing to cycle straight on. At 10.20 the patient was pronounced dead. 'I bet he regrets not taking the tube' called out Henry, one of the doctors. The others laughed.

While appearing uncaring, this doctor is using humour to deal with this stressful situation.

OMNIPOTENCE

Omnipotence is acting as if one is possessed with special powers or abilities. This defence is present in almost all doctors and bolstered by the position we hold in society as privileged professionals. Given that doctors have to believe in themselves, it is hardly surprising that they develop fantasies of omnipotence. It is partly the reason I also believe doctors struggle so much to seek out care for themselves. Relinquishing our omnipotence means accepting vulnerability, and this in turn means loosening our attachment to our medical self. Becoming a patient is a fundamental breakdown of this defence mechanism.

ALTRUISM AND SUBLIMATION

Altruistic behaviour alleviates the anxiety created by guilt, through constructive service to others that brings pleasure and personal satisfaction. It is probably ubiquitous in all doctors.

Miriam is a GP. In her personal life, her father was suffering from dementia and in a nursing home many hours' drive away. She had always been close to her father; he had encouraged her to follow in his footsteps and become a doctor. Miriam, at that time, felt intensely guilty and ashamed that she could not visit him as often as she would have hoped. Instead she was busy with her work and doing extra sessions to help ease the backlog. She also spent her spare time helping out at a local nursing home. She even offered to cover the Christmas shift for the home. She loved the company of the residents and the work she did gave her intense personal fulfilment.

Miriam has alleviated her guilt at not being able to be with her father into working harder with patients with similar problems. Unchecked, she risks becoming overinvolved with her patients, missing out socially and not being with her father during his last few years.

Closely aligned to this defence mechanism is that of sublimation, which is the channelling of unacceptable impulses into more acceptable ones, such as altruism, humour or distraction. It is perhaps the most advanced of the defence mechanisms, allowing for partial expression of unconscious drives into more socially acceptable ones. For example, imagine Miriam had had a poor relationship with her father, that he had been abusive to her when she was growing up and wishes he were dead. By working in the care home, she is sublimating murderous impulses into enriching both individuals in the home and the wider community.

PROJECTION

Projection is the process where we put our own undesired thoughts, feelings or impulses into another person, 'the pot calling the kettle black'. Projection is used when thoughts are considered unacceptable for the person to express, or they feel ill at ease having them. Projection is often the result of a lack of insight and acknowledgement of one's own motivations and feelings. A common projection doctors engage in is the feeling that their patients are the sick ones – the ones with the flaws and failures and as such they (the doctor) cannot become unwell. The psychiatrist Jeremy Holmes, who inspired me to study psychiatry when a medical student, has postulated that the most important way a doctor defends themselves is by projecting their weaknesses and vulnerabilities onto their patients, allowing them to remove diseased and vulnerable parts of themselves.[35] This helps doctors feel stronger and more powerful, fostering the fantasy of invincibility. Closely aligned to projection is the defence of splitting, which involves the complete separation into good and bad aspect of oneself or others. Splitting happens in times of distress and leads to blaming and scapegoating. For example, managers are all bad, doctors are all good.

Defences in institutions

Organisations develop structures and practices that serve to protect those within it from anxiety. As with individual ones, organisational defences give the illusion of certainty and safety and provide protection from being overwhelmed by anxiety and helplessness, and from the possibility of being overwhelmed by need. The seminal work of Isobel Menzies-Lyth helped to describe what she called social (institutional) defences, social as they are created by the organisation in which they work. Menzies-Lyth was a British academic who, from a background of economics and experimental psychology, joined the Tavistock Institute in London, where she qualified as a psychoanalyst in 1954. Her observations of student nurses showed that the anxiety created by close and intimate involvement with a patient's illness could be avoided through the development of specific social defences. She drew attention to the stress of work the nurses were engaged in; especially distasteful tasks that the nurses found so disturbing were those connected to death and sexuality. The defence mechanisms she described are similar to those seen in individuals: depersonalisation, denial and detachment. She argued that practices such as handovers, frequent ward rounds, use of rigid protocols, systems of allocating tasks and responsibilities and the practice of referring to a patient in abstract ways, such as 'the liver in Bed 10', were all defences aimed at discouraging attachment and engagement with the patient.[36] Social defences are therefore not simply an individual's way of responding to stress and anxiety, instead they become institutionalised into ways of doing things.

CONCLUSION

Considering what doctors (and other clinical staff) have to face it is amazing how well they do function. I have discussed how doctors learn and use conscious and unconscious categories to help deal with their work. These all help us deal with the emotional work of medicine. Defences can however be overdone. The surgical scrubs can become a suit of armour, a protection worn to convey power and conceal impotence and fear. At an institutional level, defences can lead to ignoring the basic needs of patients and to a dehumanising culture, and at an individual level, to a deadening of affect and a loss of compassion and caring. Overall, talking helps, and bringing back the spaces where doctors can come together with their peers and colleagues in other disciplines will go a long way to address the emotional burden of their work and protect them from the hardships of the job.

REFERENCES

1 Hale R, Hudson L. Doctors in trouble. In: Firth-Cozens J, Payne R (eds). *Stress in Health Professionals*. Chichester: John Wiley, 1999, p. 221.

2 Lief HI, Fox RC. Training for 'detached concern' in medical students. In: Lief HI, Lief VF, Lief NR (eds). *The Psychological Basis of Medical Practice*, 1st edn. New York: Hoeber Medical, Division of Harper & Row, 1963, pp. 12–35.

3 McCann CM, Beddoe E, McCormick K, *et al.* Resilience in the health professions: a review of recent literature. *Int J Wellbeing* 2013;3(1):60–81. doi:10.5502/ijw.v3i1.4.

4 Fothergill A, Edwards D, Burnard P. Stress, burnout, coping and stress management in psychiatrists: Findings from a systematic review. *Int J Soc Psychiatry* 2004;50(1):54–65. http://dx.doi.org/10.1177/0020764004040953.

5 Swetz KM, Harrington SE, Matsuyama RK, Shanafelt TD, Lyckholm LJ. Strategies for avoiding burnout in hospice and palliative medicine: peer advice for physicians on achieving longevity and fulfilment. *J Palliat Med* 2009;**12**(9):773–7. http://dx.doi.org/10.1089/jpm.2009.0050.

6 Kane L. Medscape National Physician Burnout, Depression & Suicide Report 2019 [Internet]. Medscape. 2019 [cited 18 January 2020]. Available from: www.medscape.com/slideshow/2019-lifestyle-burnout-depression-6011056.

7 Cotton E. *Surviving Work in Healthcare*, 1st edn. Abingdon: Routledge, 2017.

8 General Medical Council. Adapting, coping, compromising research – exploring the tactics and decisions doctors are applying in a system under pressure. [Internet]. 2018. Available from: www.gmc-uk.org/about/what-we-do-and-why/data-and-research/research-and-insight-archive/adapting-coping-compromising-research-exploring-the-tactics-and-decisions-doctors-are-applying.

9 Neighbour R. *The Inner Consultation*. Lancaster: MTP Press Limited, 1987.

10 Drummond D. Prevent physician burnout: 4 work-life balance tools. *Mo Med* 2016;**113**(6):450–454. Available from: www.ncbi.nlm.nih.gov/pmc/articles/PMC6139766/pdf/ms113_p0450.pdf.

11 Littlewood S, Case P, Gater R, Lindsey C. Recruitment, retention, satisfaction and stress in child and adolescent psychiatrists. *Psychiatrist* 2003;**27**(2):61–7.

12 West M, Coia D. Caring for Doctors, Caring for Patients. GMC, 2019. Available from: www.gmc-uk.org/-/media/documents/caring-for-doctors-caring-for-patients_pdf-80706341.pdf.

13 Dyrbye LN, Power DV, Massie FS, *et al.* Factors associated with resilience to and recovery from burnout: a prospective, multi-institutional study of US medical students. *Med Educ* 2010;**44**(10):1016–26.

14 Thoits PA. Mechanisms linking social ties and support to physical and mental health. *J Health Soc Behav* 2011;**52**(2):145–61.

15 Jovanovic A, Wallace JE. Lean on me: an exploratory study of the spousal support received by physicians. *Psychol Health Med* 2013;**18**(5):543–51.

16 MacLeod S. The challenge of providing mentorship in primary care. *Postgrad Med J* 2007;**83**(979):317–19.

17 Alliott R. Facilitatory mentoring in general practice. *BMJ* 1996;**313**(7060):2.

18 Berwick D. National Advisory Group on the Safety of Patients in England. A promise to learn – a commitment to act. Improving the Safety of Patients in England. 2013. Available from: https://assets.publishing.service.gov.uk/government/uploads/system/uploads/attachment_data/file/226703/Berwick_Report.pdf.

19 Martin P, Copley J, Tyack Z. 2014. Twelve tips for effective clinical supervision based on a narrative literature review and expert opinion. *Med Teach* 2014;**36**(3):201–7.

20 Launer J. 2010. Supervision as therapy. *Postgrad Med J* 2010;**86**(1021):686. Available from: http://pmj.bmj.com/content/86/1021/686.

21 Balint M. *The Doctor, his Patient and the Illness*. Edinburgh: Churchill Livingstone, 1957.

22 Salinsky J. The Balint movement worldwide: present state and future outlook: a brief history of Balint around the world. *Am J Psychoanal* 2002;**62**(4):327–35.

23 Zaher E, Ratnapalan S. Practice-based small group learning programs: Systematic review. *Can Fam Physician* 2012;**58**(6):637–42.

24 The Point of Care Foundation. About Schwartz Rounds [Internet]. [Cited 18 January 2020]. Available from: www.pointofcarefoundation.org.uk/our-work/schwartz-rounds/about-schwartz-rounds.

25 Goodrich J. Supporting hospital staff to provide compassionate care: do Schwartz Center Rounds work in English hospitals? *J R Soc Med* 2012;**105**(3):117–22.

26 Brooks N, Barr J. Evaluation of protected learning time in a primary care trust. *Quality in Primary Care* 2015;**12**(1):29–35. Available from: Google Scholar (March 2020).

27 Stevenson AD, Phillips CB, Anderson KJ. Resilience among doctors who work in challenging areas: a qualitative study. *Br J Gen Pract* 2011;**61**(588):e404–10.

28 Jensen PM, Trollope-Kumar K, Waters H, Everson J. Building physician resilience. *Can Fam Physician* 2008;**54**(5):722–9.

29 Zwack J, Schweitzer J. If every fifth physician is affected by burnout, what about the other four? Resilience strategies of experienced physicians. *Acad Med* 2013;**88**(3):382–9.

30 Johnston J, Paley G. Mirror mirror on the ward: who is the unfairest of them all? Reflections on reflective practice groups in acute psychiatric settings. *Psychoanal Psychother* 2013;**27**(2):170–86.

31 Zaher E, Ratnapalan S. Practice-based small group learning programs: systematic review. *Can Fam Physician* 2012;**58**(6):637–42.

32 Freud S. *The Ego and the Mechanisms of Defense*. New York: International Universities Press, 1936.

33 Vaillant GE. *Adaptation to Life*. Boston: Little Brown, 1977.

34 Grohol JM. 15 Common Defense Mechanisms [Internet]. Psych Central. 2019 [cited 28 September 2019]. Available from: https://psychcentral.com/lib/15-common-defense-mechanisms.

35 Holmes J. Mental health of doctors. *Adv Psychiatr Treat* 1997;**3**(5):251–3.

36 Menzies IEP. A case study in the functioning of social systems as a defense against anxiety. In: Colman AD, Bexton WH (eds). *Group Relations Reader I*. Washington: AK Rice Institute Series, 1975.

6

Resilience

CLARE GERADA

Although the risks and contradictions of life go on being as socially produced as ever, the duty and necessity of coping with them has been delegated to our individual selves.

Zygmunt Bauman, 2007, p. 14[1]

Resilience seems to be the vogue across many different sectors, including health. It is a word being used interchangeably between describing a personality trait 'is the person tough enough' and a process 'did they absorb the pressure and recover'. Given the rising number of doctors with mental distress, policy makers, educators and even regulators are beginning to question whether today's generation of doctors are 'resilient enough' to work in modern healthcare. There are even suggestions whether we need to enhance their psychological robustness, for example by including compulsory mindfulness lessons or even selecting prospective students by screening for traits that are thought to foster mental resilience.

However, I can find no evidence that today's doctors are more, nor less able to withstand pressures than those of previous generations. Despite this, there has been proliferation of 'resilience training', which seems to come in all shapes and sizes. This includes workshops, e-learning programmes and self-help manuals designed to enhance their ability to cope with adversity. There is even an online quiz.[2]

I imagine the idea that 'yesterday's' doctors were made of 'tougher' stuff is largely due to my generation not talking about mental illness or burnout and, as such, these issues remained out of sight and out of mind. While these concepts might have been discussed in academic circles, they did not make their way to the front line of day-to-day medical training. When I was training, doctors were expected to work the hours set (sometimes more than 100 per week), with strict hierarchies, often bullying consultants and the expectation of 'lumping it or leaving it'. Of course, people fell by the wayside and others were harmed by their experiences. Just as today, we were damaged by long working hours and intense fatigue. For example,

I recall a fellow junior doctor, when I was working in 1986, Chris Johnstone, having a near-fatal car accident when he fell asleep at the wheel while driving home from a weekend on-call. He has since written a book, *Seven Ways to Build Resilience*.[3] Doctors have to be able to handle pressure and bounce back from adversity, and most are able to, though obviously, some more than others. They have to be adaptable and flexible, able to move rapidly between different clinical and leadership situations. They even need to have resilient bladders and go long periods without a bathroom break. This was the same 30 years ago as it is today. The belief that today's doctors are not resilient enough, that they lack the strength to do the job expected from them, is not backed up by evidence, just conjecture.

There are many attributes accredited to individuals deemed to be resilient. So many, that one might as well pull out of a thesaurus all the positive descriptions a person could possibly have. Attributes such as: confidence, coordination, composure, commitment, able to make adversity meaningful, having an effective work–life balance, good self-management skills, able to appropriately delegate, able to prioritise work, able to express their needs, have the social skills to enlist the support of others and to form secure emotional attachments.[4,5] To have all of these characteristics in a single individual is impossible.

Studies looking at what makes an individual resilient tend to start at the end. They look at individuals who have been successful, such as in the best-selling book *7 Habits of Highly Successful People*[6] and a study that involved 13 high achievers from different professions,[7] including an individual who held two world records in their field, a Member of Parliament, those in receipt of senior national awards or who had been honoured by the Queen. All we know about those deemed to be resilient is how we see them in the public domain. We know nothing about their private demons, their anxieties behind their public persona, their struggles or how luck might have played a part in their success. I have been called 'resilient', but I have survived and even thrived in my career largely due to luck, or factors external to my control. I have been able to work and live in the same area (minimising travel), I have had two healthy children and a supportive husband (allowing me time to develop my career), I have the good fortune of being able to work in the same practice for 30 years and to have a good income. Yet I have been riddled with self-doubt, fear of failure and struggling to feel equal among my peers.

Resilience may not be a positive trait. An individual might be resilient, not through positive personality attributes, rather because they are single minded, ruthless, selfish, lack insight and prone to put work above everything and everyone else. I am struck by how similar resilience is to the concept of 'self-efficacy', a term introduced in the psychological literature by the influential Canadian psychologist, Albert Bandura. He used it to refer to an individual's belief in their ability to succeed, accomplish a task or deal with challenges. According to Bandura, people with high self-efficacy, that is those who believe they can perform well, are more likely to view difficult tasks as something to be mastered rather than something to be avoided.

The literature on resilience is messy. As it is hard to define, it becomes very difficult to study or measure it. It comes from the Latin word, 'resilire' meaning to leap back. The dictionary definition of resilience is '*the ability of a substance or object to spring back into shape (elasticity)'* and *'the capacity to recover quickly from difficulties (toughness)'.*[8] Most definitions in the healthcare environment emphasise that resilience is the ability to not only survive, but to adapt. They also imply that resilience is a dynamic process whereby one effectively negotiates, adapts and learns from adversity. This means it is more than just hardiness, the ability to withstand pressure. Health Education England, the body that organises junior doctor training, describes it as 'the capacity to absorb negative conditions, integrate them in meaningful ways, and move forward'.[9] What is certain, is that resilience is always contextual, a dynamic interplay between the stressful agent or situation, the context and environment, and individual factors.

I grew up in a city in the Fenlands, a flat windy area just off the east coast of England. My late father, who as well as being a single-handed general practitioner, also grew orchids in a small green house inside our home. I remember that little room with its tropical heat and humidity created by the twin presence of a fan heater always set to 'high' and endless bowls of water creating permanent dampness inside the house. As well as giving me a love for medicine, my father also left me with an intrigue for these flowers. He used to talk to me about a very rare local orchid, the Fen Orchid, which always struck me as strange. Here in this outwardly desolate, windy, bleak area, these small flowers were able to thrive. But of course, though bred to be robust and survive the inhospitable fenlands, the everchanging and now more toxic environment has placed this plant on the endangered species list and is facing extinction. Special measures are required to help them continue to grow in the area. This little orchid taught me about resilience. That it is much more to do with the suitability of the environment in which we are placed than some innate ability or disability. Change the environmental pressure and a previously robust, hardy and 'resilient' flower fails to survive.

Everyone and everything has its breaking point beyond which it cannot go on. This has certainly been my experience. I am probably outwardly a very resilient individual, certainly in my general practice setting I am. If needed I am able to clear a waiting room full of patients, deal with patients' distress and deal competently and efficiently with their problems. I am often asked by colleagues to see patients that others struggle with. Yet, when I was asked to cover a colleague in an unfamiliar setting, with an IT system I could not use, patients with conditions slightly outside my area of expertise and staff unable to support me, I could not cope. I found myself becoming very anxious and then tearful. I was not able to deal with the new environmental situation. Our ability to deal with, and recover from, adverse events differs both between people and even within a single person, depending on external factors. Dealing with a failed resuscitation might be possible at the start of the day. However, at the end of a long shift and 'hungry, angry, late, tired' ('HALT'), the individual will be less able to cope, be more emotionally receptive to negative events and might feel overly responsible for situations outside their control. Resilience is depleted, and they might not bounce back. It is further reduced in a hostile setting, where staff are unsupported, work is relentless and resources are limited. Resilience also changes with experience. Being involved in a traumatic event, even if appropriately dealt with, might not guarantee the person will be psychologically better prepared next time around. The suggestion that resilience can be learnt through simulation seems to be wishful thinking. Dealing with the resuscitation of a baby in a simulation suite is a far cry from the real, emotionally fraught environment of an accident and emergency department.

STUDIES OF RESILIENCE IN DOCTORS

Despite resilience being a subject of study in the educational world for over 70 years, there are surprisingly few studies that look at the issue specifically in doctors. In 2011, the psychologist Clare McCann and colleagues conducted a literature review in nurses, social workers, psychologists, counsellors and doctors.[10] Being female and maintaining a work–life balance were the only two factors consistently and positively related to resilience across all five disciplines. Only one study was specific to doctors. The results indicated that the strongest relationship to high physician well-being (the measure of resilience) was positive patient interactions, which buffered the negative relationship between high emotional demands and well-being.[11]

A systematic review of resilience by McKinley and colleagues published in 2019 included papers from the previous decade and found 24 studies that examined resilience in doctors alone.[12] Studies were undertaken in the USA, Australia, South Africa, UK and Germany. The review cited research where a formidable array of personality traits and attributes correlated with resilience. These included: being mature, responsible, optimistic, persevering and cooperative,[13] having social supports and the ability to use them, good team working, having interests outside work, engaging in continuing professional development or small reflective groups, positive past experience of dealing with adversity,[14,15] high persistence, high self-directedness and low avoidance of challenges.[16] Given the importance of the work environment (and increasing concerns about the harm it is causing), it is perhaps rather surprising that the review found very few studies that investigated environmental influences on resilience. One found a positive correlation between high resilience scores and a lighter workload.[17] Another found that resilience was positively correlated with job resources such as opportunities for career development, influence at work and degrees of freedom in the workplace.[18] In military studies, resilience is correlated to peer support and group cohesion,[19,20] and this is the same for doctors. I have touched on the need for doctors to belong to groups that can sustain them throughout their careers. These groups change during the course of one's professional career but are vital to cope with a lifetime in medicine.[17]

Resilient individuals might also turn to unhealthy behaviours. For example, a study of nurses in Australia and New Zealand found the ability to problem solve (the study's marker of resilience) was only mildly related to better mental health, while sleeping, drinking, smoking and using drugs were positively associated with being able to better deal with adversity.[21]

RESILIENCE TRAINING

There have been thousands of studies, many conducted in the last decade, trying to evaluate whether intervention X (usually a mindfulness intervention with the addition of peer group work) improves resilience.

Resilience was depicted as a variable set of self-reported measures including those for: well-being, stress, coping, resilience, burnout, depression, anxiety, mood, empowerment, engagement with work, self-awareness and happiness.[22,23] Almost all the studies recruited volunteers.[24] Some involved a single 90-minute session, others such as the Stress Management and Resiliency Training (SMART) programme, a 12-week course.[25] To date the research on whether training or other processes can improve resilience (by that I mean any measure of surviving pressure at work) is a lukewarm 'maybe', but only if the participants attend of their own free will. One study where it was made compulsory for medical students to attend a monthly mindfulness-based stress management session[26] **did not** lead to a measurable improvement in student resilience. Ironically, on free text several students found the curriculum either counterproductive (as it took time away from studying or pursuing other activities of greater personal interest) or too specific in its focus on mindfulness. A systematic review of resilience among psychiatrists published in 2019[27] concluded that while the 33 studies showed that a combination of workplace, personal and non-workplace factors were important, workplace factors were the most commonly cited aspect influencing resilience.

Where studies have been performed on changing the workplace, they tend to involve interventions to improve team working, putting in place time where the emotional impact of work can be shared as well as introducing changes to the organisational aspects of work.[28] In Chapter 21 on medical students, I mention an intervention implemented at St Louis medical school, which aimed, among other things, to de-clutter the undergraduate curriculum. This study provided a number of interventions to medical students throughout their training, including access to reflective practice groups, reduction in the amount of taught and examined aspects of their training and access to confidential help if needed. The interventions had some impact, although short-lived as their positive effects were overwhelmed by the negative effects of external factors that were outside the medical school's control. For example, the stress caused by the national medical school examination and exposure to negative attitudes of other doctors when in their clinical placements.

More studies are needed that incorporate primary prevention strategies into the workplace. For example, stopping 12-hour shifts, improving team cohesion, reducing the number of patients seen per person per day or even making changes to the onerous monitoring and inspection regimes. At present, interventions are aimed at secondary prevention, that is shoring up the individual to deal better with their stressors, or tertiary prevention, that is treating those who become unwell. To create a resilient environment will require structural changes from ward to board, something that sadly seems unlikely to happen given the mindset to blame the hard-working healthcare professional rather than the system they work in.

Overall, across the different studies and with varying degrees of statistical significance, factors associated with improving resilience can be summarised as: **finding time to think, time to meet with peers, time to reflect (with another person) on the emotional impact of one's work and time to care for oneself and have life outside work.**

Where resilience training works, I suspect it is not because the person learns how to breathe deeply, but because it is a **distraction** from their stressful working environment, and importantly it allows them to form peer groups (the by-product of the resilience training interventions) for support. It is important to have spaces to talk with each other, to discuss the impact of one's work. This should not be about 'resilience training' though, it should just be good practice. Just as it is good practice to allow people time off for breaks or space in the day to eat. I fear that we are 'scientising' resilience in a way to deflect responsibility away from the obvious: making the workplace safer to work in.

CONCLUSION

It is fair to say that factors that influence personal resilience are similar to those that contribute to overall psychological well-being. These include close relationships with family, friends and colleagues, the ability to manage strong emotions and impulses and a positive view of oneself, with confidence in one's abilities and strengths. Resilience is about bending with pressure and bouncing back; it says nothing about the individual's ability to provide high-quality empathic care. Being resilient might mean becoming hardened, developing a thick outer shell and being able to withstand any pressure – but at what cost to the individual or their patients? Are we willing to trade a battle-weary, tough doctor for one who might be more compassionate, but needs more time or space to reflect and re-charge their emotional batteries? Doctors may already be too resilient, too willing to take on more work, stay longer hours and do extra shifts. So, the problem of the rising tide of mental illness might not be too little resilience, but too much. The fear I have is that resilience training is not about training to be resilient, but training to withstand abuse.

No amount of training, yoga, deep breathing or reflection can compensate for a dangerous and flawed system.

REFERENCES

1   Bauman Z. *Liquid Times: Living in an Age of Uncertainty*. Cambridge: Polity Press, 2007.
2   Siebert A. Resiliency Quiz: How Resilient Are You? from the Resiliency Center [Internet]. Available from: https://resiliencyquiz.com/index.shtml.
3   Johnstone C. *Seven Ways to Build Resilience*. London: Robinson, 2019.
4   Jensen P, Trollope-Kumar K, Waters H, Everson J. Building physician resilience. *Can Fam Physician* 2008;**54**(5):722–9.

5 Spangler N, Koesten J, Fox M, Radel J. Employer perceptions of stress and resilience intervention. *J Occup Environ Med* 2012;**54**(11):1421–9.

6 Covey SR. *7 Habits of Highly Effective People*. Covey SR (ed). London: Simon & Schuster 1989.

7 Sarkar M, Fletcher D. Ordinary magic, extraordinary performance: psychological resilience and thriving in high achievers. *Sport, Exercise, Perform Psychol* 2014;**3**(1):46–60.

8 Lexico Dictionaries. Resilience | Definition [Internet]. 2019 [cited 16 December 2019]. Available from: www.lexico.com/en/definition/resilience.

9 Health Education England. Meeting the challenge of reducing stress and building resilience in the NHS workforce. 4 April 2019. Available from: www.hee.nhs.uk/news-blogs-events/news/meeting-challenge-reducing-stress-building-resilience-nhs-workforce.

10 McCann C, Beddoe E, McCormick K, *et al*. Resilience in the health professions: A review of recent literature. *Int J Wellbeing* 2013;**3**(1):60–81.

11 Shapiro J, Astin J, Shapiro SL, Robitshek D, Shapiro DH. Coping with loss of control in the practice of medicine. *Families, Systems, Health* 2011;**29**(1):15–28. http://dx.doi.org/10.1037/a0022921.

12 McKinley N, Karayiannis P, Convie L, Clarke M, Kirk S, Campbell W. Resilience in medical doctors: a systematic review. *Postgrad Med J* 2019;**95**(1121):140–7.

13 Eley D, Cloninger C, Walters L, Laurence C, Synnott R, Wilkinson D. The relationship between resilience and personality traits in doctors: implications for enhancing well being. *Peer J* 2013;**1**:e216.

14 Olson K, Kemper K, Mahan J. What factors promote resilience and protect against burnout in first year pediatric and medicine-pediatric residents? *J Evid-Based Complementary Altern Med* 2015;**20**(3):192–8.

15 Perez G, Haime V, Jackson V, Chittenden E, Mehta D, Park E. Promoting resiliency among palliative care clinicians: stressors, strategies, and training needs. *J Palliat Med* 2015;**18**(4):332–7.

16 Robertson H, Elliott A, Burton C, *et al*. Resilience of primary healthcare professionals: a systematic review. *Br J Gen Pract* 2016;**66**(647):e423–33.

17 Waddimba A, Scribani M, Hasbrouck M, Krupa N, Jenkins P, May J. Resilience among employed physicians and mid-level practitioners in upstate New York. *Health Services Res* 2016;**51**(5):1706–34.

18 Mache S, Vitzthum K, Wanke E, *et al*. Exploring the impact of resilience, self-efficacy, optimism and organizational resources on work engagement. *Work* 2014;**47**:491–500.

19 Jones N, Seddon R, Fear N, McAllister P, Wessely S, Greenberg N. Leadership, cohesion, morale, and the mental health of UK Armed Forces in Afghanistan. *Psychiatry* 2012;**75**(1):49–59.

20 Department of the Army. Field Manual No. 6-22.5. Combat and Operational Stress Control Manual for Leaders and Soldiers. Washington: Headquarters, Department of the Army, 2009.

21 Chang EM, Bidewell JW, Huntington AD, *et al*. A survey of role stress, coping and health in Australian and New Zealand hospital nurses. *Int J Nurs Stud* 2007;**44**(8):1354–62. http://dx.doi.org/10.1016/j.ijnurstu.2006.06.003.

22 Sood A, Prasad K, Schroeder D, Varkey P. Stress management and resilience training among Department of Medicine Faculty: a pilot randomized clinical trial. *J Gen Intern Med* 2011;**26**(8):858–61.

23 Fox S, Lydon S, Byrne D, Madden C, Connolly F, O'Connor P. A systematic review of interventions to foster physician resilience. *Postgrad Med J* 2017;**94**(1109):162–70.

24 Krasner M, Epstein R, Beckman B, *et al.* Association of an Educational Program in Mindful Communication with burnout, empathy, and attitudes among primary care physicians. *JAMA* 2009;**302**(12):1284.

25 Berkland B, Werneburg B, Jenkins S, *et al.* A worksite wellness intervention: improving happiness, life satisfaction, and gratitude in health care workers. *Mayo Clin Proc Innov Qual Outcomes* 2017;**1**(3):203–10.

26 Dyrbye L, Shanafelt T, Werner L, Sood A, Satele D, Wolanskyj A. The impact of a required longitudinal stress management and resilience training course for first-year medical students. *J Gen Intern Med* 2017;**32**(12):1309–14.

27 Howard R, Kirkley C, Baylis N. Personal resilience in psychiatrists: systematic review. *Br J Psych Bull* 2019;**43**(5):209–15.

28 Dunn P, Arnetz B, Christensen J, Homer L. Meeting the imperative to improve physician well-being: assessment of an innovative programme. *J Gen Intern Med* 2007;**22**(11):1544–52.

7

Shame in Medicine

SANDY MILES

Shame is a social emotion. It is the feeling of inadequacy we experience when we fail to meet our own, or others, expectations of ourselves. Experiences of shame in medicine are rarely discussed by doctors, yet shame is a powerful, primitive emotion that plays an important role in development of self and in one's social values. Shame differs from guilt as it is a personal and internalised emotion; 'I am bad' rather than guilt: 'I did something bad'. It is a 'quiet' emotion, resulting in withdrawal or making oneself small, so can be easily missed by colleagues and educators. It is such a distressing emotion that most strive to avoid it. However, as well as being potentially destructive, feeling shame can drive the so-called pro-social behaviour of helping others, increase doctors' awareness of their important core values and act to reinforce their commitment to caring. All of these are vital assets in a well-rounded doctor.

THE ORIGINS OF SHAME

Doctors feel shame when they fail to live up to the values that they feel are essential to maintain their professional identity. The author and comedian, Adam Kay was working as a junior doctor in obstetrics when his pregnant patient suffered a massive haemorrhage. Despite his best efforts her baby died. His experience of shame, his feeling that he had failed, is painfully documented in his book *This is Going to Hurt – A Secret Diary of a Junior Doctor*.[1] His sense of failure and shame overwhelmed him, and he left medicine. The idealised, 'omnipotent doctor' image sold to him during training was just an illusion; when things went wrong, he felt ashamed of his inability to cure his patient. He directed his shame into comedy telling and writing funny stories about his work.

Medical professionals are exposed to shame from many incidents in their daily work. These include failing to meet organisational targets, the shame of making errors and of not reaching the standards we aspire to. Doctors are also shamed by exposure to the sickness and vulnerability of patients. Shame can result in doctors becoming depressed, addicted to alcohol and drugs, self-harming or, as with Adam Kay, leaving medicine altogether. It can also lead to withdrawal from colleagues, unprofessional behaviour and even to humiliation of patients.

Causes of shame for medical professionals

Danielle Ofri, an American physician and author, in her exploration of how emotions affect the practise of medicine[2], describes an episode where she made a clinical error as a junior doctor. Her mistake potentially endangered the patient's life. In front of staff and patients she was humiliated by her senior colleague. She describes her experience as 'standing in a puddle of self-mortification'. Her inability to provide a reasonable explanation for her actions caused time to distort and, as she describes, '30 seconds clawed out to an eon'. She recovered her composure sufficiently to manage the patient's condition. She says the experience was so painful that she did not mention it again for 20 years, before writing of it in her book. Adam Kay, too, kept his pain to himself and says even his close friends would only have heard about it first on reading his book. With Ofri, the guilt of the mistake was easily dealt with. It was the destruction of her self-image, her identity, as a competent physician that haunted her all those years. She describes it as 'the shame of realising I was not the person I thought I was'. Shame distorts how doctors perceive themselves, shattering their illusion of competent, strong and trusted doctors; instead, the self-image becomes someone who is incompetent and **hurts** patients. The error leads to the doctor blaming themselves, failing in the process to consider the role of others or system factors. They distort their view of themselves as flawed and inadequate. An American doctor and author, William Bynum, experienced a devastating reaction to his serious error made during an operation. He describes his view of himself:

> I looked at myself, and I was aghast at what I saw: a broken, incompetent, unworthy resident who hurts patients. Before then, others had seen me – and I had seen myself – as a fairly strong resident, but I clearly had everyone fooled. My true colors and deeply flawed self were now on full display, and a rush of fears came into focus: What would others, particularly those I respected most, think of me? Would they trust me again? Who else would suffer from my incompetence? I plotted ways to leave the hospital completely unseen, and I wondered if I could return. In the days after, I isolated myself, disengaged from the world around me, and suffered quietly. It was brutal.[3]

He channelled his feelings into academic research to 'pull back the curtain' on shame. His work highlighted the importance of it as powerful, debilitating emotion often triggered by single events such as errors. He found doctors applied labels themselves during a shame reaction, such as: deficient, undeserving and inadequate, not smart enough and the dumbest person here, the worst, unlikeable and inferior, flawed, and like there's something wrong with me.[4]

SHAME AND IMPERFECTION

The need to be perfect can become a psychological trap as the responsibility to get things right is a heavy burden, which brings huge potential for shame when things do not go well.

SHAME OF TARGET-BASED CULTURE AND REDUCTION OF AUTONOMY

Another source of shame for doctors is the constant focus on increased productivity and meeting performance targets. This industrialisation of healthcare is shaming; it reduces doctors' autonomy to provide the care they believe is in their patient's best interest and forces them to compromise choices in order to adhere to targets. The nurse Karen Sanders has written about her experience of being rendered powerless by the impossibility of meeting UK government-set targets for treating all emergency departments patients within four hours.[5] These targets were enforced by a top-down system of surveillance and management. While acknowledging that patients need to be treated efficiently, she was faced with being unable to achieve the target without making shame-inducing compromises between meeting the target and treating patients according to their severity of condition. Her despair that the rapid treatment of someone with a mild viral illness was valued more highly because it achieved the time target, than the care of someone who was very sick, was profound. She suggested that the emergency department is a place that is prone to the dynamics of shame and humiliation. This potential is exacerbated by staff being subject to externally determined time targets and reprimanded for failing to achieve them. The result is that nurses and doctors may lose their sense of professional competence and responsibility, moral agency and integrity, to their own personal detriment and to the detriment of the patients with whom they work.

EFFECTS OF SHAME

Brené Brown, an American professor of social work who has extensively studied vulnerability and courage, proposes that shame leads to one or more of the following responses:

- Firstly, moving away, physically withdrawing, silencing the self and keeping secrets.
- Secondly, moving towards, seeking to appease and please others.
- Finally, moving against, seeking to gain power by aggression or shaming and blaming others.[6]

Her work adapts Donald Nathanson's model for describing the impact of shame, *The Compass of Shame*.[7]

One source of doctors' shame derives from struggling to meet organisational targets. The threat of this shame can be seen by employers as a useful tool to keep individuals in line and boost productivity. Undoubtedly the fear of shame can perform this role for doctors. Yet in cultures that are based on shame, it can also have the opposite effect. People behave immorally in order to court favour, to appease superiors, to avoid being rejected for not complying with requests or orders. In 2009 serious concerns were raised by relatives and patients being treated in a hospital about excessive patient deaths and deficiencies in the care provided. The subsequent investigation and public inquiry into the actions of Mid Staffordshire Hospital Trust uncovered appalling patient neglect, including patients being left to lie in their excrement and denied food and water. In this hospital basic patient care such as requests for assistance to use a bedpan or get to and from the toilet were not responded to. The barrister, Robert Francis in his investigation revealed a systematic demoralisation of staff, followed by a decline in their ethical behaviour leading to the shaming and scapegoating of patients and relatives.[8] The psychotherapist and author John Launer highlighted the inescapable link between the shameful standards of care and 'incentivising short cuts to compliance by applying career-threatening pressure – or, in plain language, bullying people'.[9] A target-focused, shame-based organisation lost its awareness of the needs of patients and humiliated and bullied staff, creating a culture of secrecy and loss of compassionate care. The shamed staff then proceeded to behave shamefully to patients and their families. Francis rightly advocated that patients who had been harmed should be offered emotional support. However, disappointingly he made no mention of the emotional needs of the staff shamed by their superiors and their subsequent involvement in the substandard care. The shame doctors feel when they are unable to meet targets is compounded by them being blamed for not being resilient enough, thereby shifting the blame and shame to the individual rather than addressing the working conditions that caused their distress.

Bearing witness to care that falls below the standard they want to provide, drives doctors to emotionally withdraw, splitting their personal and professional identities as a protective mechanism against shame. Shame, therefore, is associated with suffering – for both patients and doctors. With these negative effects it is easy to agree with June Tangney when she refers to shame as the 'ugly emotion'.[10] However, it can also have a positive, necessary and moral role to play.

Positive effects of shame

Shame also has the potential to motivate people to do good. The sociologist, Ilona De Hooge has focused on investigating shame's prosocial role, in particular its link to the promotion of the interests of others above those of the self.[11] Through empirical experiments, she and co-researchers demonstrated that individuals who experienced or imagined shame were more likely to act beneficently towards others. Experiencing the pain of shame drove moral behaviour. Shame therefore can have positive interpersonal consequences. The prosocial effect on behaviour is driven by a desire for appeasement or boosting self-esteem, and shame could therefore act as a commitment device to altruism – vital in medical professionals.

Shame also has an essential role of making us aware of what we hold dear, what our values are and what is essential to our identity. The Australian academic, Elspeth Probyn, quoting Sylvan Tomkins'[12] seminal work on affect in babies, observed that shame operates only after interest or engagement has been activated.[13] In other words, we only experience shame when our personal values are being challenged. As such, a situation that is shameful to one person may not evoke shame in another.

Another positive function of shame, promulgated by the therapist and theologian Carl Schneider, is to hide the vulnerable self.[14] Schneider's notion is that shame is not to be feared or shunned as it provides essential protection for the self and privacy to develop one's identity. Far from being an impediment to self-realisation, healthy shame emerges from Schneider's analysis as one of the distinguishing markers of our humanity. The sociologist Erving Goffman described a theory of self whereby people have the desire to control the impressions that others form of them.[15] He recognised that in all social interactions people engage in practices to avoid causing themselves, or others, shame or embarrassment. He then likened these performances to those undertaken by actors with constructed language, props and costumes. The 'front' stage represents the desired view of the self as seen by others while the 'back' stage is where that self can be further prepared or put to one side. He recognised that groups form bonds to enable them to put on the performances that they see as representing their group ideal. According to this theory, the performative links with medicine are clear with doctors speaking a specialised, technical language, wearing distinctive clothes and using props such as stethoscopes to help them play their role. Adopting the typical behaviours of the professional group that they have joined helps doctors to avoid shame, even if it means setting aside their other self, their personal identity, when they move to the 'front of stage'.

ATTENDING TO SHAME

Brené Brown promotes the benefit of individuals retaining their vulnerability to feeling shame. She explains in *Daring Greatly*[6] that it is impossible to avoid shame as it forms an integral part of the human experience. She claims, however, that it is possible to experience it without sacrificing values and identity. She calls this ability 'shame resilience' and explains that the antidote to shame is empathy from others, as well as self-compassion. The first step to helping the self and others who are suffering with shame is to recognise the phenomenology of shame, which could be withdrawal, appeasement or anger; secondly, working out what triggers it; and finally, acknowledging that shame drives disconnection. She advocates discussing the experience with others in order to neutralise the shame and rebuild a connection to the self. This is the basis of success in group discussions for those suffering from mental illness and points to the need to create a culture where the topic of shame can be discussed openly. This is why group therapy for doctors can help to address the isolation of their perceived shameful experience (such as that of being mentally ill).[16]

CONCLUSION

Shame forms a covering between the vulnerable self and the projected professional identity – between the personal and the social. However, instead of being a protective shield, the fear of the pain of shame can act as a barrier, preventing the vulnerable self from having a connection with the future doctor identity.

Doctors are now more regulated, have less autonomy and are increasingly troubled by having to meet the often-competing demands of their employers and their patients. There is a growing awareness of the mental distress suffered by doctors doing an ethically and emotionally challenging job. Increasing doctors' awareness of their emotional needs and the role that shame plays in identifying the values that form their core personal identity, can help reduce this distress and improve the compassion they afford patients.

Moral decisions required in medical practice are often made using emotional rather than rational reasoning. Therefore, we need to help doctors regulate rather than repress their emotions, understand shame and develop a resilience to it. Becoming adept at noticing shame is an important first step. Reversing the current trend for intrusive regulation and external targets, removing the culture of blame for honest errors and helping trainees to accept that some errors are inevitable, can help relieve the burden of shame from doctors. Finally, trusted seniors and peers need to be available to encourage discussion, provide empathy and neutralise experiences of shame to prevent harm.

REFERENCES

1 Kay A. *This Is Going to Hurt: Secret Diaries of a Junior Doctor*. London: Picador, 2018.

2 Ofri D. *What Doctors Feel: How Emotions Affect the Practice of Medicine*. Boston: Beacon Press, 2013.

3 Bynum W. To pull back the curtain on shame in medical education, I had to start with myself. [Internet]. AM Rounds. Available from: http://academicmedicineblog.org/to-pull-back-the-curtain-on-shame-in-medical-education-i-had-to-start-with-myself.

4 Bynum W, Artino A, Uijtdehaage S, Webb A, Varpio L. Sentinel emotional events. The nature, triggers, and effects of shame experiences in medical residents. *Acad Med* 2019;**94**(1):85–93. doi: 10.1097/ACM.0000000000002479.

5 Sanders K, Pattison S, Hurwitz B. Tracking shame and humiliation in Accident and Emergency. *Nurs Philos* 2011;**12**(2):83–93. doi:10.1111/j.1466-769x.2010.00480.x.

6 Brown B. *Daring Greatly: How the Courage to Be Vulnerable Transforms the Way We Live, Love, Parent, and Lead*. Gotham Books, 2012, p. 77.

7 Nathanson DL. Shame transactions. *Transact Analy J* 1994;**24**(2):121–9. DOI: 10.1177/036215379402400207.

8 Francis R. The Mid Staffordshire NHS Foundation Trust Inquiry: Independent Inquiry into Care Provided by Mid Staffordshire NHS Foundation Trust January 2005–March 2009. London: The Stationery Office, 2010.

9 Launer J. Bullying in the health service. *Postgrad Med J* 2013;**89**(1051):307–8. doi:10.1136/postgradmedj-2013-131983.

10 Tangney JP. Moral affect: the good, the bad, and the ugly. *J Pers Soc Psychol* 1991;**61**(4):598–607. Available from: www.researchgate.net/profile/June_Tangney/publication/21194658_Moral_Affect_The_Good_the_Bad_and_the_Ugly/links/57437bd208ae298602f0f075/Moral-Affect-The-Good-the-Bad-and-the-Ugly.pdf.

11 de Hooge IE, Breugelmans SM, Wagemans FMA, Zeelenberg M. The social side of shame: approach versus withdrawal. *Cogn Emot* 2018;**32**(8):1671–7. DOI: 10.1080/02699931.2017.1422696.

12 Sedgwick EK, Frank A (eds). *Shame and Its Sisters: A Silvan Tomkins Reader.* Duke University Press, 1996.

13 Probyn E. *Blush: Faces of Shame.* University of Minnesota Press, 2005.

14 Schneider CD. *Shame, Exposure and Privacy.* Norton, 1992.

15 Goffman E. *The Presentation of Self in Everyday Life.* Doubleday Anchor, 1959.

16 Gerada C. Healing doctors through groups. *Br J Gen Pract* 2016;**66**(651):e776–8. DOI: 10.3399/bjgp16X687469.

8

Suffering, Sacrifice and Stigma

CLARE GERADA AND ISA OUWEHAND

The most tragic thing is a sick doctor.
George Bernard Shaw, *The Doctor's Dilemma*

SUFFERING

Suffering is woven into the fabric of medicine for patients and doctors. Both groups experience pain, distress and hardship in their interaction with sickness. While patients, in the main, cannot avoid this suffering, doctors choose to be surrounded by it as a way of life. This begs the question, what drives a person to become a doctor, knowing, on some level, that their chosen work will be hard, emotionally draining, physically exhausting and filled with moments of absolute terror? Maybe these individuals conveniently downplay the potential hardships or imagine the benefits make it worthwhile. More likely, however, the choice is made so early on in life, when one might have a more idealised view of the profession, and that the full realisation of what is in store is hidden.

Often the decision to study medicine is made in pre-teenage years; for some so early in life to become anything else might never have been considered, a 'professional calling'. Though there are various reasons why individuals choose medicine as a future career, it is often linked to their previous life experiences of emotional distress. While not articulated as such, this choice may have been influenced by witnessing or experiencing suffering or seeing it relieved. This was discussed briefly in Chapter 3 when exploring the reasons why doctors might be at risk of mental illness. Everyone carries with them some psychological, emotional and physical pain from the past. The founder of psychoanalysis, Sigmund Freud, suggested that we are prone to repeat these, and this forms the basis of psychoanalytical practice. The choice of career might provide the theatre for playing out the 'wounded', unresolved parts of one's past. For example, choosing medicine may serve as a defence against past anxiety at not being able to heal or save family members. Even choosing a speciality might be based on previous experience: a doctor might become a paediatrician having suffered from serious illness during their own childhood, or an addiction specialist due to parental alcoholism. In both cases, their encounters with suffering might give them a better understanding of their patients' needs. This is especially the case in those who attend one of the authors' (CG) bereavement group (bereaved following the death through suicide of a doctor). So many of the group members deal with their experience by helping others, by setting up charities, support groups or spending their time trying to prevent the same happening to others.

A student talked about how the death of his father was the decisive motive for him:

> And then when my father died, I was like 'oh maybe if I become a doctor, I'll be able to, you know, stop people from dying'. And that was what I was thinking: if I become a doctor, I would be able to help more people. Maybe I would be able to stop and know what is [sic] wrong with my father and things like that. So there and then I started looking at the medical field.

This student, if unsupported, could be more vulnerable to mental illness, if, as is inevitable, he fails in his endeavours to help those affected by a similar condition as his father. These motives, predominantly unconscious, can be a driving force for compassion and commitment, but they can also be a foreshadowing for suffering if not understood and managed through supervision or reflective practice. This concept is corroborated by the Woodward *et al.* study, which explores the reasons junior doctors decided to study medicine, the most common given answer was a desire to help others, driven in part by previous life events.[1]

The unconscious desire to heal a loved one, and the guilt associated with failing to do so, can become channelled into a relentless drive to care more, be more altruistic and work harder. If unchecked, this may not lead to reparation or healing, but repeated failure at attempting to cure the incurable, which further feeds the associated emotional drive to apply oneself to an impossible task. This forms the basis of the 'wounded healer'.

The idea of the wounded healer dates back to antiquity. Plato, the founder of Western philosophy, considered the most skilful clinicians to be those who had suffered from all sorts of illnesses. The psychoanalyst Carl Jung considered the wounded to be one of the human archetypes. An archetype is something all humans have in common, irrespective of their culture, gender or period of history in which they live. Archetypes repeat themselves in the collective unconscious of mankind. This could be in the form of dreams, stories, art or even myths, all of which cross cultural boundaries. As such, they are universal and embody a hereditary factor in the human psyche incorporated metaphorically into our genetic make-up.

Jung traced the origins of the wounded healer to the Greek myth of Chiron (from where the word *chirurgie* is derived in French and *surgery* in English). He was a wounded centaur, and his student was Aesculapius, who later became the god of medicine and healing. Chiron was an immortal demigod who was accidently wounded with a poisoned arrow; the wound never healed and caused him immense pain. He chose to transform his suffering into helping others until he eventually renounced his immortality by exchanging his life for Prometheus's freedom.

Jung suggested that personally experiencing suffering is the best training for a physician and, therefore, only the wounded can make effective healers. However, within his archetype it was not enough for the wounded healer just to have experienced trauma and suffered themselves. Rather, central to his interpretation was the process of transformation, usually through personal therapy, to be changed and enlightened by the experience of trauma or adversity, the notion of the 'own' and the 'wise' as described by Goffman.[2] Jung believed the wound is essentially the awareness that flows from its experience:

A good half of every treatment that probes at all deeply consists in the doctor examining himself – it is his own hurt that gives a measure of his power to heal. This, and nothing else, is the meaning of the Greek myth of the wounded physician.[3]

The Canadian physician Searge Daneault considers both patient and doctor benefit from the doctor's experiences of suffering:

The physician's experience of being wounded is what makes him a brother of the patient, rather than his master. This triggers a fundamental change in perspective. The suffering patient can be cared for by the physician and be instrumental in the physician's own healing. Each encounter between physician and patient can be transforming and creative for both people.[4]

Everyone is 'wounded' in some way, even (or, maybe especially) doctors. There may be past physical or emotional traumas, illnesses, personal failure (or in medicine an error), difficult life events, addictions and a whole host of unnamed problems to deal with. While many of the 'wounds' may have preceded the feelings of 'not coping with the job' or becoming unwell, they may also arise from the ways in which the doctor manages their coping strategies prior to seeking or being referred for help.

Any of these wounds can provide knowledge and wisdom to the person suffering from them. They can help the person develop new insights or change one's trajectory of life. Accepting these wounds can also reduce stigma and shame. Daneault makes the point that:

There is no reason for physicians to be ashamed of their suffering. Viktor Frankl, a psychiatrist who managed to survive the Nazi concentration camps, teaches us that, just like destiny or death, suffering is a fundamental human experience.... The new focus on physicians, their health, and their suffering, speaks in a profound and fundamental way of Western medicine. It offers the possibility that physicians' health is a function of the creative potential of medicine.[4]

Working with and transforming suffering into understanding is both purposive and therapeutic and as Daneault mentioned, can be immensely creative.

There are many wounded healers in medicine, as evidenced by the large number of personal narratives in the literature. For example, the psychiatrist, Linda Gask, writes poignantly about her experience of suffering from severe depression in her memoir, *The other side of silence*;[5] in *Doctors as Patients*, edited by the general practitioner Petra Jones, each chapter is a personal account of mental illness (many written anonymously);[6] and Ahmed Hankir, who writes under the name 'The Wounded Healer', about his experience of bipolar disorder (see Chapter 14).[7] There is another genre of books (re-)emerging, those that are not so much about an individual's own experience of mental illness, rather perhaps a wish by the author to redress the discrepancy between medicine as imagined and the reality of practice, such as those by Adam Kay,[8] Paul Kalanithi,[9] Sue Black[10] and Joanna Cannon.[11] These are all largely derived from the authors' lived experiences of doctoring and each, in their own way, removes the gloss of doctoring and exposes the suffering that lies below. Finally, there are those whose experiences of suffering as doctor-patients has put them in touch with the suffering their own patients experience. Robert Klitzman's *When Doctors Become Patients* is a series of interviews with doctors with life-threatening illnesses.[12] For many their experiences changed the way they treated their own patients. Their suffering led to more compassion for, and connection with, their patients. It also led to better understanding of minor indignities that lead to suffering, such as waiting, as one interviewee said, 'A person waiting is a person suffering' and 'Waiting can be one of the most difficult parts of being a patient'. The vignettes and interviews demonstrate how suffering can be transforming, if the doctor is willing to be reflective and contemplate their own vulnerabilities. There was much more empathy because, as Klitzman points out, 'Confronting one's own mortality can make it easier to confront that of others'.

SACRIFICE

All jobs require a degree of sacrifice, but there are few where it is enshrined in their code of practice as with medicine. The first line of the Declaration of Geneva 1949[13] (the modern-day equivalent of the Hippocratic Oath) reads:

> I solemnly pledge myself to consecrate my life to the service of humanity.

The socialisation of medical students into 'Medicine' goes beyond learning the knowledge and skills necessary to do the job and includes mastering the largely unwritten rules needed to be inculcated into the profession. Self-sacrifice is one of these rules and is as expected of a doctor as washing one's hands. The academic Frederick Haffertey suggests medical students undergo an intense form of adult 're-socialisation'.[14] This is through a series of encounters underpinned by the tension between lay and medical norms and values, with the latter (medical norms) emerging as 'superior' to the former. For example, during dissection the student learns the 'feeling rules' and as such must not react as a lay person might do to the cadaver. Learning to sacrifice oneself is part of these rules as discussed in Chapter 1 as becoming a doctor is marked by immense personal sacrifice. From the outset, medical students have to work harder, longer and under more constant scrutiny than other students. Once qualified, they must endure endless postgraduate exams, studied for alongside busy jobs. Even following these examinations, the requirement to stay on the medical register means that they must continue to perform academically until retirement. This requires sacrifices in one's family and social life and extracurricular activities. In the main, they are worth it, set against the rewarding nature of the job. However, there is therefore a moral and ethical duty of the 'system' to take care of them. Evidence suggests this is not the case.[6]

On paper, today's doctors might have it easier. After all, they no longer work the onerous 120 hours per week, they have much stricter working hours and their employer can even be fined if they work over the allocated shifts. Yet a doctor starting out in the late 1970s had hospital accommodation, hot food provided day and night and protected time for training. They had flexibility over shifts, which were easier to change, and could book annual leave rather than take what was allocated. Doctors today must work extra shifts when gaps appear in rotas and they have little flexibility over their working life or taking time off – try planning your own wedding when it is uncertain whether you can get the day off as annual leave. They no longer get hospital accommodation when on-call and can be reprimanded if they have 'micro-naps'. Some junior doctors working today do not even have a place to hang their coat, let alone somewhere to rest their bodies or even get their legal breaks to eat. Sustenance outside daytime hours is most likely crisps and sandwiches obtained from a vending machine or a pre-prepared meal heated in a microwave.

When sacrifice becomes martyrdom and the individual is willing to risk their own personal well-being then this signifies their loss of perspective on what it means to be a doctor. It means they are continuously ignoring the needs of themselves, their families and friends. By caring for others, perhaps they hope to appease the guilt for not caring for those closest to them, both past and present.

Martyrdom can create a vicious cycle. It can make the doctor dependent on their patients for validation, who are in turn likely to view the doctor with overvalued idealisation. This might bolster the doctor's self-esteem, leading them to seek more validation through harder work and more self-sacrifice. The end result, when the cycle inevitably breaks down, is exhaustion, burnout and depression. The dependence generated by the distortion of a realistic doctor–patient relationship moves, as the GP David Zigmond wrote, from one of 'helping the needy' to 'needing the helpless'.[15] This brings to mind Emile Durkheim's seminal work on suicide, in particular his typology of suicides and what he saw as the underlying factors and where these apply to medicine. For example, 'altruistic' suicide arising from excessive social integration, or 'sacrifice' as arising from becoming excessively integrated into the culture and norms of medicine, internalised beliefs that good doctoring means giving oneself totally to others. Durkheim also illustrates the significance of social support and integration for mental well-being.[16] Jung talked about self-awareness being a vital prerequisite for anyone who cares for patients. An important part of learning to be a good-enough doctor is to understand our shadow self, which might lead us to become entrenched in accepting suffering and sacrifice as a way of life.

Closely aligned to martyrdom is what the British psychoanalytic psychotherapist David Malan has referred to as the 'helping profession syndrome' or compulsive caregiving. In this he refers to where the professional compulsively gives to others what he would like to have for himself.[17] Helping is therefore often in the form of altruistic self-sacrifice, such as working harder and longer hours, which doctors engage in to overcome feelings of incompetence or inadequacy. Malan speculates that such professionals perceive other people's needs as demands, which they try to satisfy. If their attempts are unsuccessful, they render themselves susceptible to depression, anxiety and, alongside added vulnerabilities, increased risk of suicide.

More and more doctors feel that it is their duty to 'save' their patients from the inadequacies of the health system, as if it is their fault for the underfunding, long waiting times and failures of a stressed service. A survey of doctors undertaken by the medical indemnity provider, the Medical Protection Society (MPS), found nearly three-quarters suffered from what they called the 'Superdoctor syndrome'.[18] This refers to doctors saying they will always come into work even though they are too unwell, fatigued or stressed to be productive. Healthcare professionals try to live up to this superdoctor expectation, which can lead to burnout, mental health issues, longer-term sickness and increased medico-legal risk, as doctors who continue to work while unfit are more likely to make mistakes. In the MPS survey, one-quarter of the doctors suspected that their emotional exhaustion contributed to an irreversible clinical error, with the remainder saying this was due to lack of concentration. The Superdoctor is possibly an opposing archetype to that of the Wounded Healer.

STIGMA

In the sociological literature stigma invariably appears as part of a trinity, that is deviance, labelling and stigma. It is worth looking at these before examining the issue of stigma in doctors specifically. Being 'normal' is a socially constructed and negotiated process, via norms of conduct, values and behaviours. It is through adherence to these that individuals obtain membership of their social groups. There is undoubtedly tremendous variability in social norms, but the designation of stigma involves the boundaries between membership and non-membership based on conformity. Becker observed:

> Social groups create deviance by making the rules whose infraction constitutes deviance and by applying these rules to particular people and labelling them as outsiders ... deviance is not a quality of the act the person commits but rather a consequence of the application by others of the rules and sanctions to an offender.[19]

The deviant is one to whom the label of deviant has been successfully applied; deviant behaviour is behaviour that people choose to label as such. Edwin Lemert advanced Becker's ideas in developing the notion of primary and secondary deviance,[20] primary deviance being the initial act and secondary deviance being the societal reaction, that is the response of the public and influential groups (for example doctors, clergy) to that act. It is the societal reaction that sets in train the labelling process, the creation and amplification of deviance and the alteration of deviance perceptions. Labels take two forms, informal and formal. What differentiates them is the amount of power, the credentials and social status of the individual or group applying the label and the prevailing discourses, ideology, norms and values. Certain labels when applied to individuals or groups can be highly potent, inasmuch as they cloud or colour judgments about the individual and impact upon our interactions with them, typically in a negative manner. The same label will have variable potency depending on the prior status of the individual, and the status of the person applying the label; for example, it is 'worse' to be an 'addict' doctor than an addict 'office worker'. Such are the rules of medicine, that there is added stigma when labels such as mental illness or addict are applied to a doctor.

Stigma is a sign of disgrace or discredit and has been defined as:

> Any condition, attribute, trait or behaviour which symbolically marks the individual as 'culturally unacceptable' or 'inferior', and has, as its subjective referent, the notions of shame and disgrace which sets a person apart from others.[21]

The 'weaponising' of stigma is most noticeable in welfare reforms (deserving and undeserving poor) but is also seen where medical practitioners make errors.[22] The difference between blaming and shaming, when shame is added to blame is often an act of 'political will' making it easier to 'abandon' certain people or sections of the population. This was the case of Hadiza Bawa-Garba, the paediatrician who was found guilty of, and given a suspended prison sentence for gross medical manslaughter. She was erased and expunged from the medical profession, made the scapegoat of the failings for the hospital in which she was working.

Stigma also adds 'blame', whereby the stigmatised individual is held to be culpable when mental illness, injury or disease is cast as (self-perpetuated or self-inflicted) deviance, and as such is particularly prevalent in mental illness.[22] From colloquially describing someone as 'crazy' to excluding them socially on account of a mental health diagnosis, society perpetuates mental health stigma. The internalisation and acceptance of these experiences, described as *self-stigma* or *internal stigma* may create further issues for those struggling with mental illness.

While the problem of stigma might be lessening for the general population (with national anti-stigma campaigns), it doesn't appear to be so for doctors. It is at the heart of why doctors do not seek help when mentally unwell. They suffer from personal (internalised), professional and institutional aspects of stigma. Mental illness among doctors is probably one of the last taboos, despite a massive drive from policy makers, politicians, professional leaders and even royalty to de-stigmatise it. A doctor may stigmatise himself with respect to mental illness.[23] Being unwell makes them feel ashamed, blaming themselves for not being resilient enough to cope with the pressures of work. They fear being seen as weak by their colleagues. The adaptive response to private and public stigma is secrecy and concealment of illness, mediated either consciously or unconsciously. Secrecy acts as a major barrier to help seeking, meaning the individual is then denied help from other health professionals and from colleagues, friends and peers. This leads to doctors thinking they must portray a healthy image to the outside world (including other doctors) and feeling embarrassed and even ashamed at adopting the patient role. This is borne out by a study of doctor's attitudes to personal illness, which found that many linked their health to his or her professional competence. This attitude even affected their approach to attending for routine screening tests.[24] Embarrassment at adopting the patient role extended towards their families, manifesting as an inability to seek help for one's own children. An example of stigma by association.

Stigma was one of the reasons the psychiatrist Daksha Emson took her own life and before doing so killed her three-month-old baby. The report into their deaths concluded that:

> Daksha was afraid of being stigmatised if others knew of her illness... Her fear would seem well justified.[25]

The psychiatrist Aashish Tagore wrote a poignant, honest and insightful personal account of his psychotic illness that culminated in a hospital admission. He wrote:

> It was my worst nightmare realised... when the stigma of my illness came to the fore. Not only was I embarrassed to be there, the staff with whom I used to work alongside appeared equally embarrassed for me. The pity was written all over their faces. And I must confess that my own prejudice towards mentally ill patients surfaced. I felt the need to distance myself (both physically and psychologically) from the other patients – I needed to reassure myself that I was not one of them. But, alas, I was. I was no better than or different to them – I was just as unwell, and just as human as the rest of them. I was no longer this superior being, the 'doctor' to their 'patient', I was their equal. In the immediate aftermath of my episode, I felt a sense of deep-seated shame and guilt.[26]

Tagore talked of stigma rearing its ugly head in subtle ways, even in situations where people mean no ill will, such as collecting a prescription for antidepressants at a pharmacy. I am also surprised that many doctors I see with depression are reluctant to take medication 'in case someone finds out'.

> And so, it is with the concept of 'self-stigmatisation', where the stigmatised individual actually relates to others' negative attitudes towards themselves and their illness. If you yourself share the negativity you might endure, and view such attitudes as 'understandable', then where is the motivation to fight it?... It's strange how the stigma of mental illness affects one's self-identity so profoundly.[26]

Stigma has many manifestations, including shunning the individual with the 'disease'. Being away from work leaves such doctors feeling lost, isolated and sad; these emotions are amplified by the negative reactions of friends and family making them feel failures, guilty and ashamed.[27] Stigma is ingrained into the profession early on in training. A junior doctor's account of her experience with mental health illustrates the significance of personal stigma:

> pathetic… particularly because it's mental illness and that I couldn't 'cut it'. That I'm not the right sort of personality to be doing the job.[28]

The view of 'not cutting it' is professional stigma. Separating personal and professional stigma is challenging as they are so interlinked. Doctors feel bad for becoming unwell, and their colleagues treat them differently. There is an increasingly popular attitude to conflate a doctor's professionalism, delivering excellent patient care despite external pressures, with their *resilience*, their ability to deal with adversity. From this, we can extrapolate that failing to cope could be interpreted as lacking competency and 'being weak', which of course it is not. One GP reported overhearing colleagues talk about patients with mental illness saying that 'they just need[ed] to pull themselves together'.[29]

This reasoning and account of stigma among medical practitioners is consistent with the *stiff upper lip* attitude in the medical profession; the concept of getting on with the job, struggling in silence and sacrificing oneself for their work.[30] Thus, it is unsurprising that being mentally ill as a doctor can be professionally stigmatising, as it may call your proficiency into question:

> I do feel like there's stigma attached to it. Not being able to cope and like stress and depression and things… I mean I'm sure I've perpetuated it; you know everyone feels the same probably about it.[28]

The hidden message is that being mentally unwell lacks legitimacy within the medical community. Although overt stigma is uncommon, the attitude doctors hold towards colleagues with mental illnesses manifests itself in a non-accepting culture. There exist cultural expectations from the general population for doctors to remain healthy. Patients do not expect doctors to become sick. They describe feeling less comfortable with the doctor, less confident of the doctor's ability and less trusting of those they think of as unwell.

Cultural stigma refers to discrimination against individuals due to personal characteristics that differ from societal norms and, despite being very common, is largely ignored. In many cases discrimination towards minority groups, such as the lesbian, gay, bisexual, transgender and queer (LGBTQ) community, people of colour, women and many others, complicates the already challenging minefield of mental health stigma in the medical profession. As mental health treatment is often most effective when provided by a practitioner who understands the cultural stigma the patient faces, these minorities can struggle even more to seek out appropriate care from the limited resources available.

CONCLUSION

The notion of the 'wounded healer' allows us to examine the impact both sacrifice and stigma can have on a doctor, and consequently their vulnerability to mental illness. For many practitioners, suffering, whether it is personal or witnessing it in others, is the origin of their motivation to pursue a career in medicine. It sadly can also be the reason, if left unchecked, that doctors are more vulnerable to the stressors inherent to medical practice. If, however, doctors are adequately supported in the processing of these experiences they can transform suffering into a therapeutic and beneficial experience for both them and their patients. Further to this suffering, the medical profession fosters a culture that expects altruistic self-sacrifice even at the cost of personal wellbeing. This is most clearly demonstrated by the initial section of the Hippocratic Oath and more subtly by professional socialisation of students before they even start work. Doctors are expected to work long hours, 'save' their patients and continue to do so productively despite exhaustion or sickness. This high level of pressure and expectation, set by both the professional environment and wider societal culture, means that doctors are more susceptible to burnout and mental health issues. This feeds into a larger problem of institutional and professional stigma in regard to mental health illness, further supplemented by personal stigma. The healthcare profession perpetuates the idea that mental health diagnoses are less legitimate than physical problems. This belief directly impacts on a physician's experience of mental illness and health seeking behaviours, which may be further complicated by personal attributes outside of their control such as sexuality. Suffering, self-sacrifice and stigma collectively contribute to the struggles of a 'sick doctor', and without these we cannot fully comprehend the process by which they experience mental illness.

REFERENCES

1 Woodward A, Thomas S, Jalloh M, Rees J, Leather A. Reasons to pursue a career in medicine: a qualitative study in Sierra Leone. *Global Health Research and Policy* 2017;**2**(1):34.

2 Goffman E. *Stigma: Notes on the Management of Spoilt Identity*. London: Penguin, 1990.

3 Stevens A. *Jung: A Very Short* Introduction. Oxford: Oxford University Press, 2001.

4 Daneault S. The wounded healer. Can this idea be of use to family physicians? *Can Fam Phys* 2008;**54**(9):1218–19.

5 Gask L. *The Other Side of Silence. A Psychiatrist's Memoir of Depression*. Chichester: Vie Books, 2015.

6 Jones P (ed). *Doctors as Patients*. Oxford: Radcliffe Publishing Ltd, 2005.

7 Ahmed H. [Internet]. Ahmed Hankir Physician, Senior Research Fellow & Author of The Wounded Healer. [cited 18 January 2020]. Available from: www.ahmedhankir.com.

8 Kay A. *This is Going to Hurt: Secret Diaries of a Junior Doctor*, 1st edn. London, Picador, 2017.

9 Kalanthi P. *When Breath Becomes Air*, 1st edn. London: Bodley Head, 2016.

10 Black S. *All That Remains: A Life in Death*. London: Transworld Publishers Ltd, 2019.

11 Cannon J. *Breaking and Mending: A Junior Doctor's Stories of Compassion and Burnout*. London: Profile Books Ltd, 2019.

12 Klitzman R. *When Doctors Become Patients*. New York: Oxford University Press, 2008, p. 118.

13 Declaration of Geneva. International code of medical ethics. Available from: www.wma.net/wp-content/uploads/2018/07/Decl-of-Geneva-v1948-1.pdf.

14 Haffertey F. Reconfiguring the sociology of medical education: emerging topics and pressing issues. In: Bird CE, Conrad P, Fremont AM (eds). *Handbook of Medical Sociology*, 5th edn. Upper Saddle River: Prentice Hall, 2000, pp. 238–57.

15 Zigmond D. Physician heal thyself: the paradox of the wounded healer. *British Journal of Holistic Medicine* 1984;**1**:63–71.

16 Durkeim E. *Suicide*. Oxford: Routledge Classics, 2002.

17 Malan D. Individual psychotherapy and the science of psychodynamics. Oxford: Butterworth-Heinemann, 1979.

18 Medical Protection Society. 72% of UK doctors facing 'Superdoctor Syndrome' [Internet]. 2019 [cited 18 January 2020]. Available from: www.medicalprotection.org/uk/articles/72-of-uk-doctors-facing-superdoctor-syndrome.

19 Becker H. Reprinted from *The Outsiders: Studies in the Sociology of Deviance*, 1963, pp. 1–18. Copyright 1963 by the Free Press.

20 Lemert E. Secondary deviance and role conceptions. In: Herman NJ. *Deviance: A Symbolic Interactionist Approach*. Oxford: Rowman & Littlefield, 1995, pp. 111–13.

21 Monaghan L, Williams S. *Key Concepts in Medical Sociology*. London: SAGE Publications; 2016, p. 59.

22 Scambler G. *A Sociology of Shame and Blame*, 1st edn. Cham: Palgrave Pivot, 2020.

23 Cohen D, Winstanley S, Greene G. Understanding doctors' attitudes towards self-disclosure of mental ill health. *Occupational Medicine* 2016;**66**(5):383–9.

24 Thompson W, Cupples M, Sibbett C, Skan D, Bradley T. Challenge of culture, conscience, and contract to general practitioners' care of their own health: qualitative study. *BMJ* 2001;**323**(7315):728–31.

25 North East London Strategic Health Authority. Report of an independent inquiry into the care and treatment of Daksha Emson and her daughter Freya. London, 2003.

26 Tagore A. Personal experience: coming out – the psychotic psychiatrist – an account of the stigmatising experience of psychiatric illness. *The Psychiatric Bulletin* 2014;**38**(4):185–8.

27 Henderson M, Brooks S, del Busso L, *et al*. Shame! Self-stigmatisation as an obstacle to sick doctors returning to work: a qualitative study: Table 1. *BMJ Open* 2012;**2**(5):e001776.

28 Fox FE, Doran NJ, Rodham KJ, Taylor GJ, Harris MF, O'Connor M. Junior doctors' experiences of personal illness: a qualitative study. *Medical Education* 2011;**45**(12):1251–61.

29 Spiers J, Buszewicz M, Chew-Graham CA, *et al.* Barriers, facilitators, and survival strategies for GPs seeking treatment for distress: a qualitative study. *Br J Gen Pract* 2017;**67**(663):e700–8. DOI: https://doi.org/10.3399/bjgp17X692573.

30 Balme E, Gerada C, Page L. Doctors need to be supported, not trained in resilience. *BMJ Clin Res* 2015;**351**:h4709.

SECTION II

Doctors and Their Illnesses

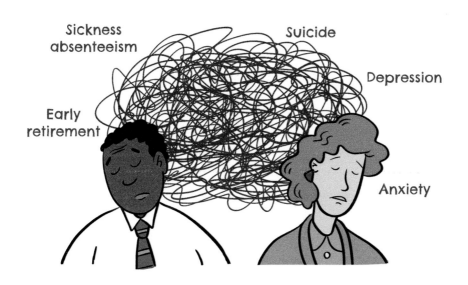

Sickness absenteeism

Suicide

Depression

Early retirement

Anxiety

9

Doctors and Mental Illness

An Overview

CLARE GERADA

A medical degree does not give protection from the normal vicissitudes or hardships of life. Doctors have the same mental illnesses as the general population. Where doctors do differ, is not in the illnesses they get, but rather in *how* they present, their prevalence, potential impact and outcome. Perhaps the most significant difference, as I have already touched on in this book, is how hard it is to cross that invisible boundary from professional to patient, even when that boundary is for a physical, rather than a psychological disorder. I am guilty of this myself. When knocked off my bike enroute to my evening surgery, instead of abandoning ship and going to the accident and emergency department, I hailed a taxi, completed the clinic (with blood oozing from my foot and in great pain). It did not cross my mind that I could have cancelled and sought help. This was a physical illness. It is even harder for doctors to seek help for mental illness. For doctors, mental illness is their shameful secret, hidden from sight. This means large numbers of depressed and anxious doctors are denied help (usually through their own reluctance to seek it). It is vital that this 'secret' comes into the open and that they are able to receive appropriate treatment. This is not just for the doctor's sake, but also for their patients, since untreated mental illness is linked to more medical errors.[1,2] This chapter gives an overview of doctors and their mental illnesses.

DOCTORS AND THEIR ILLNESSES – AN OVERVIEW

Some headlines from the UK:

- Nearly 43% of doctors have considered leaving their careers.[3]
- 55% of 417 UK doctors 'meet the criteria' for burnout and emotional exhaustion. The study, conducted by Birkbeck, University of London, and University College London, also found that one in 20 doctors are alcohol dependent, with

more than one-third admitting to drinking alcohol 'to cope with work-related stress'. Overall, one in five said they used 'substances' (alcohol or drugs) as a 'stress coping strategy'.[4]

- One-quarter of doctors in training said that their job leaves them burnt-out to a high or very high degree, up from 24% in 2018, the General Medical Council's (GMC) national training survey found.[5]

High rates of mental illness in doctors are a global phenomenon. In every system, whether privately, insurance or nationally funded, and across all specialities, ages, gender, levels of seniority and training grades, doctors are at risk of mental illness.[6] As with the general population, common mental illnesses (such as depression and anxiety) are more frequent, and less common ones, such as bipolar disorder, less so. Eating disorders might be more prevalent in doctors than the general population given the number of young women who enter medicine (and this might explain the large numbers of female doctors we see who have taken up triathlons). There are other conditions, such as schizophrenia that, given the intensity and working conditions, might not be compatible with a career in medicine. Whether doctors have higher, lower or the same levels of alcohol and drug misuse depends on when and where the study was conducted.

Studies that compare prevalence rates of mental illness in doctors with the general population tend to focus on the more common illnesses, and, as this chapter will discuss, reach conflicting conclusions. Overall, higher quality studies (with better research methodology, larger cohorts or validated instruments) tend to show **lower** prevalence rates.

Generally speaking, overall prevalence of mental illness in doctors has been found to be at least comparable, if not higher, than in the general population and other professional groups. In one of the largest surveys of mental illness, the level of both general distress and specific mental health diagnoses were high and significantly greater in doctors in comparison to the general population and other professionals in Australia.[7] In particular, high levels of psychological distress were found in doctors aged under 30 years old, significantly higher than in aged-matched individuals and other professional groups. Other studies have reported prevalence rates of psychiatric morbidity ranging from 17% to 52%.[8-11]

Depression

Depression is more than merely feeling down for a few days. It is a persistent low mood that can go on for months or even years. It is accompanied by feelings of hopelessness and helplessness and loss of interest in things that would normally have given pleasure. There is often sleep disturbance (either early morning wakening or oversleeping). Depressed individuals have problems concentrating and lack energy to do even the simplest of tasks. Doctors, even those with a training in mental health, do not always recognise 'tell-tale' signs of depression in themselves. They can, and in my experience caring for doctors do, attribute symptoms such as insomnia, poor appetite and generalised anxiety to the normal 'cut and thrust' of working in a stressful environment. As with the general population, depression is the most common mental illness in doctors, and it appears to be more common in doctors than the general population, though by how much, varies considerably across studies.

A systematic review in 2010 identified 19 papers on depression and anxiety in doctors. The reported rate varied from 14% to 60%.[12] Current levels of depression, as determined by the Australian survey, showed similar rates to the general population, but higher than for other Australian professionals. Approximately 21% of doctors reported having ever been diagnosed with or treated for depression and 6% had a current diagnosis.[7] Another review published in 2014 found 112 articles on depression in American doctors. Rates of depression ranged from 1% to 56%, an enormous variance, reflecting sample size, methodology used and cut-off limits for 'caseness'.[13] The larger and more robust studies included in this review found between 22% and 35% of doctors reported between four and five symptoms of depression.[14] A similar figure was found in another systematic review, which included 54 cross-sectional and longitudinal studies involving 17,560 hospital trainees from 18 countries across the world.[15] Similar levels of depression were found regardless of the country in which the study was done, and gave a pooled prevalence of around 30%. There is a trend for newer studies to find higher rates, which, while modest, is notable given the reduction in duty hours and improved working conditions over the last decade.

A study of American interns (doctors doing their first job post qualification) found the percentage of doctors meeting the diagnosis of severe depression increased from 4% before starting work to 27% one year later.[14] Overall, over the 12 months, 42% of the doctors met the criteria for depression at one or more of the quarterly assessments, though only 23% sought help.[16] This study found a direct association between number of hours worked and increased depressive symptoms.

When researching for this chapter, I have been surprised to learn that Chinese doctors have some of the highest rates of mental illness in the world. I wrongly assumed that given the economic success of the Chinese economy that this would translate into more protective working environments for health staff. I was wrong. For example, a study published in 2019 from Hangzhou, the capital of the Zhejiang Province and an economically advanced city, found nearly 70% of hospital doctors screened positive for anxiety and 72% for depression.[17] Even given the figures mentioned in this chapter, these rates of psychiatric morbidity are extraordinarily high (and higher than the background rates of anxiety and depression in the general Chinese population) and might suggest a sampling bias or that the doctors were over-reporting their symptoms, or indeed that these are the true rates. While using different methodology, the authors cite other studies of Chinese doctors and find ranges between 65% (depression) and 28% (anxiety). As with doctors across the world (though probably more so in China given their rapid economic growth and demand for health care), the pressure to address overwhelming medical needs, intensity of workload, difficult clinical encounters and being sued or facing complaints, are all contributors to high rates of mental distress.

As depression is more likely to emerge in anyone before the age of 30 years of age it is unsurprising that it is also more prevalent in younger doctors. What we can conclude from all the research is that depression is at least as common in doctors as an aged-matched group; around one-fifth have been depressed and around 7% currently are; that it is probably more common in younger doctors; and that there is some evidence that women doctors have higher rates of depression than men (similar to the general population).

Anxiety

Everyone is familiar with the term 'anxiety' and no part of our daily lives can be free from it. Where anxiety becomes a problem is when it becomes pervasive and the symptoms begin to interfere (for the worse) with our work, life and relationships. Three of the most common anxiety disorders doctors suffer from are generalised anxiety disorder (GAD), panic disorder and post-traumatic stress disorder (PTSD), with GAD being the most common. GAD is characterised by out-of-control, intrusive anxiety present for most days, about several subjects for more than six months.

Anxiety is less well studied among doctors than depression has been, and studies are of lower quality as they do not tend to use formal diagnostic instruments, and therefore 'anxiety' tends to encompass a range of different diagnoses, from 'stress', 'psychological distress', generalised anxiety or phobic anxiety states. The academics Valerie Hope and Max Henderson reviewed depression, anxiety and distress among medical students, including papers published between 1948 to 2013. Of the 11 studies that were included in the review for anxiety, seven different tools were used (some specifically developed by the researchers).[18] Prevalence ranged from 8% to 66%. With the exception of a study conducted in New Zealand,[19] few examined specific anxiety disorders such as GAD in any formal way.

Around 9% of doctors in an Australian survey reported having been diagnosed or treated with an anxiety disorder at some point in their lives; female doctors had higher rates compared to men (11% vs. 7%, p.3);[7] around 9% of women and 5% of men are reported to have a current diagnosis of anxiety (p. 5). In a separate systematic review the prevalence of anxiety among doctors was found to be between 18% and 55%, with evidence to suggest that doctors had higher scores compared to the general population, though not compared to other professions.[13] Other studies suggest that anxiety in doctors is as high as 24%.[20]

Evidence wise, it is not possible to say whether rates of anxiety are more, less or the same as in the general population. Experience wise, generalised anxiety is a common finding in the doctors we see in our service, either presenting alone or alongside a depressive disorder. I would suggest that anxiety is almost pathognomonic of being a doctor in todays' healthcare system. There are so many anxiety-provoking events in clinical practice that it has become normal for doctors to ignore their racing heart, fearful thoughts or the vague feeling of constant nausea in their everyday lives.

POST-TRAUMATIC STRESS DISORDER (PTSD)

Exposure to traumatic events is generally unavoidable in medicine, but more so for those who work at the front line of acute care such as accident and emergency, intensive care, anaesthetists, surgeons and obstetricians. For all doctors though, contact with dying patients, serious injury, patients with intense pain and distress is commonplace in their everyday clinical lives. Outside their consulting rooms, doctors also experience further traumatic events from being subjected to bullying, complaints, assault or racism.

Most people who are exposed to a traumatic event have no adverse long-term problems and resume their normal functioning. Some may even have an increase in well-being, confident that they handled the event or themselves well. A small number, however, will experience a range of adverse psychological effects, including PTSD. Symptoms include persistent thoughts, images, flashbacks or dreams in response to reminders of the event, the desire to avoid discussion or reminders of the trauma and a host of other symptoms such as loss of interest, withdrawal and anger. Symptoms need to be present for more than one month and not caused by medication, substance use or other illness.

While most of the literature on PTSD is from the Armed forces, service personal and emergency staff (ambulance, fire and police), awareness is increasing that those working in the front line of healthcare also suffer from this disorder. As I mentioned when discussing resilience, a past Chair of the General Medical Council once remarked that doctors should take a leaf out of army personnel and learn to be resilient. He was referring to dealing with complaints and referrals to the regulator, but his comments were taken as a general view that doctors were not resilient enough to survive the rough and tumble of a career in medicine. I imagine he now regrets this comment, but the sentiment behind it, that working in the NHS is akin to serving in the armed forces, seems a good analogy given the prevalence of PTSD in healthcare staff. Slade *et al.* found that two-thirds of trainees and consultants in obstetrics and gynaecology were exposed to traumatic events at work, and of these 18% reported clinically significant PTSD symptoms.[21] However, a study of emergency department doctors found that the incidence of PTSD was in the range of 12–22%,[22] around the same rate as those exposed to a traumatic event in the general population.[23]

Alcohol and drug misuse

Over the decade my service has cared for hundreds of doctors with various forms of addiction, mainly alcohol and drug, but also others too, including gambling, sex and porn addiction. I will discuss this in more detail in Chapter 10. I am often struck how far doctors need to fall before they reach out for care. Often, they continue drinking and using drugs despite serious relationship difficulties, problems at work, loss of livelihood, housing and physical illness. This is the nature of addiction, compulsion to use, despite harm done to self and others. Untreated, the doctor is likely to present in a crisis, potentially following a drink-drive offence, being caught stealing drugs from work or having an accident. Some die before they get the chance to present at all, whether through accident or suicide. Overall, drug and alcohol use are probably lower in doctors than in the general population, though in the absence of large studies it is not possible to be certain.

Personality disorder

An individual with a personality disorder thinks, feels, behaves or relates to others differently. There is scant research into doctors with this disorder, possibly due to it being uncommon but also because of the difficulty of diagnosing it. It is likely to be even less common in medicine, as medicine selects against some traits common in people with personality disorders (such as poor impulse control, lack of empathy) and for ones such as resilience and obsessiveness. In my experience, where personality disorder does present, it is accompanied by performance issues at work or professional misconduct, such as boundary violations. When you look back into these doctors' histories, often there are repeated complaints the doctor was 'not a team player', they become angry when stressed and elicited fear, shame and rage in others, and consequently distress in their teams. Not all disruptive behaviour is due to an underlying personality disorder, some might be just bad behaviour.

CONSEQUENCES OF MENTAL ILLNESS FOR THE INDIVIDUAL, THE PATIENT AND THE PROFESSION

Whether doctors have the same, lower or higher rates of mental illness than the general population is not the main issue. What is important is ensuring that this group, who after all have a critical role to play in the care of millions of people, receive timely help such that they do not pose a risk, not just to themselves but also to the patients they manage. Doctors with mental illness are more likely to stay at work than not, a term called *presenteeism* and working at suboptimal levels due to their symptoms. There is evidence that medical errors are more common in depressed doctors, both an increase in self-reported errors and also when objectively measured. Depression is closely correlated with fatigue, which might explain the higher levels of medical errors found in doctors with this condition.[24,25] One study found depression had a greater negative impact on time management and productivity than any other health problem.[26]

Mental illness matters as it has a significant macroeconomic impact too. In the UK the total cost to employers of mental health problems among their staff is estimated at nearly £26 billion each year: £8.4 billion from sickness absences and £15.1 billion from reduced productivity at work.[27] While these figures are for all staff, doctors are an expensive resource and their absenteeism will place a large hole in health services finances. A mentally unwell doctor is likely to enter a downward spiral, as feelings of hopelessness and worthlessness lead to declining performance and a greater risk of errors, causing further despair. Patient care and professional standing can then be placed at risk, possibly leading to more complaints and concerns. This is why it is so important to minimise the barriers to accessing care.

CONCLUSION

In this chapter I have given the evidence for the extent of mental illness among doctors. Despite this area being the subject of interest for decades, it is telling how few robust studies there are to guide us in answering the simplest questions as to rates, comparisons across different groups or to other non-medical populations. Given these problems it does appear that doctors do have higher rates of mental illness, certainly in the more common conditions, such as depression and anxiety. It is perhaps not surprising that doctors do have high rates given the nature of their work. I will discuss these risks further in subsequent chapters.

REFERENCES

1 Fahrenkopf A, Sectish T, Barger L, et al. Rates of medication errors among depressed and burnt out residents: prospective cohort study. *BMJ* 2008;**336**(7642):488–91.

2 West C, Huschka M, Novotny P, et al. Association of perceived medical errors with resident distress and empathy. *JAMA* 2006;**296**(9):1071.

3 Medical Protection Society. The increasing level of burnout amongst doctors is extremely troubling. Medical Protection is calling for organisation wide interventions to safeguard the wellbeing of doctors. Available from: www.medicalprotection.org/uk/hub/breaking-the-burnout-cycle-keeping-doctors-and-patients-safe.

4 Medisauskaite A, Kamau C. Does occupational distress raise the risk of alcohol use, binge-eating, ill health and sleep problems among medical doctors? A UK cross-sectional study. *BMJ Open* 2018;9(5). Available from: http://dx.doi.org/10.1136/bmjopen-2018-027362.

5 GMC. National training surveys 2018. Available from: www.gmc-uk.org/-/media/documents/dc11391-nts-2018-initial-findings-report_pdf-75268532.pdf.

6 Brooks S, Gerada C, Chalder T. Review of literature on the mental health of doctors: are specialist services needed? *J Ment Health* 2011;20(2):146–56.

7 National Health Survey of Doctors and Medical Students [Internet]. 2013 (updated 2019). Beyond Blue. Available from: www.beyondblue.org.au/docs/default-source/research-project-files/bl1132-report---nmhdmss-full-report_web.

8 McManus I, Jonvik H, Richards P, Paice E. Vocation and avocation: leisure activities correlate with professional engagement, but not burnout, in a cross-sectional survey of UK doctors. *BMC Med* 2011;**9**: 100.

9 McManus I, Keeling A, Paice E. Stress, burnout and doctors' attitudes to work are determined by personality and learning style: a twelve-year longitudinal study of UK medical graduates. *BMC Med* 2004;**2**:29.

10 Taylor C, Graham J, Potts H, Richards M, Ramirez A. Changes in mental health of UK hospital consultants since the mid-1990s. *Lancet* 2005;**366**:742–4.

11 Imo U. Burnout and psychiatric morbidity among doctors in the UK: a systematic literature review of prevalence and associated factors. *B J Psych Bull* 2017;**41**(4):197–204.

12 Elliot L, Tan J, Norris S. The Mental Health of Doctors: a systematic literature review [Internet]. 2010. Beyond Blue. Available from: http://resources.beyondblue.org.au/prism/file?token=BL/0823.

13 Joules N, Williams D, Thompson A. Depression in resident physicians: a systematic review. *Open J Depression* 2014;**03**(03):89–100.

14 Sen S, Kranzler H, Krystal J, *et al*. A prospective cohort study investigating factors associated with depression during medical internship. *Arch Gen Psychiatry* 2010;**67**(6):557.

15 Mata DA, Ramos MA, Bansal N, *et al*. Prevalence of depression and depressive symptoms among resident physicians: a systematic review and meta-analysis. *JAMA* 2015;**314**(22):2373–83. doi: 10.1001/jama.2015.15845. https://jamanetwork.com/journals/jama/fullarticle/2474424.

16 Guille C, Speller H, Laff R, Epperson CN, Sen S. Utilization and barriers to Mental Health Services among depressed medical interns: a prospective multisite study. *J Grad Med Edu* 2010;**2**(2):210–14. www.jgme.org/doi/full/10.4300/JGME-D-09-00086.1.

17 Xi X, Lu Q, Wo T, *et al*. Doctor's presenteeism and its relationship with anxiety and depression: a cross-sectional survey study in China. *BMJ Open* 2019;**9**(7):e028844.

18 Hope V, Henderson M. Medical student depression, anxiety and distress outside North America: a systematic review. *Med Educ* 2014;**48**:963–79.

19 Samaranayake CB, Fernando AT. Satisfaction with life and depression among medical students in Auckland, New Zealand. *NZ Med J* 2011;**124**(1341):12–17.

20 Ruitenburg MM, Frings-Dresen MH, Sluiter JK. The prevalence of common mental disorders among hospital physicians and their association with self-reported work ability: a cross-sectional study. *BMC Health Serv Res* 2012;**12**:292–8.

21 Slade P, Balling K, *et al*. Work-related posttraumatic stress symptoms in obstetricians and gynaecologists: findings from INDIGO a mixed methods study with a cross-sectional survey and in-depth interviews. *BJOG* 2020. Available from: https://doi.org/10.1111/1471-0528.16076.

22 Vanyo L, Sorge R, Chen A, Lakoff D. Posttraumatic stress disorder in emergency medicine residents. *Ann Emerg Med* 2017;**70**(6):898–903.

23 Ursano RJ, Goldenberg M, Zhang L, *et al*. Posttraumatic stress disorder and traumatic stress: from bench to bedside, from war to disaster. *Ann N Y Acad Sci* 2010;**1208**:72–81.

24 De Oliveira GS, Chang R, Fitzgerald PC, *et al*. The prevalence of burnout and depression and their association with adherence to safety and practice standards. *Anesth Analg* 2013;**117**(1):182–93. doi:10.1213/ane.0b013e3182917da9.

25 West C. Association of resident fatigue and distress with perceived medical errors. *JAMA* 2009;**302**(12):1294.

26 Burton W, Pransky G, Conti D, Chen C, Edington D. The association of medical conditions and presenteeism. *J Occup Environ Med* 2004;**46**:S38–S45.

27 Sainsbury Centre for Mental Health. Mental Health at Work: Developing the Business Case. Policy Paper 8. SCMH, 2007.

10

Doctors and Substance Misuse Disorder

SHIVANTHI SATHANANDAN AND CLARE GERADA

In 2017 an anaesthetist was jailed after stealing codeine. He had opiate addiction. The trial judge accepted his problems were genuine, but stated as a doctor, he should have known where to get help.[1] For a host of reasons, many of which have been discussed in this book, doctors with mental illness, and especially those with addiction, do not know where to get help. They have poor access to confidential, accessible and supportive care. Doctors are often in denial, terrified of acknowledging to themselves, let alone to others, that they have a problem. Colleagues tend not see the obvious and ignore the unmistakable and unpleasant stale smell of alcohol, the pinpoint pupils of someone using opiates or the bizarre behaviour of colleagues using stimulants.

THE HISTORY OF ADDICTION IN DOCTORS

Addiction in the medical profession is not a modern phenomenon, and if anything, it is less prevalent and less acceptable today, than in the past. In 1869, the English surgeon and pathologist James Paget wrote a report of the outcome of 1000 medical students. He commented that ten of these students had to be failed 'through their continuance in habits of intemperance or dissipation as had made us, even while they were students, anticipate their failure'.[2] In 1894, a standard medical text by the Canadian doctor William Osler, *The Principles and Practice of Medicine,* suggested that doctors formed one of the major group of addicts.[3] In the main, these doctors were able to continue with their career. William Stewart Halsted, considered one of the greatest and most influential American surgeons of all time, is such an example.[4] In 1884, Halstead developed addiction to cocaine after experimenting on its anaesthetic properties[5] and was treated with morphine as a substitute, not surprisingly leading to opiate addiction. While he continued working as the chief of surgery at John Hopkins Hospital for 30 years until 1922, his addiction was unremitting throughout his life.[4] In the late 19th century, former doctor-addicts were recruited to be part of the new and growing speciality of addiction medicine. Between 1891 and 1894, the Keeley Institute, an 'inebriate asylum' originally founded in Illinois America, employed doctors who had been addicted to alcohol or drugs, including morphine, opium or cocaine. Many were less than one year from being in receipt of treatment themselves.[6] Employing these doctors caused controversy, with superintendents of asylums denouncing the use of former addicts in such a way, voicing concerns that these physicians would be 'incompetent by reason of organic deficits of the higher mentality' and working with addicts would lead them to inevitable relapse into substance misuse.[7] Doctors with previous addiction continued to be employed; for example, of the 475 physicians who participated in addiction training at the Long Beach Naval Regional Centre between 1974 and 1978, 44 signed themselves into treatment before continuing to work in addiction medicine.[8] By 1982, more than 200 recovered physicians in the USA had entered the field of addiction medicine.[9]

The psychiatrist Max Glatt, who set up one of the first treatment services for alcoholics in the UK, published a letter in the *Lancet* in 1975 about a group of doctors he was treating. He wrote how hard it was for them to present for treatment, but once they did (much the same as today), they had very good outcomes. He also noted how supportive other doctors could be in their recovery, saying they 'can often be the greatest assistance to other alcoholics' and wrote about a group that doctors in recovery had set up:

> Not unexpectedly, some alcoholic doctors find it easier to attend these meetings than ordinary Alcoholics Anonymous meetings, in the knowledge that all those attending it are professional men who had, or still have, to face similar problems. There is, thus no fear of others sitting in judgement or talking down to the new-comer. who can but receive very helpful, constructive advice and support from colleagues who, because of their own experiences, are in full empathy.[10]

This group was the beginning of the formation of the British Doctors and Dentists Group (BDDG), which still has regular meetings across the UK today, providing support for doctors with addiction. They are affiliated to the International Doctors in Alcoholic Anonymous (IDAA). Both work using the 12 steps methodology created by the founders of Alcoholic Anonymous as one of the best ways to overcome an addiction to alcohol.

In the present day, doctors in recovery still play an important role in the addiction field. They help engage doctors into treatment, support their early first steps into recovery and contribute education, research and development. One does have to be mindful though of the warning given by the superintendents of the inebriate asylums. Addiction is a chronic relapsing condition and working closely with active patients might make the doctor more, not less, susceptible to relapse. One such doctor, Torin Finver, in Buffalo, USA, was working as the medical director of a community addiction treatment centre. He is open about his own battles with drug addiction saying that 'it lessens the shame' and 'my past makes me a stronger person'. However, after 9 years in recovery, in 2018, he was arrested having admitted to using the dark web to buy cocaine and heroin.[11]

PREVALENCE

Unlike our understanding of substance misuse disorders in the general population, current knowledge of substance misuse or dependence in doctors is comparatively poor. There are a number of reasons for this. There is an inevitable response bias and under-reporting in self-report surveys. Those who no longer practise are frequently excluded or simply not captured by studies. Some studies do not include addiction to self-prescribed benzodiazepines or intermittent use of drugs such as methamphetamines. Others use a broad definition of addiction, such that any use of recreational illegal drugs or self-prescription is included rather than adhering to the definition given by ICD (International Classification of Diseases) or DSM (Diagnostic and Statistical Manual). Most prevalence figures use data obtained from licencing boards, mortality studies, hospital statistics, treatment programmes and surveys, rather than well-designed research.[12-14] Figures that do exist can be conflicting. Some show the same rates of addiction as in the general population (15%),[12,15-17] others higher[18] and some lower rates.[14] Overall, there is a dearth of robust epidemiological studies on prevalence; the available research comes mainly from the USA and Canada and most of this is now 20–30 years old.

There are no large-scale prevalence studies carried out in the UK, although the British Medical Association has reported that one in 15 doctors (around 7%) may be addicted to drugs or alcohol at some point in their career.[17] Prevalence rates in American doctors are generally reported to be in the range of 8–15%, which is similar to that in the American general population.[12,19] A survey of American physician substance use was published in 1992 and reported an 8% lifetime rate of a substance-use disorder.[16] Overall, doctors had lower rates of substance misuse compared to college and high school graduates. The authors found lower proportions than in the general population used illicit substances, such as marijuana, cocaine and heroin. The only exception was that physicians were more likely than the general population to misuse two kinds of prescription medications: opiates and benzodiazepines – doing so for purposes of self-treatment, whereas their use of illicit substances and or alcohol was for so-called recreational purposes. A further study, this time of Australian doctors, examined the link between hazardous alcohol use and psychiatric morbidity.[20] Potentially hazardous use for the total cohort was 15% (8% for women, 17% for men).

A systematic review of problem-related drinking among medical doctors published in 2005 found a breadth of prevalence of problem-related drinking – from heavy drinking and hazardous drinking (12–16%) to misuse and dependence (6–8%) – within the population-based samples of doctors. An increased risk was positively related to male doctors, doctors of 40–45 years and older and to some factors of work, lifestyle and health.[21] Overall, no evidence was found that alcohol abuse was more common in doctors or medical students. In fact, the limited evidence suggested that alcohol abuse was actually **less** common in the medical profession and other than benzodiazepine use, no evidence of increased drug use.

An American study published in 2015 has bucked the trend and found higher rates of alcohol misuse in female doctors compared to men and the general population.[18] As well as assessing alcohol use (using the AUDIT), doctors were asked to indicate use and frequency of use of prescription drugs (not prescribed by their physician) and illicit substances. Overall, 15% had an AUDIT score consistent with alcohol abuse or dependence, females had higher rates than males (21% vs. 13%). The rate for the general population was 13%. Abuse of prescription and illicit drugs were both rare. The most common was cannabis (3%). One percent of physicians did acknowledge the abuse of opiates either illicitly or abuse of a medication prescribed by a physician for a legitimate purpose. Use or abuse of other substances was uncommon. That women doctors drank more heavily than men has not been found in other studies, nor the finding in our sick doctor service. It might be women are more honest about their drinking habits in surveys.

Within our own service (which as a treatment service only has data on doctors who have stepped forward with problems), we have seen a change in the percentage of addicted doctors attending, which might suggest that the level of substance misuse disorder in doctors is reducing. At the start in 2008, 30% of our caseload was related to addiction. Over the years this percentage has changed, falling to 12% in 2014 and 5% in 2019 (averaging out over the decade to 7%). This might be related to doctors having fewer opportunities to unrestricted access to potential drugs of abuse, since stricter prescribing rules have been implemented following the Shipman Inquiry, which is discussed in Chapter 25.[22] Nowadays, even the ability to self-prescribe drugs such as benzodiazepines raises concerns. This means that the opportunity for doctors to become addicted through better access to drugs has been significantly curtailed, except in certain fields such as anaesthetics, surgery and emergency medicine (where there is access to onsite drugs at work, albeit with strict monitoring protocols). This drop might be due to doctors presenting earlier before their use becomes problematic and entrenched. In recent years we have seen the age group change to a younger cohort.[23] The earlier high prevalence is likely to be unmet need, especially as the first cohorts of doctors tended to be male, over 50 years old, with long-standing alcohol dependence.

Where we have seen an increasing number of doctors coming for help are those engaged in so called 'chemsex'. This is when people take drugs that enhance sexual performance and make them feel uninhibited. It is more often a feature in gay men communities and involves the drugs, crystal methamphetamine, GHB (gamma hydroxybutyrate) or mephedrone. A survey of gay men found that one-fifth had had chemsex in the last five years and 10% in the past month.[24] Some users report using these drugs to manage negative feelings, such as a lack of confidence and self-esteem, internalised homophobia and stigma about their HIV status.[25]

These individuals are at risk of sexually transmitted infections through unsafe sexual practices and needle sharing. There are also problems with forming and sustaining relationships that are predicated on chemsex, as well as higher rates of sexual assault. Doctors engaged in chemsex find it difficult to present to sexual health clinics as taking drugs is illegal and they fear being referred to the regulator if they admit their problem. The doctors who attend our service also have an immense sense of shame associated with their out-of-control behaviour and the dissonance between being a doctor and living this lifestyle.

DOCTORS, ADDICTION AND STIGMA

In 1973, the American Medical Association (AMA), looking at the question of addicted doctors, concluded that a balance needed to be struck between being too lenient, which may endanger patient lives, and being too harsh, which could lead to doctors going into 'hiding', not seeking help and the possibility of suicide as a consequence.[26] The AMA encouraged the expansion of Medical Professionals Health Programs (now called Physician Health Programs) to 'improve physician wellness and eliminate any barriers that stand in the way of physicians accessing needed mental health-care services'.[27]

In the UK, it was Max Glatt, in 1975 who identified the difficulties alcoholic doctors had in accessing care and that '[they] often apparently shy away from asking a doctor for help'.[28] Publicly funded practitioner services as we recognise them now, did not appear for a further 40 years in the UK, though self-help ones have been in operation for many years. Addiction is contaminated with stigma and despite decades of trying to establish it as a medical problem, it is, more often than not, viewed as a moral failing, a lifestyle choice or lack of self-control or will power. This view is amplified when doctors become addicts. Doctors are not meant to transgress, certainly not into addiction. Addicted doctors endure almost universal negative attitudes from colleagues, the public and those who have jurisdiction over them. This leads to secrecy for fear of punishment (which is not uncommon). In our view, this fear and the isolation doctors endure leads to them coming late for help.

Denial of having a problem is common. For example, a GP who reports '*I don't drink much more than anyone else*', can hold onto this belief despite being caught on a drink-drive charge. Or the junior doctor 'dabbling' in club drugs '*all my friends do it, it's just to let off some steam, only at the weekends*', but has to miss work on a Monday due to the 'come down'. Or the anaesthetist '*it was only once, I was stressed, the fentanyl calmed me down. It won't happen again*', but finds they can't resist the open medicines cabinet at work. Stigma and shame may lead doctors to hoping the problem will just goes away: '*when I swap rotations I won't be as stressed and I'll stop taking codeine*', '*if I just have a week of annual leave, I'll get over it and be okay*'.

Even once in treatment these automatic defences can make it difficult to engage with treatment. Often doctors say in their first assessment, '*My nightmare in coming here is that you'll tell me to go on sick leave... to stop on-calls... to take a break*'. Doctors have to be told, clearly and emphatically, the worst-case scenario is that they could overdose and die, or their employer could find they have stolen medication, and this might lead to a criminal charge and termination of their employment. Colleagues too are often reluctant to identify problems in their peers.

OVERVIEW OF PATTERNS WITH ADDICTED DOCTORS

The aetiology of addiction in doctors is multi-factorial, with contributory factors including genetic predisposition, personality factors, work-related stress, co-morbid mental illness, family stress, bereavement and/or an injury or accident at work.[29] These are similar to the risk factors in the general population. However, doctors are unique in the ease of access to prescribed and non-prescribed medication[14] and their work environment, which attracts high stress, low tolerance for failure and a culture of blame.[30,31]

The addicted professional is in an interesting conundrum. Doctors come with a set of conscious and unconscious expectations, some internal and others from the public. They are seen as stalwart citizens, with a sense of responsibility and reliability, with the ability to be self-reliant and capable. There is a sense they are often in 'service' to others.[32] All of these factors, along with personality factors common in the 'medical self', can make them spectacularly bad at accepting the patient role.[33] As doctors we are used to achieving, and to hit a brick wall of perceived 'failure' as large as addiction can be a difficult thing to fully accept and come to terms with.

While no one speciality is 'above' developing an addiction, studies have consistently shown certain specialities to be over-represented. Comparative studies from North America show that there is an over-representation of emergency doctors and psychiatrists in abusing multiple substances.[34] In another study, general practitioners (GPs), internal medicine doctors, anaesthetists, emergency medicine doctors and psychiatrists accounted for over 50% of addicted doctors. Anaesthetists alone accounted for 10.9% of cases,[35] confirming that access is an important risk factor.[36] A higher proportion of anaesthetists compared to other doctors also report intravenous drug use.[37] Across the numerous prevalence studies in America, anaesthetists and GPs consistently appear as vulnerable groups. This could be due to the isolated nature of their work and increased clinical patient demand, as well as easier access to drugs.[38] The over-representation of psychiatrists in some studies could be due to the increased risk of being exposed to high levels of trauma and emotional burden.

The majority of literature has focused on doctors with established addiction; there are few longitudinal studies looking at these doctors and whether there were earlier signs of 'chemically coping' or historical recreational use in their teenage years/early 20s that might act as risk predictors for developing addiction.[38] There is a link between substance misuse and criminality, especially in those using heroin and crack cocaine, as often use can spiral to the point of people losing their homes and families and becoming embroiled in the murky world of drug dealers. As far as we can see in the literature, and in our experience at our service, doctor addicts have the advantage of often having stable families and financial situations, which prevent them going down the overt criminal route, though there are cases of doctors who do steal drugs from hospitals, drive under the influence or are found guilty of possession charges. However, it is rare to see a doctor present with 'street heroin/crack' use. When opiates are the problem, they are more likely to be self-prescribed or stolen from hospital stock. The doctors we see using club drugs, stimulants and novel psycho-active substances are obviously sourcing them illegally, either through the internet or through dealers.

Our doctors often have the advantage of a wide network of non-drug using friends and family, with a structured, meaningful and purposeful life to return to once they have sought help. While this is a clear advantage, sometimes, within professionals' families, it can make spotting the addiction harder. Even when it is identified, often more can seem at stake than just the health of the individual, such as financial and societal security. The addiction can become a 'closely guarded secret' and spouses/family members may end up adopting co-dependent behaviours that revolve around keep the 'secret safe'.[39]

TREATMENT

Mario is a GP. He had been encouraged to come for help by his practice partner who was worried about his drinking. He had recently had a complaint from his practice nurse after he had uncharacteristically become irritated with her at work. Reluctantly he came. At the assessment he described how he had begun to drink heavily to help deal with insomnia relating to exhaustion after long working days. He was now regularly drinking a least ten units of whiskey every day, including on his way to work, and topping up during the day. His alcohol use had been creeping up over many years and he cannot remember the last time he had an alcohol-free day. He admits to getting the shakes in the morning and having to start most days with a small drink. He was convinced that he would lose his job and faced with the wreckage of his life, he began to cry.

Mario is fairly typical of the doctors we see at our service. After presenting to our service and having an assessment, he will be offered a place at a six-week residential unit or a community detoxification programme. The choice will be largely his. Both will likely involve initial detoxification using benzodiazepines (we use a five-day tapering course of chlordiazepoxide). For community detoxification we involve a close family member to supervise. We would see him on a daily basis for the duration of the reduction. Once through the initial detoxification stage, he will be encouraged to attend 12-steps orientated (abstinence) base groups (AA, BDDG), one-to-one therapy and will address with his case manager any underlying and residual health issues. He might require antidepressants and psychological therapy. He does not need to be referred to the regulator as though he was drinking heavily, he is engaged in treatment and is fully compliant with future abstinence. His follow-up would involve regular (weekly, then monthly) consultations with his case manager. Together with his case worker, a return to work plan will be put in place, which might require reduction in the number of hours or sessions worked.

Josette is an anaesthetist. Severe neck pain resulted in her receiving tramadol from her GP. The pain initially responded to the drug, though returned soon after stopping her treatment. She increased her dose, not just to control the pain, but also to stop withdrawal symptoms. She was asking her GP for repeat prescriptions earlier, and he continued to prescribe, oblivious to her overuse. Her dose increased more, which she covered through self-written private prescriptions, though she was careful to go to different pharmacies each time. She then began to take fentanyl from the anaesthetic room. This went on for months until eventually an anaesthetic nurse noticed her slip a used ampoule of fentanyl into her pocket. The police were called, she was referred to the GMC and the Trust instituted disciplinary processes.

Josette is again similar of the doctors with addiction who come to our service. She did not present for care before 'the balloon went up' and her dependence was discovered. Her recovery would now be complicated by needing to go through various disciplinary, criminal justice and regulatory processes, which would run in sequence and take years to complete. Treatment for Josette would be based on addressing the underlying addiction and health issues (physical, psychological or other problems) and then maintaining recovery through follow-up, and monitoring, as well as supporting her to return to work or training. Abstinence is always the aim, though we have a small number of doctors on opiate maintenance treatment (buprenorphine) and a small number where we 'allow' controlled, non-problematic drinking.

Our service is unique internationally at the time of writing, in that it is the only physician health service that is wholly independent of the regulatory bodies and provides treatment. The North American PHPs do not strictly speak provide treatment, but they do have a clear treatment pathway that they expect their clinicians to adhere to. A brief summary and comparison of American PHP and my own service is presented. Bear in mind that for doctors in the NHS system who require more detailed and careful monitoring, they may also have the GMC involved. The GMC does not provide treatment but will have their own monitoring protocol pathway.

	USA PHP The figures are based on a study of 904 doctors enrolled into 16 PHPs in USA 1995–2001[40]	NHS Practitioner Health The figures are based on ten years of caring for doctors with addiction[23] and an in-depth analysis of eight years of patient outcomes[41]
Referrals	55% of doctors are mandated to enter the PHP by a licencing board, hospital, or other agency 45% are also 'mandated', but informally by employers or colleagues Self-referral is unusual	100% self-referrals though can be encouraged to attend by others
Assessment	Detailed assessment covering many aspects of the individual's physical, psychological health and past history Typically two to five days multidisciplinary, multimodal evaluation	In the main, 90-minute assessment by PH clinician, which addresses precipitating, perpetuating and protective factors Formulation and care plan are arrived at

Multidisciplinary team (MDT)	MDT involved in care planning, assessing risk and any other issues based on the assessment	MDT involved in care planning, assessing risk and any other issues based on the assessment
Contract	Will have to sign a contract that stipulates, for example, abstinence, sharing of information, adhering to treatment, requirements to work under supervision, testing	None
Treatment	Clear, mandated pathway involving approved providers Providers based on care specific needs	NHS provider made up of doctors (psychiatrist, GPs), nurses, therapists and other support staff Patients given choice of treatment options
Residential rehab	30–90 days of intensive residential treatment or community-based treatment Around 70% doctors have residential care	6 weeks of other intensive community-based treatment or residential treatment Around 25% have residential care
Testing	Intensive random, unannounced, drug and alcohol testing for 20 drugs or more, including alcohol Testing is weekly or twice weekly at start (e.g. first two years), then reduced (20 times per year) for around five years 75% of all urine samples are supervised Testing is urine (92%), saliva (0.1%), hair (0.2%), breath (0.6%)	Only tested if clinically indicated – typically at the start of treatment No observed urine testing Testing is urine (70%), blood (10%), hair (20%)
Work	Workplace monitoring	Cannot stipulate any monitoring Some doctors require stricter monitoring and/or clinical supervision than NHS PH can provide. For these doctors we encourage them to self-refer to the GMC

Confidentiality	Requirement for information sharing	Memorandum of Understanding with GMC with respect to needing to breach confidentiality
Supervision/ follow-up	Must meet, with frequency determined by case manager	As necessary based on each individual case
12 Steps	Required AA or NA	Recommended Mostly AA or NA or BDDG
Other treatment	Must attend individual and group work as required by contract	As determined by individual care planning All voluntary
Funding	Self-funded	NHS
Abstinence based	Uniformly abstinence based	Allows some controlled drinking
Adjunctive medication	Unusual, but prescribed as needed, for example, 1 out of 904 doctors were placed on methadone for opiate-dependence	Unusual, but prescribed as needed 2 out of 400 placed on buprenorphine for opiate-dependence

OUTCOMES

Treatment works. Once addicted doctors are in treatment, they have excellent recoveries. As part of a review of outcomes, doctors in the first eight years of our service were examined in detail.[23] Between 2008 and 2016, 255 doctors presented with addiction. Of these, 27% were female and 73% male. Mean age at presentation to the service was 42.31±10.00 years. GPs made up 28% of the cohort, the emergency specialities (anaesthetics, emergency medicine and acute medicine) 25% and psychiatrists 15%. The remainder comprised medical specialities (15%), surgeons (6%) and other medical fields or specialities (paediatrics, public health, occupational medicine, sports medicine) (11%). Over half of doctors with substance misuse disorder attending the service were involved in regulator or disciplinary processes at the time of starting treatment. Of the remaining doctors we recommended 12 to self-refer to the GMC or to disclose their substance use to their workplace. The recommendation was based on a concern for their safety and the safety of the patients they saw. This may include, for example, doctors who had frequent relapses, or where extra support and stricter monitoring would be necessary for them to be able to continue to practise medicine. Nearly 80% of the cohort had alcohol dependence. The remainder misused opiates (10%), stimulants (4%), club drugs and novel psychoactive substances (NPS) (6%) (including synthetic stimulants and hallucinogens), non-opiate prescribed medication (4%) and 3% had behaviour addiction (for example, gambling, porn). Of all doctors, 34% were admitted for a six-week residential detoxification and rehabilitation, while the remainder were treated in the community.

At the time of data collection (with follow-up periods between 12 months and 9 years), 78% of the doctors were abstinent and 68% of the cohort had completed treatment and were discharged. Thirty-four doctors were lost to follow-up or had an unplanned discharge (six of these doctors were abstinent from all substances before being lost to follow-up). Doctors stayed an average of 2.7 years with the service, though this ranged from six months to five years. As well high rates of abstinence of drugs and/or alcohol, doctors were also able to return to work. At presentation, only 43% were working; by the end of treatment this increased to 85%. Our results are comparable with those of other studies of addicted doctors in treatment, which give five-year abstinence rates of between 78%[36,39] and 85%.[42] This is a higher rate of sustained abstinence compared to non-medical cohorts, which report abstinence rates of around 40–60% for standard addiction treatment in the general population.[29]

Within general addiction services, it is not uncommon to hear patients, especially patients in professional work, say *'I don't want this on my record'*, *'Can you not tell my GP'*, *'What happens if I want to work abroad and my employers know about it? I'll never get insurance again'*. When we see addicted doctors this anxiety about 'who else knows' becomes immense, so much so, it often paralyses doctors from seeking help in the first place. Most of the fear centres on the GMC, other regulatory bodies and employers finding out rather than worries about police involvement. The doctors ruminate 'I'll be struck off', 'What will my consultant or GP partners think?', 'Will anyone trust me again?' 'I can't do anything else but be a doctor', 'People will think twice about hiring me'. It is with these weighty questions bearing down that the addicted doctor has to grapple with their recovery. Once in recovery there will be on-going questions about who, how, whether and when to tell future employers. Addiction marks the doctor for the rest of their professional life. When we see doctors in our service, it is not uncommon when they attend programmes like AA, that they often feel their stories are vastly different: 'My life hasn't got so bad', 'I'm not in as much as trouble as those people', 'I still have a job and family'. This can sometimes give a false sense of security that a doctor's 'problem' might not be a 'problem' after all. At these times, I find discussing the AA mantra of finding similarities rather than differences in the stories useful. While the outward dressing of their situation is often (thankfully) different, their internal struggles are the same.

It is always better to be treated, abstinent and in recovery, than hiding the problem. There is more risk to life, professional reputation and career prospects from not admitting to the habit.

CONCLUSION

Looking at the evidence as it appears, it would be safe to say that doctors have no higher, if not lower use of alcohol and prevalence of alcohol dependence than the general population. Prevalence rates of drug dependence are likely to be considerably lower. That doctors drank considerably more than the general population might have resulted from earlier studies, involving doctors practising in the 1970s and 1980s, when heavy drinking was more prevalent.[43,44] In my early working days, hospitals had bars on site (especially in the doctors' mess) and some served free alcohol, either in the mess or with meals in the doctors' dining room. During my first surgical house job at University College Hospital, when not on the ward, myself and the team would be in the pub opposite, which was even equipped with a dedicated on-call telephone connected to the hospital switch board. This meant doctors who were on-call could spend their time in the pub. Alcohol seemed to be more integral to the day-to-day working of a doctor when I was a junior doctor than today, enhanced probably, by the preponderance of male doctors. Men (doctors or otherwise) are more likely to drink more, have problems with alcohol and create more of an alcohol-centric culture.

While doctors might drink less than the general population, this does not mean that we have nothing to worry about. In the UK, it is estimated that there are as many as 13,000 doctors with an addiction problem.[45] This is a large number of potentially impaired doctors making a lot of decisions. While alcohol is the commonly used substance, anecdotal reports suggest that the use of cocaine and other stimulants has increased over the last decade.

FINAL WORDS FROM A DOCTOR

I first started to realise I had a problem with alcohol when I was working out in Australia. I had moved there straight out of my registration in the UK. I didn't realise it at the time, but my mood had become low and I gradually started to drink more often. It was just a glass of wine to start with, but it crept up each day, two glasses, then three, then to a whole bottle every night. It wasn't really the amount I was drinking that bothered me. It was that feeling I had, driving home from work. I would be willing the journey to be over so I could get through the front door, not have to go out again and start drinking. I knew the first thing I would do would be to throw my bag in the hall and head straight to the kitchen to get some wine. Even before a single drop had passed my lips, just in the act of opening the bottle I felt a huge sense of relief. And so, it continued, night after night, sitting alone in my room watching cheesy TV shows, with my bottle (or two) imagining I was happy. My flatmates started to notice that I was more withdrawn. But more, they noticed the empty wine bottles building up throughout the week. When one confronted me, I felt so ashamed and angry. How dare he! I didn't have a problem! I was a doctor. I knew about alcohol; I knew about alcoholism. I was not one, I was still in control of it. Of course, I knew deep down that I couldn't stop. I was in too much pain, I just didn't realise it.

I was eventually able to see my GP and tell him about my low mood. I never mentioned the alcohol because I was embarrassed and ashamed and wanted to keep it a secret, and the thought of stopping drinking scared me so much. Thankfully, once I started in treatment (medication and therapy) for my depression I began to drink less. But it didn't stop. Even after I returned to the UK, I could only stop drinking for short periods of time, but it would always creep back in, and it would build up faster than ever before. I just couldn't imagine life without alcohol. How would I cope? How would I get through a tough day? How would I have fun and celebrate good times? I went into work for an on-call shift one day, topped up from my evening's drinking. But instead of being able to take over the on-call bleep, I crumpled to the floor. Within minutes, the helping hands of my colleagues were with me. I was being comforted with a cup of tea, replaced for the shift and sent home and that was the true beginning of my journey of recovery from alcoholism. My colleagues were as shocked as I was, I think, they hadn't seen it coming. Like many doctors I hid my drinking behind the smiling face of someone who was 'coping'. Looking back, it was clear to see the cracks were starting to show at work. I was becoming more anxious, checking my letters obsessively and scared I had missed something when interpreting blood results or an ECG. I was foggy headed from hangovers most days and was thinking about my next drink well before lunchtime. I was staying later and later at work although I was desperate to get home for that first drink.

When I did finally go off sick from work and start to drink less, I still only spoke to colleagues about my 'depression'. I never spoke about my drinking. It took me six years to accept I was an alcoholic and to stop drinking completely, and I have just celebrated my first five full years of sobriety. What helped me to become and stay sober were understanding colleagues, the support of other alcoholics in a group, taking things one day at time and the daily practice of a few simple principles around my emotional and spiritual well-being, as well as helping other doctors who were struggling too. In Alcoholics Anonymous they say about sobriety that 'you have to give it away to keep it' and I have definitely found that to be true for me. Part of my work with The Joyful Doctor (an organisation I founded to support the well-being of doctors) is to speak openly about my alcoholism and mental health problems. I hope to reduce the stigma for doctors who are struggling as I was, to offer support to them through various means (writing, speaking, coaching, training and events), and one day at a time to keep 'giving it away to keep it'. If you are reading this and you are wondering if your own relationship to alcohol may not be that healthy, please speak to someone about it . There is help out there and it doesn't have to be the end of your world. In fact, my life has just got better and better since I put down that last drink.

Caroline Walker, Psychiatrist and founder of the Joyful Doctor

REFERENCES

1   Dyer C. Anaesthetist is jailed after stealing codeine from hospital where he no longer worked. *BMJ* 2017;359: j4841.

2   Paget J. What becomes of medical students? *St Bartholomew's Hosp Rep* 1869;**5**:238–42.

3   Davenport-Hines R. *The Pursuit of Oblivion: a Social History of Drugs.* London: Weidenfeld and Nicolson, 2001, Ch 4, p. 81.

4   Lathan SR. Dr. Halsted at Hopkins and at high Hampton. *Bayl Univ Med Cent Proc* 2010;**23**(1):33–7. doi:10.1080/08998280.2010.11928580.

5   Rankin JS. William Stewart Halsted: a lecture by Dr. Peter D. Olch. *Ann Surg* 2006;**243**(3):418–25. doi: 10.1097/01.sla.0000201546.94163.00.

6   White WL. The role of recovering physicians in 19th century addiction medicine: an organizational case study. *J Addictive Dis* 2000;**19**(2):1–10.

7 Crothers TD. Reformed men as asylum managers. *Q J Inebriety* 1897;**19**:79–81.

8 White WL. The history of recovered people as Wounded Healers: II. The era of professionalization and specialization. *Alcoholism Treat Quart* 2000;**18**(2):1–25.

9 Bissell L. (1982). Recovered alcoholic counselors. In: Pattison E, Kaufman E (eds). *Encyclopaedic Handbook of Alcoholism*. New York: Gardner Press, 1982, pp. 810–17.

10 Glatt M, Doctors with drinking problems. *Lancet* 1975;**305**(7900):219.

11 Becker M. Arrested addiction doctor has had long struggle with drugs [Internet]. The Buffalo News, 2018 [cited 18 January 2020]. Available from: https://buffalonews.com/2018/12/24/addiction-doctor-had-long-drug-struggle-of-his-own.

12 McAuliffe W, Rohman M, Breer P, Wyshak G, Santangelo S, Magnuson E. Alcohol use and abuse in random samples of physicians and medical students. *Am J Pub Health* 1991;**81**:177–82.

13 Vaillant G, Brighton J, McArthur C. Physicians use of mood-altering drugs: a 20-year follow-up report. *N Engl J Med* 1970;**282**:365–70.

14 Hughes P, DeWitt C, Baldwin MJ, Sheehan D, Conard S, Storr C. Resident physician substance use, by speciality. *Am J Psychiatry* 1992;**149**:1348–54.

15 Brewster J. Prevalence of alcohol and other drug problems among physicians. *JAMA* 1986;**255**:1913–20.

16 Hughes P, Brandenburgh N, Baldwin DJ, *et al*. Prevalence of substances use among US physicians. *JAMA* 1992;**267**(17):2333–9.

17 British Medical Association. The misuse of alcohol and other drugs by doctors, Report of a Working Group. London: British Medical Association, 1998.

18 Oreskovich MR, Shanafelt T, Dyrbye LN, *et al*. The prevalence of substance use disorders in American physicians. *Am J Addict* 2015;**24**(1):30–8.

19 Baldisseri MR. Impaired healthcare professional. *Crit Care Med* 2007;**35**(2 Suppl):S106–16.

20 Nash LM, Daly MG, Kelly PJ, *et al*. Factors associated with psychiatric morbidity and hazardous alcohol use in Australian doctors. *Med J Aust* 2010;**193**(3):161–6.

21 Rosta J. Prevalence of problem-related drinking among doctors: a review on representative samples. *Ger Med Sci* 2005;**3**:Doc07. ISSN 1612-3174.

22 Field R, Scotland A. Medicine in the UK after Shipman: Has 'all changed, changed utterly'? *Lancet* 2004;**364**(Suppl1):s40–1.

23 NHS PHP. The wounded healer; report on the first 10 years of Practitioner Health Service. 2018. Available from: http://php.nhs.uk/wp-content/uploads/sites/26/2018/10/PHP-report-web.pdf.

24 Bourne A, Reid D, Hickson F, Torres Rueda S, Weatherburn P. The chemsex study. London: Sigma Research, 2014. Available from: http://sigmaresearch.org.uk/files/report2014b.pdf.

25 McCall H, Adams N, Willis J. What is chemsex and why does it matter? *BMJ* 2015;351:h5790. doi: https://doi.org/10.1136/bmj.h5790.

26 AMA Council on Mental Health. The sick physician. *JAMA* 1973;**223**(6):684–7.

27 AMA Announces New Approach to Physician Mental Health Care. AMA press release, 13 June 2018. Available from: www.ashclinicalnews.org/news/ama-announces-new-approach-physician-mental-health-care-2.

28 BDDG. Dr Max M Glatt, Lancet 1975. Available from: www.bddg.org/dr-max-m-glatt-lancet-1975.

29 Brooks D, Edwards G, Andrews T. Doctors and substance misuse: types of doctors, types of problems. *Addiction* 1993;**88**:655–63.

30 Pedersen A, Sorensen J, Bruun N, Christensen B, Vedsted P. Risky alcohol use in Danish physicians: associated with alexithymia and burnout? *Drug Alcohol Depend* 2016;**160**:119–26.

31 Mayall RM. Substance misuse in anaesthetists. *BJA Educ* 2016;**16**:236–41.

32 Nace EP. *Achievement and Addiction: a Guide to the Treatment of Professionals.* New York: Routledge, 2013. ISBN 1134861702.

33 Gerada C, Wesley A. When doctors need treatment; an anthropological approach to why doctors make bad patients. *BMJ* 2013;347.

34 Myers T, Weiss E. Substance use in interns and residents: an analysis of personal, social and professional differences, *Br J Addiction* 1987;**82**:1091–9.

35 McLellan AT, Skipper GS, Campbell M, DuPont RL. Five-year outcomes in a cohort study of physicians treated for substance use disorders in the United States. *BMJ* 2008;**337**:a2038.

36 Oreskovich MR, Caldeiro RM. Anaesthesiologists recovering from chemical dependency: can they safely return to the operating room? *Mayo Clin Proc* 2009;**84**:576–80.

37 Lefebvre LG, Kaufmann, M. The identification and management of substance use disorders in anaesthesiologists. *Can J Anesth/J Can Anesth* 2017;**64**:211–18.

38 Nace EP. *Achievement and Addiction: a Guide to the Treatment of Professionals.* Routledge, 2013. ISBN 1134861702.

39 Cermak T. *Diagnosing and Treating Codependence.* Minneapolis, MN: Johnson Institute, 1986.

40 DuPont RL, McLellan AT, White WL, Merlo LJ, Gold MS. Setting the standard for recovery: Physicians' Health Programs. *J Subst Abuse Treat* 2009;**36**:159–71.

41 Sathanandan S, Abrol E, Aref-Adib G, Keen J, Gerada C. The UK Practitioner Health Programme: 8-year outcomes in Doctors with addiction disorders. *Res Adv Psychiatry* 2019;**6**(2):43–9.

42 Brewster JM, Kaufmann IM, Hutchison S, MacWilliam C. Characteristics and outcomes of doctors in a substance dependence monitoring programme in Canada: prospective descriptive study. *BMJ* 2008;**337**:a2098.

43 Harrison D, Chick J. Trends in alcoholism among male doctors in Scotland. *Addiction* 1994;**89**(12):1613–17.

44 Brooke D, Edwards G, Taylor C. Addiction as an occupational hazard: 144 doctors with drug and alcohol problems. *British Journal of Addiction* 1991;**86**: 1011–16.

45 Addiction [Internet]. Sick-doctors-trust.co.uk. 2019 [cited 12 September 2019]. Available from: http://sick-doctors-trust.co.uk/page/addiction.

11

Autism in Doctors

MARY DOHERTY

I am an anaesthetist; I am also autistic. From as far back as I can remember I have always felt 'different', which is an experience common to late diagnosed autistic adults.[1] It wasn't until my son was diagnosed with autism that I realised that I also view the world through the same autistic lens, and that I have had to deal with the same challenges as he has. The greatest difficulty of an undiagnosed autistic adult is not knowing what we are dealing with, not knowing *why* things seem so difficult, or why other people seem so odd. Now that I understand it, life is so much better and I love being autistic.

Autism is not a mental illness though autistic people are more likely to develop mental health problems. It is a complex, lifelong neurodevelopmental condition that changes the way an individual experience the world and communicates with others. Autistic spectrum conditions (including what was previously termed Asperger syndrome), occur in around 1–2% of the population.[2]

People are surprised to learn that doctors can be autistic. We don't fit into the neat diagnostic criteria learnt at medical school, or the stereotypes of boys preoccupied with train timetables or of profoundly disabled individuals requiring full time care many of us see in our clinical practice. Believe me, doctors can be autistic. I am, and so are lots of my colleagues. By its nature, medicine may actually select for autistic traits, including obsessionalism and perfectionism. There are no published prevalence rates for doctors or individual specialities, although anaesthetists appear to be over-represented in an online network of neurodivergent doctors. Personality traits of anaesthetists seem different to other specialities[3] and anaesthesia is one of the specialities particularly attractive to autistic doctors, where autistic traits can be beneficial. It is an exacting speciality, with little room for error and a great deal of reliance on systems, protocols, standardised working and checking. Without realising it at the time, I can see that's why I chose the speciality. However, I know autistic doctors in almost every speciality I can think of. We learn to cope in medicine by learning the skills, communication and social interactions needed to engage with patients and colleagues. Doctors can be, by their nature, perfectionists. Add autism to the mix and we get perfectionism in spades. We are intensely focused, have great attention to detail and strengths in pattern recognition; skills that are clearly advantageous in anaesthesia. Generally, we deal with patients one at a time, in a sequential order. Anaesthetics is procedure based and solution focused, which is attractive to innovative but concrete thinkers. Adherence to routines and repetitive behaviours are key traits of autism, and these tend to feature heavily in anaesthetic practice, so it can be a good choice for us. Autism is associated with co-occurring psychiatric disorders in up to 80%,[4] most often anxiety and depression. Suicide rates are higher in the autistic population than in the general population,[5] and coupled with the increased risk of suicide in doctors, the author surmises an even greater risk for autistic doctors, particularly those who remain unsupported and possibly undiagnosed. Increased recognition of autistic spectrum conditions means more students are entering medical school with a pre-existing diagnosis. For others, it is when the demands of training or independent practice, perhaps coupled with adverse life events, overwhelm existing coping strategies that the diagnosis is first made. The recurrent narrative among those who have been diagnosed late is of personal distress, career difficulties and a truncated career or early retirement.

Diagnosis can be challenging as autism is rarely considered in the differential diagnosis when a doctor presents with a mental illness, and a lifetime of masking to fit in can often obscure the signs. Missed and misdiagnosis is common, particularly in women.[6] Anxiety, depression, or substance misuse are often the presenting conditions. Patients with autism are often misdiagnosed as having bipolar disorder, obsessive compulsive disorder, schizophrenia or personality disorders (particularly borderline personality disorder).[7] Autistic adults commonly use alcohol or illicit drugs to manage mental health difficulties,[8] so increased rates of substance misuse could be expected in autistic doctors.

We have difficulties in training. Social challenges and sensory differences are the main issues for autistic people. Difficulties with communication can be overcome with training and autism specific tutoring, ideally delivered by autistic specialists. Communication with patients is relatively structured and task focused, which is ideal for autistic doctors, and the skills required can be easily learnt and indeed are specifically taught in modern medical training. In contrast, interactions with colleagues are more socially based. This is where an autistic doctor may struggle most, and we are often found on the periphery of the team or may even be excluded entirely from the social group. Overliteral interpretation of instructions, miscommunications, misunderstandings and unintentional use of non-verbal communication or misinterpretation of body language can all cause difficulties. This may lead to interpersonal conflicts, resulting in social isolation, social anxiety and depression. An autistic colleague may appear anxious, emotional and easily upset, or in contrast may be reserved, aloof or distant. Alternatively, autistic people can learn appropriate social skills and can appear to interact well and become popular and valued members of a department. However, such interaction is learnt, not intuitive, and the intense effort required to maintain it is difficult in the longer term. The health effects of such 'masking' have recently been highlighted,[9] and therefore it is vital to find a balance between social inter-action and restorative solitude.

Executive functioning challenges are a feature of autism and may present as a disorganised 'scattered' doctor who struggles with paperwork, deadlines and time keeping. Specific support strategies targeting executive functioning are particu-larly helpful in such cases, and the best professional to advise on an individual basis may be an occupational therapist familiar with autistic spectrum conditions. A monotropic thinking style, in which a small number of interests pull the autistic person more strongly and use up a good deal of the person's processing resources, can lead to sustained intense interest in a particular topic, leading to great expertise in that area. However, this can also lead to difficulty switching focus and possibly idiosyncratic practise in a socially isolated doctor. This high degree of focus can be particularly beneficial in research, but executive functioning challenges may mean an autistic trainee may be unable to juggle research interests alongside a busy clinical role. A period of dedicated research might be sensible, if this is a spe-cific interest or training requirement.

Sensory issues can be particularly disabling for autistic people and the degree of discomfort should not be underestimated. Noise is a common sensory trigger, as is bright light, particularly fluorescent light. The typical operating theatre environment can be a sensory nightmare for an autistic trainee, who may take longer to acclimatise than peers. Multiple beeps, alarms, music, smells, tangled lines and tubes and challenging communication from behind surgical masks all add up to a significant extra cognitive load, which should be taken into account when evaluating an autistic trainee. Coupled with the difficulty making transitions, negotiating new social relationships means that the early days of a new rotation will be particularly stressful for an autistic trainee, and unfortu-nately this can have negative consequences as first impressions are formed just at the point of greatest stress. Fostering a culture of tolerance and acceptance of diversity will offset this and allow a trainee to perform optimally more quickly. Autistic people who have succeeded to complete medical school training have made monumental efforts to learn communication and social skills, and any attempt to reciprocate on the part of colleagues is hugely beneficial and always appreciated. Specific advice for communication with an autistic colleague would include being explicit with directions and avoiding hints or mixed messages. The degree of clarity required to accurately transmit a message may seem blunt or even rude, but this is usually gratefully received. If interpersonal conflicts continuously occur between a consultant and trainee, the best approach may be to follow the procedure in aviation and 'do not pair' a trainee and consultant who have difficulty working with each other. Such situations are usually due to a communication style that is particularly difficult for an autistic person to inter-pret. It is important to recognise that a frazzled brain cannot learn, and if too much effort is going into decoding a colleague's non-verbal communications, little else can be processed.

Polarised impressions of a trainee may be a clue to an underlying neurodevelopmental condition. Where possible, there may be a great benefit in allocating a trainer for the whole rotation. The value of a supportive and understanding mentor cannot be overestimated. Feedback must be clear and unambiguous. We don't intuitively understand figurative language or hints and it is easy for us to miss the meaning behind the message. In the event of an unexpected response or behaviour, check for misunderstanding as literal interpretation of rules or instructions may cause confusion. We need to be told explicitly if there is a change to plans, which others may pick up instinctively. For example, if an event is re-scheduled from its usual location to somewhere else, an autistic trainee might not notice colleagues going in a different direction and may not be included in online groups where key information is shared.

Doctors with autism struggle with simulation-based teaching techniques and objective structured clinical examinations. We find it hard in a group training session where the response expected from us is ambiguous. Change is hard for us and we need time to readjust. An autistic trainee might have an inconsistent, 'spiky' profile, displaying excellence in some domains while underperforming in others. This might all add up to a prolonged or stepwise progression through training and this should be acknowledged and positively encouraged.

Challenges are situational and often transient. Sensory overload is real. Beware of assuming that a trainee who is struggling in a stressful sensory nightmare of a theatre with a colleague who communicates in a non-autistic friendly style, is simply a trainee struggling with the job itself. Understanding, acceptance of difference and minimal adjustments to the environment can have disproportionate effects in such circumstances. Be aware of the additional effort it takes to socialise and appear part of the team and be understanding when someone needs solitude. It can be confusing when a colleague happily chats one day but sits in silence appearing to ignore people other days. Be understanding, be tolerant. A high degree of social masking often means the condition remains hidden. It may be that a doctor's professional life is unremarkable but personal life is chaotic. Life events and unexpected changes may mean that demands exceed an individual's capacity to cope, which can result in a sudden and catastrophic decompensation. This may require a period away from practice, but with awareness of the specific challenges arising from autism, in my view many of those doctors can be supported to return to practice. It is my opinion that an autistic spectrum condition should be specifically considered whenever a doctor presents in difficulty, particularly when the difficulties arise after any sudden change to professional or personal life.

If you are considering that autism may be an issue for you, I would suggest you seek an opinion from a professional experienced in diagnosing autism, as the benefit of diagnosis is enormous. There are online resources available such as the AQ10, which is recommended by the NICE guidelines as a screening tool,[10] or the more comprehensive AQ 50.[11] The *Ritvo Autism Asperger Diagnostic Scale – Revised*[12] is particularly useful for those who have learned to mask effectively, but none of these can replace a formal diagnostic process. There is also a supportive online network of autistic doctors, and having a formal diagnosis is not a requirement to join the private group.[13]

CONCLUSION

Autism among doctors is a hither-to unexplored area. However, it does exist and given the experiences of the author, in not insignificant numbers. This chapter has outlined the problems doctors with autism face in the workplace and ways of overcoming these.

REFERENCES

1 Stagg SD, Belcher H. Living with autism without knowing: receiving a diagnosis in later life. *Health Psychol Behav Med* 2019;**7**(1):348–61.

2 CDC. Data and Statistics. Autism Spectrum Disorder. Resource Document. [Accessed 27 January 2020]. Available from: www.cdc.gov/ncbddd/autism/data.html.

3 Kluger MT, Laidlaw TM, Kruger N, Harrison MJ. Personality traits of anaesthetists and physicians: an evaluation using the Cloninger Temperament and Character Inventory (TCI125). *Anaesthesia* 1999;**54**:926–35.

4 Lever AG, Geurts HM. Psychiatric co-occurring symptoms and disorders in young, middle-aged, and older adults with autism spectrum disorder. *J Autism Develop Disord* 2016;**46**(6):1916–30.

5 Hirvikoski T, Mittendorfer-Rutz E, Boman M, Larsson H, Lichtenstein P, Bölte S. Premature mortality in autism spectrum disorder. *Br J Psychiatry* 2016;**208**(3):232–8.

6 Gould J, Ashton-Smith J. Missed diagnosis or misdiagnosis: girls and women on the autism spectrum. *Good Autism Pract* 2011;**12**(1): 34-41.

7 Tebartz van Elst L, Pick M, Biscaldi M, Fangmeier T, Riedel A. High-functioning autism spectrum disorder as a basic disorder in adult psychiatry and psychotherapy: psychopathological presentation, clinical relevance and therapeutic concepts. *Eur Arch Psychiatry Clin Neurosci* 2013;**263**(2):189–96.

8 Doherty M, O'Sullivan JD, Neilson SD. Barriers to healthcare for autistic adults: consequences and policy implications. A cross-sectional study. 2020. Available from: www.medrxiv.org/content/10.1101/2020.04.01.20050336v1.full.pdf.

9 Mandy W. Social camouflaging in autism: is it time to lose the mask? *Autism* 2019;**23**(8):1879–81.

10 NICE. Autism spectrum quotient (AQ-10) test. Available from: www.nice.org.uk/guidance/cg142/resources/autism-spectrum-quotient-aq10-test-143968.

11 ARC. Downloadable tests. Available from: www.autismresearchcentre.com/arc_tests.

12 RAADS-R. Available from: www.aspietests.org/raads.

13 www.facebook.com/AutisticDoctors.

Burnout in Doctors

CLARE GERADA

INTRODUCTION

Burnout is now a public health crisis. It is the single most prevalent psychological complaint found in those who work in the caring professions, with counsellors, doctors, nurses and social workers all at high risk. It is formally defined and subjectively experienced as a state of physical, emotional and mental exhaustion caused by long-term involvement in demanding situations. For me it conjures up an image of 'destroyed' individuals, shells of their former selves, damaged by the 'fire' of their work that has raged all around them. It leads them to lose their joy and zest for work. Work instead becomes mundane, routine and a burden. Burnout strikes those who have been most idealistic, enthusiastic and engaged.

Burnout is thought to be distinct from depression, but I prefer to think of them as part of the same process. There is a considerable overlap between symptoms (in particular around hopelessness, poor self-esteem, sleep disturbance) and it might be more acceptable to call oneself 'burnt-out' than 'depressed'. Cleary the two are linked. A study from Finland found a relationship between burnout and depression, with each predicting subsequent developments in the other.[1] High levels of burnout predict high level of antidepressant medication.[2]

Compassion fatigue is also closely linked to burnout and again the two could be considered to be part and parcel of the same thing.

BURNOUT

Burnout is a psychological and behavioural syndrome in which emotional exhaustion is a major feature. It has been defined as long-term, unresolvable job stress, a sense of being overwhelmed and lacking in personal accomplishment. First described in 1974 by the psychologist Herbert Freudenberger in his seminal work looking at why those working with drug addicts experienced a gradual depletion in energy and loss of motivation and commitment,[3] he labelled this state of exhaustion as 'burnout'.[4]

The World Health Organization International Classification of Diseases (ICD) recognises burnout as an **occupational** rather than a **medical** condition. The most recent ICD-11 (2019) describes burnout as 'resulting from chronic workplace stress that has not been successfully managed'.[5] While linked, stress and burnout are not the same. Stress is a general term referring to temporary adaptation (with positive as well as negative connotations) accompanied by physical and mental symptoms (*'flight or fight responses'*). In contrast, burnout is the final stage in a breakdown of the person's ability to adapt, which results from the long-term imbalance between demands and resources.

ICD-11: Burnout is characterised by three dimensions:

- Feelings of energy depletion or exhaustion (*emotional exhaustion*).
- Increased mental distance from one's job, or feelings of negativity or cynicism related to one's job (*depersonalisation and cynicism*).
- Reduced professional efficacy (*diminished personal accomplishment*).

The measure of burnout most often used is the Maslach Burnout inventory (MBI), though there are many others. It was originally designed by the social psychologist Christina Maslach and consists of a 22-item questionnaire in three areas: emotional exhaustion, EE (loss of enthusiasm for work); depersonalisation, DP (negative, unfeeling and impersonal responses towards recipients, lack of empathy and sometimes viewing people as objects); and personal accomplishment, PA (feeling ineffective at work).[6]

It is important to notice that the term depersonaliation with respect to burnout *differs from that used in psychiatry and psychoanalytic literature*, which refers to a person's extreme alienation from oneself and from the world.

Problems with studying burnout

Despite thousands of studies, the exact prevalence of burnout is hard to pin down. This is due to the variation in how it is measured, different instruments used and cut-off points for diagnosis, as well as studies using different sampling frames. Perhaps though, the main reason is because despite attempts over the years to define, measure, study, address and reduce it, burnout is not a disease as such, rather it is dis-ease, a discomfort with oneself and one's place, value and efficacy at work. It is probably as hard to measure as nostalgia, stoicism, fear, hate or love.

We also have little idea about the epidemiology or natural history of burnout. Even now, 50 years on from when it was first defined, we cannot answer basic questions such as, who gets it, who is more at risk, how much of it is there, let alone what interventions work in reducing it. Even the impact of burnout is not clearly known. Of course, the cause is known – chronic, unremitting emotionally stressful jobs. But this does not really help in studying it, as one might be able to study the link between smoking and lung cancer. Burnout involves the 'painful realisation that we have failed to make the world a better place, to help the needy, to have a real impact in the organisation, that all of our efforts are for nothing'.[7] For me, this feels a much better, more honest and a less clinical definition to describe that hopeless feeling, when you know (hopefully temporarily) you cannot go on caring for others and when you realise you cannot make a difference to your patients' lives or to the system you work in.

I have had experience of losing interest in the wellbeing of my patients, of becoming bored and, worse still, of losing my compassion for them. Exhausted from juggling work and two young children, I felt an overwhelming desire to resign, to pack it all in and leave medicine completely. It came to a head after a particularly busy and stressful morning surgery. I felt washed out, didn't want to return for the evening clinic and resented patients having more of my time than my own family. Many were my regulars, patients with longstanding, intractable problems and I felt disillusioned. What could I do to help them? I couldn't find them jobs or rehousing. I couldn't repair their broken relationships. I couldn't fix their lives. Medicine had lost its spark. I knew I needed a break from clinical practice. These emotions are so much harder to quantify than the multiple questions in burnout questionnaires and studies would imply.

Although the intensity, duration, consequences of burnout may vary between different individuals and across time in the same person, it always has the combination of the three components: physical, emotional and mental exhaustion. After I ran the London marathon in 2004 (in a time of 4 hours 20 mins before you ask), I was exhausted, but elated. This is clearly not burnout.

It is not just following intense clinical work that places someone at risk of burnout, it can occur in those who have non-clinical leadership roles. As part of my position as head of the Royal College of General Practitioners I had to lead my profession's response to the Government's proposal to reorganise the NHS. This meant balancing the needs of my profession and yet not being overly critical of the Government. I worked extremely hard to raise concerns about the proposed changes and was subjected to personal attack, intense media interest and political pressure. I worked incredibly long hours (up to 18 hours per day) and had to portray the outward façade of a confident individual the role demanded. This all took a toll on my psychological health. Outwardly I was the strong, determined, powerful leader. Inwardly I lived in a state of anxiety; I lost weight, could not sleep and was concerned that I was being watched (this turned out to be true but not to the extent I believed). I became disillusioned and demoralised and felt I had let my profession down. At the same time, I continued with my clinical work, caring for doctors with mental illness, all of us archetypal wounded leaders. My symptoms matched theirs. I was physically, emotionally and mentally exhausted. The day the NHS Bill passed through the House of Lords, meaning an unimpeded passage to becoming law, I became unwell and developed influenza (I am rarely unwell). Only in retrospect did I realise I had the classic features of burnout, brought on by my real sense of failure. It is not uncommon for physical exhaustion to increase susceptibility to illness and accidents. I have written about my experience in the *Art and Science of Working Together*.[8]

RESEARCH INTO BURNOUT

There are thousands of studies on burnout. Most use questionnaires to 'diagnose' it, that is saying it is either present or not, based on any single positive response, rather than scores across the different constituents of burnout. Others shorten the questionnaires (in the hope of improving completion rate) and risk undermining the validity of the instrument. There are also other problems such as bias when filling in questionnaires to measure burnout that are not blinded (essentially leading the responder to give the answer the researcher is trying to find). Almost all studies rely on self-report and largely poorly constructed cross-sectional surveys. I worry that, by constantly measuring burnout we might be perpetuating the problem rather than finding solutions. We might also risk exaggerating the level of distress through contagion of misery. Furthermore, by measuring *individual* burnout we risk shifting the focus away from where it truly resides, the organisation.

Examples of studies

I have included a few studies mainly those that are systematic reviews. Not surprisingly given what I have already said, there are few consistent findings. Examining some of these studies shows how variable the rates are of burnout. Some find it so high that it should be considered to be the norm, rather than the exception. For example, a 2015 survey of hospital residents at the University of North Carolina found all scored above 50% from baseline.[9] Another from British Columbia reported 80% of doctors suffered from moderate to severe emotional exhaustion, 61% from moderate to severe depersonalisation and 44% had moderate to low feelings of personal accomplishment.[10] The Medscape Physician's Lifestyle Survey is an annual study of more than 15,000 American doctors across 29 different specialities. It measures rates of burnout, depression and suicidal ideation.[11] In the 2019 survey, 44% of responders reported burnout. Rates were highest in doctors working in critical care, neurology and family medicine and lowest in plastic surgeons. When asked what the doctor attributed their symptoms to, unsurprisingly 'the job' was the most common response. The majority of doctors had neither sought help nor had any intention of seeking professional help for their symptoms. A review conducted by Udemezue Imo of studies published between 1993 and 2013 of psychiatric morbidity in doctors in the UK, found across all specialities the rate of burnout was 31% (ranging from 17% to 52%). General practitioners (GPs), newly qualified doctors and consultants had the highest scores.[12] Even the medical regulators have now taken to measuring burnout. For example, in 2018 the General Medical Council included questions on burnout in their annual survey of doctors in training. One-third of doctors felt exhausted at the thought of another day at work, on a regular basis. The survey found that one-sixth of doctors fell into the category of high risk of burnout, with GPs at highest risk (25%).[13] The risk of burnout was closely related to dissatisfaction with work. Two-thirds of doctors in the highest risk for burnout group were also dissatisfied in their day-to-day work, compared with 9% of the doctors with very low burnout risk. There's no individual measure of burnout that appears to be a particularly strong indicator of dissatisfaction, rather it is the compounding effect of multiple experiences that lead to dissatisfaction. A study involving GPs across 12 European countries found rates varied between 20% and 35% on all dimensions of burnout.[14] Southern European countries had significantly lower levels of 'emotional exhaustion' but higher levels of 'personal accomplishment'. Finally, studies by Tait Shanafelt and colleagues enable us to compare burnout over different years and compared to the background population. These researchers have been conducting surveys of burnout and satisfaction with work–life balance in American physicians relative to the general American population since 2011, repeated in 2014 and 2017; all found higher rates of burnout than in the general population. In 2011, 46% of physicians reported at least one symptom of burnout.[15] The highest rates were found among those at the front line of care (family medicine, general internal medicine and emergency medicine). In 2014 just over one-half of doctors had at least one symptom of burnout.[16] The latest study was published in 2019; 44% had at least one symptom of burnout.[17] In a recent study of doctors practising in the UK around 32% had high burnout scores.[18] Emergency medicine and GPs had the highest scores.

What can be gleaned from these studies is that:

- Burnout is common.
- Prevalence reduces with better designed and larger studies.
- It is probably more prevalent in younger versus older doctors, though this is not entirely clear.
- It is probably more prevalent and more intense in those specialities working with patients who present with undifferentiated problems (general practice, accident and emergency) or where workload is harder to control (such as general medicine).
- Rates tend to be lower in those specialities that have less on-call commitments and are more containable in terms of hours and workload (and are more highly remunerated), such as plastic surgery and dermatology.
- It is probably increasing in the medical workforce.

CORRELATES AND CAUSES OF BURNOUT

Just as there are numerous studies measuring burnout, there are probably equal numbers trying to find causation or correlation. In the main, those who are most at risk of burnout share three characteristics. The first is that their work is *emotionally demanding*. The second, that the individual has certain *personality characteristics* that draws them to 'public' service as a career, and finally these individuals share a *'patient centred'* approach to their work. All three are equally important.

Looking at the *emotionally demanding* nature of our work, in public service professions (be they teaching, medicine, social work) people are exposed to emotionally demanding situations over a long period of time. Each job has its particular stressors depending on the demands of the job. Doctors have to deal with pain, helplessness, despair, death and accept the limits of science. I have written about this throughout this book, but it is important to keep reminding myself, being a doctor is not easy. Even 40 years later I am amazed at the trust patients give me, how they open up unconditionally and believe that I can 'sort them out'. This is hard, emotional work. This is not the same as saying the job is 'stressful'. All jobs are stressful, and many of us thrive on stress (and remember the opposite of no stress is boredom). It is the emotional aspect of our work that makes us most at risk of burnout. Working long hours, seeing many patients in a single session, having no time between patients, working double shifts, in highly emotionally charged or uncertain areas of medicine (such as cancer care, general practice) magnifies the risk because they act to increase our exposure to this emotional toil. I worked 100-hour weeks when I was a junior hospital doctor. Yet, I did not become burnt-out (not then anyway). I had the time and space to talk to others, my senior medical colleagues, the nurses on the ward and colleagues as we met in the doctor's mess or dining room. I had spaces during the day to catch my breath. I wasn't watched day-in day-out by on-line minders and I could make errors and be human. Patients' medical problems were not as complex as today and the demands on me where fewer. Yet one day as a GP, sometimes having more than 100 patient encounters in single day, leaves me emotionally, physically and mentally exhausted, that is, burnt-out. Work overload contributes to burnout by reducing the capacity to meet the demands of the job. When this kind of overload is a chronic job condition, there is little opportunity to rest, recover and restore balance.

The second characteristic common in those professional groups with burnout is that individuals share a *common set of personality characteristics, attitudes and values* that has drawn them to their role, and which makes them more at risk. Simply put, we become doctors because we think we can make a difference to people's lives and are willing to sacrifice parts of ourselves to do this. This links back to the reasons why people choose to study medicine, as discussed in Chapter 3, which can make them vulnerable to the emotional stressors of their job. These include wanting to care for others in the hope of being cared for oneself, choosing medicine in part as reparation for past traumas and having personality traits that might predispose to mental illness, especially, altruism, perfectionism and obsessionalism.

The third factor common in burnout is that of having a *patient (or person) centred* approach to one's work. This means, making others *one's first concern* (as in the GMC Good Medical Practice). Most relationships are reciprocal, but the therapeutic relationship is not: the professional gives, the patient receives. This asymmetry is a source of stress. This was the finding of Leiter and Maslach who formulated a model focusing on the degree of match or mismatch between the person and six domains in their job.[19] The greater the gap, the greater the likelihood of burnout. The areas were workload, professional control, reward, community, fairness and values. Lack of recognition devalues both the work and the worker. Doctors have always worked hard and made sacrifices in their personal and professional lives to care for patients. Sadly, in the modern healthcare system the needs of the 'workers' are often ignored, leading to an imbalance of reciprocity and increasing burnout.

On top of these three factors, we each bring our own vulnerabilities derived from our unique experiences, supports and personalities. However, other than working with people, there are surprisingly few demographic factors that have been associated with an increased risk of burnout. Burnout is present in younger and older doctors, men and women, those in training and those who have achieved final accreditation status, those who work in hospital or general practice.

CONSEQUENCES OF BURNOUT

Given that burnout is by definition a state of disengagement with patients and a loss of interest in work, it is unsurprising that it correlates with: wanting to leave the profession early or reduce hours, [20,21] reduction in patient satisfaction,[22] increased risk of errors[23] and a reduction in quality of care.[24] There is considerable overlap between burnout and depressive symptomology, especially with feelings of hopelessness, worthlessness, fatigue and loss of interest in activities. I am aware of patients in my service who present with 'burnout' who in fact have depression. Burnout is contagious and can be spread through social interactions at work with those experiencing burnout having a negative impact on their colleagues.[25]

ADDRESSING BURNOUT

I do not believe we can prevent burnout, rather we have to manage it, recognise it, minimise it and deal with it when it occurs. Anyone working so close to human suffering will, at some point in their career, develop some aspects of it. Just as aging is the end result of a successful healthcare system, so burnout is the inevitable consequence of caring. We all have ebbs and flows in job satisfaction and years of being in the psychological trenches with our patients will have its effects. Emotional depletion, negative attitudes towards patients and the feeling we cannot achieve more are not uncommon, and hopefully fleeting symptoms.

What is important is recognising:

- When we can go on no longer.
- When negative attitudes turn to loss of compassion.
- When our sense of futility becomes a feeling of hopelessness and helplessness.
- When our work loses its sparkle, day-in, day-out.
- When we need to remove ourselves from the stressor.

I am not suggesting that we should not try and reduce levels of burnout; as it is an occupational hazard, the best place to start is in the workplace and in particular reduce the pressured environment in which staff work. This quote from a doctor interviewed for a study describes how practising in an intensely pressurised system has now become the norm:

> It's a common thing that people talk about that it's stressful, they don't get breaks, the rotas are awful. I think it kind of comes with the territory of working there. So, perhaps yes, it's become so normalised that they are just accepting of it [in A&E].[26]

Research tells us what we probably all know from working in different organisations. We feel and perform better in those that have good internal communication systems, where we feel supported by management, where there are opportunities for professional development and where leaders are competent.[27] On the other hand, environments where excessive workload, long work hours, fatigue, intense emotional interactions, restricted autonomy and where constant structural and organisational changes become the norm, lead to increased risk of burnout.[28] In a classic essay (later included in his book *Narcissistic Process and Corporate Decay*, New York University 1990), Howard Schwartz distinguishes between two different types of organisations: clockwork (running smoothly, cooperative, low anxiety) or snake pit (everything is falling apart, high levels of anxiety, little pleasure or joy at work).[29] Organisations with more 'snake pit' features are likely to create the risks for burnout. This means that underfunded, understaffed environments and ones that demand high productivity at all costs, place the staff at greatest risk.

At a population level, the most important interventions should be at addressing the workplace stressors, including work pressure, resources (time, people and money) and creating the opportunities for team working. On a larger scale, it means amending external factors, such as regulatory requirements, political influences and media pressures, which all contribute to chronic workplace distress.[30] Treating burnout as a public health crisis might mean we use the same prevention strategies as with any other threat to the public's health. These would include:

Primary prevention (preventing the problem arising in the first place). This largely needs to involve modifying the working environment in which doctors work, especially reducing direct patient contact. What is needed is not to provide doctors with more resilience training but instead to address the environment in which they work. Just as mine owners have a responsibility to ensure a safe working mine for miners, so too do those who employ doctors have a responsibility to create a physical and psychological safe place to work. A dangerous coal mine is not made less so by teaching miners how to relax! The leading drivers for burnout include excessive workload, chronic work stress and a lack of control over one's day-to-day work. It is a problem of the healthcare organisation as a whole, rooted in issues related to the working environment and organisational culture.[31]

Secondary prevention (aimed at reducing the impact of environmental or individual stressors). This might include address resilience, providing time-out for doctors, improving the systems in the organisation to release time to think, providing group work, improving rest periods and so on.

Tertiary prevention (aimed at those with burnout). This is about improving the quality of life and reducing the impact of burnout on the individual. It means providing easy access to confidential services, a culture where it is 'OK' to admit you have had enough and opportunities to take time out.

No measure to prevent burnout will be effective unless attention is paid to enhancing a positive work environment and strategies directed at individuals will be of limited benefit.

I have created a short, easy mnemonic to help me remember what I need to do:

B: Balance my work and play times.
U: Understand my limitations – I am not a superhero.
R: Recognise, prevent and treat burnout in myself and my teams.
N: Nurture the next generation – bring the fun back into work.
T: Teamwork – rest, play and reflect together.

Finally, burnout can be a trigger for change and personal growth. The experience of burnout always involves pain and suffering, but it can then force someone, as it did for me, to examine priorities, learn and be more aware of one's vulnerabilities. I was lucky – my sympathetic and progressive partnership and opportunities outside the consulting room meant I could take time out, return when ready and restructure my working life to refresh my psychological self. I modified my working practices, especially decreasing the time spent on face-to-face clinical work. My experience of burnout led to growth, change and further challenges that sustained me for the years to come.

CONCLUSION

Burnout is ubiquitous among all healthcare providers. It really should be considered as not 'if', but 'when' will a doctor become burnt-out. As I have discussed in this chapter, anyone who works so closely to suffering will eventually find themselves no longer able to give more of themselves. This does not mean that I am suggesting that nothing can be done to reduce its impact or address the obvious antecedents (especially intensity of direct patient contact) and it is important that policy makers allow clinicians to re-charge their emotional batteries and design safe working practices (such as shorter hours, limits on patient facing work, opportunities for reflective practice and so on).

REFERENCES

1 Ahola K, Hakanen J. Job strain, burnout, and depressive symptoms: a prospective study among dentists. *J Affect Disord* 2007;**104**:103–10.
2 Leiter MP, Hakanen J, Toppinen-Tanner S, *et al.* Changes in burnout: a 12- year cohort study on organizational predictors and health outcomes. *J Organizat Behav* 2013;**34**:959–73.
3 Freudenberger H. Staff burn-out. *J Soc Issues* 1974;**30**(1):159–65.
4 Schaufeli W. Burnout. In: *Stress in Health Professionals*. Firth-Cozens J, Payne RL (eds). Chichester: John Wiley, 1999, p. 17.
5 Burn-out an 'occupational phenomenon': International Classification of Diseases [Internet]. World Health Organization. 2019 [cited 18 January 2020]. Available from: www.who.int/mental_health/evidence/burn-out/en.
6 Maslach C. Burnout: a multidimensional perspective. In: Schaufeli WB, Maslach C, Marek T (eds). *Professional Burnout: Recent Developments in*

Theory and Research. Washington: Taylor & Francis, 1993. Available from: www.statisticssolutions.com/maslach-burnout-inventory-mbi.

7 Pines A, Aronson E. Career burn out. In: Pines A, Aronson E (eds). *Causes and Cures*. New York: Free Press, 1989, pp. 10–11.

8 Gerada C. Using groups in leadership: bringing practice into theory. In: Thornton C (ed). *The Art and Science of Working Together*. London & New York: Routledge, 2019, pp. 87–96.

9 Holmes EG, Connolly A, Putnam KT, *et al*. Taking care of our own: a multispecialty study of resident and program director perspectives on contributors to burnout and potential interventions. *Acad Psychiatry* 2017;**41**:159–66.

10 Thommasen H, Lavanchy M, Connelly I, Berkowitz J, Grzybowski S. Mental health, job satisfaction, and intention to relocate. Opinions of physicians in rural British Columbia. *Can Fam Physician* 2001;**47**:737–44.

11 Kane L. Medscape National Physician Burnout, Depression & Suicide Report 2019 [Internet]. Medscape. 2019 [cited 18 January 2020]. Available from: www.medscape.com/slideshow/2019-lifestyle-burnout-depression-6011056?faf=1#1.

12 Imo U. Burnout and psychiatric morbidity among doctors in the UK: a systematic literature review of prevalence and associated factors. *B J Psych Bull* 2017;**41**(4):197–204. PMCID: PMC5537573 doi: 10.1192/pb.bp.116.054247 PMID: 28811913.

13 General Medical Council. The state of medical education and training in the UK 2019, p. 30. Available from: www.gmc-uk.org/-/media/documents/somep-2019---full-report_pdf-81131156.pdf?la=en&hash=B80CB05CE8596E6D2386E89CBC3FDB60BFAAE3CF.

14 Soler JK, Yaman H, Esteva M, *et al*. Burnout in European family doctors: The EGPRN study. *Fam Pract* 2008;**25**:245–65. doi: 10.1093/fampra/cmn038.

15 Shanafelt TD, Boone S, Tan L, *et al*. Burnout and satisfaction with work-life balance among US physicians relative to the general US population. *Arch Intern Med* 2012;**172**:1377–85.

16 Shanafelt TD, Hasan O, Dyrbye LN, *et al*. Changes in burnout and satisfaction with work-life balance in physicians and the general US working population between 2011 and 2014. *Mayo Clin Proc* 2015;**90**:1600–13. doi: 10.1016/j.mayocp.2015.08.023.

17 Shanafelt T, West C, Sinsky C, *et al*. Changes in burnout and satisfaction with work-life integration in physicians and the general US working population between 2011 and 2017. *Mayo Clin Proc* 2019;**94**(9):1681–94.

18 McKinley N, McCain RS, Convie L, *et al*. Resilience, burnout and coping mechanisms in UK doctors: a cross-sectional study. *BMJ Open* 2020;**10**:e031765. doi:10.1136/ bmjopen-2019-031765 https://bmjopen.bmj.com/content/bmjopen/10/1/e031765.full.pdf.

19 Leiter MP, Maslach C. Six areas of worklife: a model of the organizational context of burnout. *J Health Hum Serv Admin* 1999;**21**(4):472–89.

20 West C, Dyrbye L, Erwin P, Shanafelt T. Interventions to prevent and reduce physician burnout: a systematic review and meta-analysis. *Lancet* 2016;**388**(10057):2272–81.

21 Shanafelt T, Raymond M, Kosty M, *et al.* Satisfaction with work-life balance and the career and retirement plans of US oncologists. *J Clin Oncol* 2014;**32**(11):1127–35.

22 Halbesleben JRB, Rathert C. Linking physician burnout and patient outcomes: exploring the dyadic relationship between physicians and patients. *Health Care Manage Rev* 2008;**33**:29–39.

23 Shanafelt T, Balch C, Bechamps G, *et al.* Burnout and medical errors among American surgeons. *Ann Surg* 2010;**251**(6):995–1000.

24 Salyers M, Bonfils K, Luther L, *et al.* The relationship between professional burnout and quality and safety in healthcare: a meta-analysis. *J Gen Int Med* 2016;**32**(4):475–82.

25 Bakker AB, LeBlanc PM, Schaufeli WB. Burnout contagion among intensive care nurses. *J Adv Nurs* 2005;**51**:276–87.

26 Community research. Adapting, coping, compromising research. Available from: www.gmc-uk.org/-/media/documents/adapting-coping-compromising-research-report-79702793.pdf.

27 Wiskow C, Albreht T, de Pietro C. How to create an attractive and supportive working environment for health professionals. WHO; Copenhagen, Denmark, 2010, pp. 1–37. Available from: www.euro.who.int/__data/assets/pdf_file/0018/124416/e94293.pdf.

28 Wallace JE, Lemaire JB, Ghali WA. Physician wellness: a missing quality indicator. *Lancet* 2009;**374**:1714–21. doi: 10.1016/S0140-6736(09)61424-0.

29 Schwartz HS. (1987). The clockwork or the snakepit: an essay on the meaning of teaching organizational behavior. *Organiz Behav Teach Rev* 1987;**11**(2), 19–26. Available from: https://doi.org/10.1177/105256298701100202.

30 Kumar S. Burnout and doctors: prevalence, prevention and intervention. *Healthcare* 2016;**4**:37. doi:10.3390/healthcare4030037.

31 Maslach C, Leiter M. Understanding the burnout experience: recent research and its implications for psychiatry. *World Psychiatry* 2016;**15**:103–11. Available from: www.ncbi.nlm.nih.gov/pmc/articles/PMC4911781.

13

Suicide in Doctors and Its Sequelae

CLARE GERADA

INTRODUCTION

For a number of years, I have led a group that no-one wants to belong to, a group for those bereaved following the death of a doctor through suicide. The members meet every two months. They come from across England, ranging in age from early 20s to their mid-70s. Fathers, mothers, sisters, brothers, wives and husbands. Other than all having been doctors, the dead differ in age, gender, marital status, years since qualification, speciality, mode of suicide and whether they did or did not write a suicide letter. Some had an underlying mental illness, many did not. A few seemed to have decided to kill themselves as an impulsive act, others appear to have made meticulous plans and others had even carried out a dress rehearsal, stopping short of the final act. Yet, similarities do exist. Two families share the same (unusual) surname; two of the deceased had the same first name; two died on the same day; and a further two had chosen to kill themselves in the same way. That unconscious web of communication that connects doctors past, present and even into the future came into play. I have wanted to set this group up for a while. As the head of my service for many years I had been approached by bereaved relatives of doctors asking for help. I had linked families together and found that it allowed them, in some small way, not to feel so alone. The bereaved experience an overwhelming sense of surprise and shock that their loved ones, whom they thought they knew so well, could have killed themselves. This struggle for understanding continues for years. Their grief is compounded by guilt that they could have done more to stop their deaths. This guilt is intensified if the bereaved is a healthcare professional themselves (which is very common) and by feelings that they failed as a clinician as well as a family member or friend. These family members have taught me a lot about suicide, which I will talk about in this chapter.

SUICIDE IN DOCTORS

Suicide is a rare event and as such trying to ascertain comparisons between different occupational groups, age, gender or other factors is difficult except over long periods of time or large populations. It has been estimated that in the USA one doctor dies per day through suicide[1] and the overall suicide rate has been reported to be higher than most other professional groups and higher than in an aged-matched population.[2,3] The relative risk of suicide for doctors has been variably estimated as 1.1–3.4 for men and 2.5–5.7 for women compared with the general population, and 1.5–3.8 for men and 3.7–4.5 for women compared with other professionals.[4-7] More recent figures from the UK (2011–2015) suggest that male doctors have a significantly lower risk of suicide (standardised mortality rate [SMR] 63) and female an elevated risk (SMR 124).[8] A meta-analysis published in 2020 again confirmed the higher rate of suicide amongst women doctors compared to men, though the rate had decreased over time in both groups.[9]

In a Danish-based study, doctors were found to have a higher risk of suicide than any of the 55 occupations included in the analysis, with risks increased when other sociodemographic factors were taken into account.[10] The risk of suicide ranged from 2.73 for doctors to 0.44 for other professional groups. Much, but not all, of the excess risk in doctors and nurses is due to their increased use of self-poisoning. Occupation has little association with suicide among people who suffer from a psychiatric illness, except for doctors, where the excess risk is 3.62.

A meta-analysis conducted in 2019 again confirmed that doctors are an at-risk group for suicide, with women at particular risk, with almost double that of the general population.[11] The rate of suicide in physicians has decreased over time, especially in Europe. A UK study conducted a *'psychological autopsy'* of working doctors who died by suicide in England and Wales between January 1991 and December 1993.[12] During this period there were 56 who had died through suicide. The 38 of these who at the time of death were either working or very recently retired or had the possibility of returning to medicine after a temporary absence formed the study sample. The cases included 28 men and 10 women. The age range was 23 to 71 years, 14 were under 35 years old. Three had qualified overseas. Of the means of death, self-poisoning was more common than self-injury (74% vs. 29%). One doctor used both methods. The most common drugs used for self-poisoning were opiate analgesics, obtained through work. The three anaesthetists in the sample had used intravenous anaesthetic agents. Most of the deaths appeared to have been planned. Two-thirds of doctors had left a suicide note. One-third of doctors were known to have made a verbal suicidal communication before their deaths, most within the week beforehand. The study found that psychiatric illness was present in 25 of the doctors at the time of their death. Depressive illness and drug misuse were the most common diagnoses. Eight had primary or secondary diagnoses of alcohol and/or drug abuse, all of several years' duration. Since the majority of individuals with psychiatric disorders do not kill themselves, it is likely that mental illness in isolation is a risk factor, rather than a cause, of suicide.

While doctors who kill themselves are more likely to involve poisoning[13,14] than other methods, unlike the general population, I am struck by the violent methods the doctors used to kill themselves and where they chose to play out the drama of their death. It is not uncommon for doctors to die where they have been 'wounded', in hospital car parks, in on-call rooms or in their own consulting room or in their old medical school. This adds to the complexity of grieving for those left behind.

Suicide in doctors is not a new concern. A publication in the *British Medical Journal* in 1964 found that from 1949 to 1953 there had been 61 suicides among male doctors aged 25–64 and a further 13 among older doctors.[15] No figures were given for female doctors, though doctor's wives also showed an increased suicide risk above other wives. At the time, more than one in 50 doctors took their own life and around 6% of all deaths among doctors were through suicide (the same rate as for lung cancer). Anaesthetists, general practitioners (GPs), and psychiatrists appeared to be associated with higher risk, a trend that continues today. This article also cited a 1903 paper where the UK Registrar-General (equivalent to the GMC) drew particular concern to the high rate of suicide among the medical profession.

CORRELATION AND CAUSATION FOR SUICIDE

Suicide is the result of a complex set of events, though there are some risk factors that increase the likelihood that someone will kill themselves. The World Health Organization has classified these into different groups and doctors share many of these risk factors:[16]

Societal

- Difficulties accessing or receiving care.[17]
- Access to means of suicide.[18]
- Inappropriate media reporting.
- Stigma associated with mental health, substance abuse or suicidal behaviour, which prevents people from seeking help.

Community

- Poverty.
- Experiences of trauma or abuse.
- Experiences of disaster, war or conflict.
- Experiences of discrimination.

Relationships

- Isolation and lack of social support.
- Relationship breakdown.
- Loss or conflict.

Individual

- Previous suicide attempts.
- Self-harm behaviours.

- Mental ill-health.
- Drug and alcohol misuse.
- Financial loss.
- Chronic pain.
- Family history of suicide.

Mental illness

Mental illness increases the risk of suicide,[19-22] especially conditions such as bipolar disorder, schizophrenia and substance misuse. In my service, of the 14 deaths through suicide, nine had pre-existing mental illness, most often bipolar disorder or drug misuse. Most individuals with mental illness do not kill themselves and most people who kill themselves do not have pre-existing mental illness.

Life events

Life events are common. It is impossible to avoid them and events such as moving to a new house, divorce, illness and so on contribute to the pathogenesis of mental illness. Doctors have to move frequently due to training rotations and career progression. Moving not only causes disruption to social networks but also increases the risk of doctors feeling isolated and unable to know where to seek help and support.

Being female

The incidence of suicide is higher in female doctors than other women in the general population, and rates of suicide are more or less the same for male and female doctors. The researcher Keith Hawton and his colleagues speculated that rates of suicide by female doctors would decline as more women entered the medical profession, postulating that higher rates were perhaps related to isolation of women in a male-dominated industry.[23] Unfortunately, since this paper was written (2001), rates have not declined. Women working in medicine face additional problems, including barriers that hinder their career advancement and additional roles in the home.[24-26]

Access to drugs

Analysis of suicide risk by specialities is somewhat limited, due to relatively small numbers of deaths in most categories. However, many studies find a higher risk in anaesthetists and psychiatrists and lower risk for paediatricians. This is predicated on anaesthetists and also other doctors, such those working in critical care or emergency department, having easy access to potent drugs.

Impact of disciplinary processes

Suicide is a particular risk for doctors undergoing any disciplinary investigation. This is not new. For example, in 1976 the Oregon Board of Medical Examiners (equivalent to the GMC) became uneasy about the high rate of suicide among doctors who were under regulatory supervision. In a 13-month period, eight out of 40 doctors involved with their processes had killed themselves. All the doctors had a past history of serious, undiagnosed mental illness, namely depression and were not from the county and tended to be socially isolated.[27] Decades later, in the UK concerns were raised about the high rates of suicide among doctors passing through regulatory processes. An independent study was commissioned by the GMC to look at the 28 deaths of doctors due to suicide (or suspected suicide) for a doctor who was also involved in fitness-to-practise processes between 2005 and 2013.[28] The case reviews of these doctors showed that many suffered from a recognised mental health disorder or had drug and/or alcohol addictions. Other factors that often follow from those conditions, may have also contributed to their deaths. These include marriage breakdown, financial hardship and in some cases police involvement, as well as the stress of being investigated by the GMC. Tom Bourne and colleagues looked at the impact of complaints on the mental health and risk of suicide on doctors.[29] Doctors who had recently received a complaint of any kind were found to be 77% more likely to suffer from moderate to severe depression than those who had never had a complaint. They were also found to have an increased number of suicidal thoughts, sleep difficulty, relationship problems and a host of physical health problems compared to doctors who had not been through a complaints process. Of doctors without a complaint, around 2.5% had suicidal thoughts, which increased to around 9% for those with a current or recent complaint and 13% for those with a past complaint. Poorly handled complaints often result in dysfunctional behaviours, such as failure to disclose all events, blaming of self and others and arguments, which can contribute to doctors killing themselves. Even trivial complaints can have a major impact on doctors and can be a powerful trigger for mental illness and even suicide.

> Emma, recently qualified, was 27 years old when she left her morning clinic, went home, wrote a suicide note to her parents, took a massive overdose and killed herself. Emma had had a history of mental illness in the past, but she had been well and there was nothing to predict what she was planning to do. In the previous month, she had received a complaint. In retrospect, this had been a trivial complaint that probably would have gone nowhere. But she confided to a friend that she felt humiliated, ashamed and that she had failed as a doctor. She ruminated on the complaint and magnified its impact.

Emma was unsupported as she held a locum position at the time, and her hospital did not provide doctors in non-training grades with the same access to educational supervisors or trainers as trainees received.

In my own service over a 9-year period from 2008 to 2017, 21 doctors who were or had been patients have died. Among living patients, the GMC is involved in around 10% of cases, compared with over 50% of the patients who had died from unnatural causes (suicide or 'accidents', which were likely to be due to suicide (e.g. falling out of a window, self-emollition, infusion of opiates).

Although correlation does not equal causation, being under regulatory or disciplinary processes or having a complaint nevertheless increases the risk of mental illness among doctors. This is not just due to the complaint or referral itself, but it's protracted nature. A serious complaint can take years to pass through the various processes, and multiple jeopardy is not uncommon.[30] The process can take years, exacerbating any pre-existing mental health problem alongside being a major precipitant for new-onset mental illness.

For some doctors, the fear of transgressing any existing GMC conditions can also be a risk for suicide. For example, in 2015 a newly qualified GP who had been voted 'Trainee GP of the Year', James Halcrow, hanged himself. The inquest heard how he feared erasure from the medical register due to his relapse of drinking, as the conditions set down by the GMC dictated that he abstained from alcohol.

WHY DO DOCTORS KILL THEMSELVES?

None of us really understands why someone chooses death over life; not the relatives in my group, or experts and no more, I imagine, than the relatives of another 800,000 people across the world[15] and over 6,000 individuals in the UK[31] lost to suicide each year. Our collective lack of understanding is shared by some of the greatest philosophers in history, as through the ages suicide has been the subject of study by priests, poets, philosophers as well as doctors and politicians. The Nobel Laureate and French writer Albert Camus contemplated the issue of suicide in one of his best works, *The Myth of Sisyphus*. The final chapter of his book reads:

> There is but one truly serious philosophical problem and that is suicide. Judging whether life is or is not worth living amounts to answering the fundamental question of philosophy.[32]

Camus is suggesting that if one judges the importance of a philosophical problem by its consequences, then whether we choose to live or die is the important issue we need to consider. Camus uses the mythological figure, Sisyphus to understand why people kill themselves. Sisyphus was infamous for his trickery and twice escaped death. This led Zeus to sentence him to rolling a boulder up a steep mountain, only for it to fall back down again, repeating this action for eternity. What Camus was interested in was the state of Sisyphus's mind in the moment when the rock rolls away from him at the top of the mountain. Camus postulates that as Sisyphus heads down the mountain, briefly free from his toil, he is for that moment happy. When Sisyphus acknowledges the futility of his task and the certainty of his fate, he is freed to realise the absurdity of his situation and to reach a state of contented acceptance. Camus tells us that 'The struggle itself... is enough to fill a man's heart. One must imagine Sisyphus happy.'[32] Sisyphus is above his fate precisely because he has accepted it. The instinct to live far outweighs our desire to die and through what Camus calls an 'act of eluding' we avoid the consequences of an otherwise meaningless life.

Camus wrote philosophical essays to try to understand why someone makes the choice of death. Others have also grappled with this question from a professional and personal perspective. The psychiatrist Rachel Gibbons shines some light on the antecedents that might lead someone to kill themselves. She examined 39 coroners' records of deaths following a verdict of suicide.[33] Her examination of the notes has led her to postulate a pathway to suicide. Starting with an individual predisposition (for example, poor early family attachments, pre-existing serious mental illness or personality disorder), the final act of suicide is usually preceded by two loss events. The first is often a significant loss, such as a bereavement, unemployment or break up of a relationship. The second trigger can be something as ordinary as having an extra patient at the end of a list or a poor patient encounter. This second trigger event therefore serves to provide 'permission to act', the final proof that life is not worth living. The individual then enters a dissociative, delusional state, with their psychotic mind grappling with their rational mind in an intensely ambivalent state to stop their death. This ambivalence is aptly illustrated by CCTV footage showing people walking up and down bridges, or staring at their chosen point of death, for hours, apparently wrestling with themselves whether to complete the final act. The time between the two events can be hours, weeks, or even years, and during the interregnum the individual enters into what Gibbons refers to as a 'pre-suicidal' state. Campbell and Hale define this as a split state where the individual:

> is influenced, in varying degrees, by a suicide fantasy which reflects the self's relation to its body and an other. The fantasy may or may not become conscious, but at the time of execution it has the power of a delusional conviction and has distorted reality. The suicide fantasy is the motive force. Killing the body fulfils the fantasy.[34]

The American psychiatrist Michael Myers, who has written an account of his work with suicidal doctors *Why Physicians Die by Suicide*, talks about the act of suicide being a complex phenomenon involving the 'convergence of genes, psychology and psychosocial stressors that come together in a perfect, albeit horrific storm'.[35]

At my service we have had doctors who have killed themselves. When we get the call to tell us the news, sometimes we are not surprised. But other times, we are totally and utterly shocked, there would have been no warning (or nothing we could, even with hindsight, have identified). We have learnt that the final act can seem impulsive and unexpected or, conversely, a well-planned, premeditated and sometimes even rehearsed event. This explains why it is so difficult to predict suicide, as sometimes not even the individual knows that they are about to kill themselves, let alone those closest to them or indeed health professionals.

Philippa was a recently qualified GP who had made plans to meet friends that evening and her sister that weekend. She had signed up to attend a course the following week. At the end of her Wednesday afternoon surgery, she stopped off at the local hardware store and bought the rope she was to use to take her own life. Her death came as a shock to everyone close to her, with nothing in her demeanour to suggest what she had been planning. Looking back, her mother had died 18 months previously; she had been particularly close to her and had felt her loss immensely. In recent weeks she had seemed tired and rather grumpy at work, but nothing more. Her personal diary found after her death showed that she had been ruminating for weeks about not being good enough as a doctor, daughter and now as a practice partner. She wrote about the futility of the job and the endless need to care. She had complained to the practice manager about her workload and, on the morning of the day she took her own life, she had had a disagreement with the senior partner about always being expected to do the extra home visit.

Following his wife Louise's death, Gary Marson began to uncover his wife's meticulous pre-suicide planning. She had left him a farewell letter, as Gary writes:

thoughtfully prepared on her laptop as a hard copy tends to be taken by the police, her wedding and engagement rings and a pack of papers about her financial affairs.

However, despite her planning, her writings and emails to friends in the days immediately before her death illustrated the intense ambivalence described earlier. Louise had scribbled her thoughts on numerous pieces of paper and had sent emails to herself at various times during the final day. Some of these indicated that she was planning to live, others that she was planning to die. It appeared that she had abandoned an attempt earlier in the day as remnants of railway tickets were found in her pockets after her death as well as a letter to the railway authorities apologising for her actions (she killed herself later that day at her home).

I urge anyone interested in why people kill themselves to read Gary's book *Just Carry On Breathing: A Year Surviving Suicide and Widowhood*,[36] not just because it explains in its raw horror the grief following the suicide of a loved one, but because he writes from Louise's perspective. Her voice shines through. He uses her notes and words to try to understand why such a talented, successful, physically fit and much-loved married woman voluntarily gave up everything, seemingly for the sake of a handful of extremely bleak days. Within his book, Gary grapples with both her motive and, more so, the method she chose.

PREVENTING SUICIDE

Preventing the very rare event of suicide by identifying those who will complete a suicide act from those who only express suicidal thoughts is extremely difficult, if not impossible.

Suicidal thoughts are common. However, having such thoughts does not mean that a person will kill themselves.[37] Suicidal thoughts can vary from fleeting ideas such as musing '*I wonder what if...*' to strategically pre-meditated suicidal plans. The literature on suicidal thoughts does not discriminate between the two extremes. Having suicidal thoughts does not also necessarily mean that the individual is in a 'pre-suicidal' state. The skill of a healthcare practitioner is to try to determine the depth of their desire to die. Asking the individual '*do you intend to kill yourself?*' is rarely helpful and not reliable in determining true suicidal intent. The intensity of suicidal fantasies is made more difficult by feelings of guilt and shame and the need for the individual to protect suicide as a means of escape. In addition, many doctors know how to give the right answers to mask their true feelings.

I am struck by how common suicidal thoughts are in doctors[38,39] and wonder whether they serve a defensive purpose, perhaps against omnipotence or narcissism. They could also act as a container for painful events, instead of ruminating around the losses, suffering, failure of one's work, they are instead redirected into suicidal thoughts. This I believe helps doctors with their mourning processes. Clearly there is an overlap between suicide and suicidal thoughts (everyone who has killed themselves will have had thoughts of suicide). However, the vast number of people who have suicidal thoughts do not go on to take their own life.

Using suicidal thoughts as a screening tool for suicide is largely unhelpful. A systematic review of risk assessment for suicide concluded that the overwhelming majority of people who might be viewed as high risk for suicide will not kill themselves, and about one-half of all suicides will occur among people viewed as 'low risk'.[40] Other researchers have found similar results in reviewing questionnaires aimed at predicting high risk of suicide; none were clinically useful.[41] This does not mean we cannot try and identify who might be more at risk. Campbell and Hale identify danger signals (pp. 75–76) in their book about suicide *Working in the Dark*.[34] They group the risks into those associated with: past behaviour, for example, a previous suicide attempt or family history of suicide; current life situation, such as a recent failure or loss and those linked to the transference – that is how the person appears in the consultation (withdrawn, cut-off, given up). In my clinical experience, it is when suicidal thoughts are constantly present, when they become a pervasive part of one's daily thoughts or even enter into dreams that I become very concerned. Better to ask the patient, not just 'do you have suicidal thoughts', but '**tell me about** your suicidal thoughts'

Even with all the time, tools and treatments possible and even with permanent incarceration and 24-hour observation, if an individual is determined to kill themselves, they will find a way. I think the only real way of reducing the number of people who kill themselves is to make sure we talk about suicide, that the issue comes into the open in the hope that those who are seriously thinking of it as an option are able to seek help.

The second suicide prevention strategy is about making sure there are easily accessible services, including crisis lines and emergency respite for those who can think of no way out but to die. We are fortunate at my service in that we have a Crisis text line available 24 hours per day (www.practitionerhealth.nhs.uk). The Samaritans provide a listening ear for those in need (www.samaritans.org).

Not everyone who kills themselves has a mental health problem, but some do and as such, for doctors, access to confidential services available to provide confidential help without fear of sanction, is important. Removing or addressing some of the obvious antecedents to suicide (which I feel the GMC have been doing) also might stop someone becoming so distressed as to want to die. Small things might push someone over the edge and removing these small risks might mean the individuals lives, not dies. The one intervention that won't work, and might actually make things worse, is more mandatory training, this time in suicide prevention. Talking about suicide is important, this means talking with, not talking at.

The solutions to suicide must be multidimensional. They require us to alter, where possible, the social antecedents to suicide (for doctors this means addressing the culture of blame, rise of complaints, inspection and workload pressures), reducing the pressures faced by individuals, so supporting them when in distress, reducing the impact of unavoidable negative events and life events as well as restricting access to the means of taking one's own life (such as dangerous drugs). This is not just the remit of healthcare, but the whole system's responsibility – educators, regulators and policy makers.

THE 'AFTERMATH' OF SUICIDE

Little can prepare someone for the death through suicide of a loved one. Each death leaves those remaining to face many unanswered and unanswerable questions and the anguish of losing a loved one. Suicide and suicide attempts can have lasting effects on individuals and their social networks and communities. As clinicians, when we lose patients we can be left feeling guilty, sad, fearful and ashamed, followed by having depressive and paranoid guilt thoughts. Family members feel they have contributed to their loved one's death.

The impact of death through suicide ripples out beyond the immediate close circle of friends and family. At a conference for health professionals I held in 2018, I asked the 400 strong audience to raise their hand if they knew a colleague who had died through suicide. Almost all hands went up. Rather more scientifically, anaesthetists were invited to participate in an online survey; nearly 40% had experienced a colleague's death through this means.[42]

As mentioned previously, suicide is a rare event but has profound and long-lasting psychological effects on those left behind. The stigma of suicide runs deep. In living memory, it was considered a criminal event, hence the term 'committed'. Even today, phrases such as 'coward's way out' or 'selfish act' are used to describe those who kill themselves. For those who survive an attempt, they might be described as 'acting out' or 'attention seeking'. Unlike a normal bereavement, bereavement following suicide is marked by what the American researcher William Feigelman[43] calls 'a wall of silence'; an absence of caring or interest or a shower of unwelcome and awkward advice from friends and relatives. The bereaved often develop symptoms of post-traumatic stress disorder, re-examining the event and suffering higher rates of mental illness and suicide themselves.[44] They are prone to feelings of guilt and blameworthiness, feeling responsible for their loved one's act. After all, how could they have 'allowed' their relative, friend or colleague to die in such a way? This feeling is especially prevalent if the bereaved is also in the medical profession.[45] Suicide survivors are a highly stigmatised group.[46] During the Middle Ages, a suicide's family was denied a church burial for their lost loved one;

the kinfolk of the deceased was often forced to dispose of family property to settle church debts and were often later shunned by fellow residents. Social disapproval still remains today.

Feigelman compared stigma following the death of children through trauma (murder or suicide) vs. natural causes and found that the parents of the former group experienced significantly higher levels of stigma, rejection and shunning by significant others.[43] Importantly, the study also found that, even after controlling for time since the death, stigmatisation was associated with grief difficulties, depression and suicidal thinking.

Bereavement is a lonely experience, more so following a suicide. It is made more complex if those bereaved following the suicide of a doctor work in the same health system as their dead friend, colleague or relative. All parties (the dead and the survivors) might have both a personal and professional relationship with local services. This makes it difficult to untangle where responsibility might lie, especially if the lead clinician is also a personal friend or close colleague. Saying this, it is amazing how many bereaved individuals channel their grief into creativity – helping to prevent others from being in a similar situation.[47]

I am often asked by organisations who have experienced the suicide of a member of staff what they should do in the aftermath. The first piece of advice I always give is obvious: **acknowledge that the suicide of a colleague will have a significant impact on the psychological health of the organisation.** Emotions will be especially heightened where the suicide is thought to be connected to work issues. As with any bereavement, people's individual feelings will vary, but the overwhelming ones will be of guilt and sadness. People in positions of authority, such as managers, supervisors, human resources staff and medical directors, often feel responsible and fear being blamed for the death. Wherever possible, and within the bounds of confidentiality, seniors can help to dispel rumours and misinformation by providing accurate information, ideally presented to the whole team, and allowing staff to ask questions. Arranging one or more reflective events, led by experienced group facilitators and involving as many staff as possible, can also be very helpful. Allowing colleagues to gain some feeling of closure by attending the funeral or memorial service can help with healing, as does organising a workplace tribute. The people most affected in an organisation are not necessarily those who were closest to the colleague who died. The very fact that someone has died by suicide may reopen old wounds or add an additional stressor to existing ones. For most individuals, simply lending an ear or providing a space to talk, grieve and be among like-minded, caring colleagues will often be sufficient. However, for a minority the grief, guilt, or shame can be prolonged; in some, this can lead to depression or anger about the people in authority. This minority may require additional help. Senior managers have a vital part to play in dealing with the aftermath of a colleague's suicide. Compassion, kindness, and an open-door policy to provide a place to talk will all go a long way in helping their staff to come to terms with the loss of a co-worker.

CONCLUSION

It is important to remember that the vast majority of doctors do not kill them-selves. Most doctors thrive in their working environment. But each death is a tragedy that sends repercussions through the system, posing the risk of creating contagion. Going forward, we must halt the decline in morale among doctors. This will mean addressing many systemic issues that are creating unhappiness: tackling the culture of naming, blaming and shaming; allowing doctors to maintain a sens-ible work–life balance; and not ignoring the basic needs of staff who give their all to patients. We must restore doctors' collective self-esteem by creating a culture in which their skills can flourish. We need to ensure doctors have access to early intervention and confidential support services.[48] Finally, we have to ensure that all health staff receive the same compassion that they, rightly, are expected to give to their patients.

REFERENCES

1 Center C, Davis M, Detre T, et al. Confronting depression and suicide in physicians. A consensus statement. JAMA 2003;**289**(23):3161–6.
2 Council on Scientific Affairs. Results and implications of the AMA-APA Physician Mortality Project. Stage II. JAMA 1987;**257**(21):2949–53.
3 Pitts FN, Schuller AB, Rich CL, Pitts AF. Suicide among U.S. women physicians, 1967–1972. Am J Psychiatry 1979;**136**(5):694–6.
4 Milner A, Maheen H, Bismark M, Spittal M. Suicide by health professionals: a retrospective mortality study in Australia, 2001–2012. Med J Aust 2016;**205**(6):260–5.
5 Schernhammer ES, Colditz GA. Suicide rates among physicians: a quantitative and gender assessment (meta-analysis). Am J Psychiatry 2004;**161**:2295–2302.
6 Lindeman S, Laara E, Hakko H, Lonnqvist J. A systematic review on gender-specific suicide mortality in medical doctors. Br J Psychiatry 1996;**168**:274–9.
7 Hawton K, Agerbo E, Simkin S, et al. Risk of suicide in medical and related occupational groups: a national study based on Danish case population-based registers. J Affect Disord 2011;**134**:320–6.
8 Windsor-Shellard B, Gunnell D. Occupation-specific suicide risk in England: 2011–2015. Br J Psychiatry 2019;**215**:594–9.
9 Duarte D, El-Hagrassy MM, Couto TCE, Gurgel W, Fregni F, Correa H. Male and female physician suicidality: a systematic review and meta-analysis. JAMA Psychiatry Published online 4 March 2020. doi:10.1001/jamapsychiatry.2020.0011.
10 Agerbo E, Gunnell D, Bonde JP, Mortensen PB, Nordentoft M. Suicide and occupation: the impact of socio-economic, demographic and psychiatric differences. Psychol Med 2007;**37**(8):1131–40.
11 Dutheil F, Aubert C, Pereira B, et al. Suicide among physicians and health-care workers: a systematic review and meta-analysis (05/30/2019 20:47:04). Available from SSRN: https://ssrn.com/abstract=3397193.

12 Hawton K, Malmber A, Simkin S. Suicide in doctors a psychological autopsy study. *J Psychosom Res* 2004;**57**:1–4.

13 Kolves K, De Leo D. Suicide in medical doctors and nurses: an analysis of the Queensland Suicide Register. *J Nerv Ment Dis* 2013;**201**:987–90.

14 Skegg K, Firth H, Gray A, Cox B. Suicide by occupation: does access to means increase the risk? *Aust NZ J Psychiatry* 2010;**44**:429–34.

15 Suicide among doctors. *BMJ* 1964;**5386**:789–90. Available from: www.ncbi. nlm.nih.gov/pmc/articles/PMC1815019/pdf/brmedj02621-0011.pdf.

16 World Health Organization. Preventing suicide: a global imperative [Internet]. 2014. Available from: www.who.int/mental_health/suicide-prevention/world_report_2014/en.

17 Gerada C. Doctors, suicide and mental illness. *BJPsych Bull* 2018;**42**(4):165–8.

18 Department of Health. (2009). Mental health and ill health in doctors. Available from: www.em-online.com/download/medical_article/36516_DH_083090[1].pdf.

19 Beghi M, Rosenbaum J, Cerri C, Cornaggia CM. Risk factors for fatal and nonfatal repetition of suicide attempts: a literature review. *Neuropsychiatr Dis Treat* 2013;**9**:1725–35.

20 Chesney E, Goodwin G, Fazel S. Risks of all-cause and suicide mortality in mental disorders: a meta-review. *World Psychiatry* 2014;**13**(2):153–60.

21 Hawton K, Zahl D, Weatherall R. Suicide following deliberate self-harm: long-term follow-up of patients who presented to a general hospital. *Br J Psychiatry* 2003;**182**(6):537–42.

22 Brådvik L. Suicide risk and mental disorders. *Int J Environ Res Pub Health* 2018;**15**(9):2028.

23 Hawton K, Clements A, Sakarovitch C. Suicide in doctors: a study of risk according to gender, seniority and specialty in medical practitioners in England and Wales, 1979–1995. *J Epidemiol Community Health* 2001;**55**(5): 296–300.

24 Antoniou ASG, Davidson MJ, Cooper CL. Occupational stress, job satisfaction and health state in male and female junior hospital doctors in Greece. *J Manag Psychology* 2003;**18**(6):592–621.

25 Riska E. Towards gender balance: but will women physicians have an impact on medicine? *Social Sci Med* 2001;**52**(2):179–87.

26 Boulis A, Jacobs J. *The Changing Face of Medicine: Women Doctors and the Evolution of Health Care in America*. Ithaca: Cornell University Press, 2008.

27 Crawshaw R, Bruce JA, Eraker PL, Marvin G, Lindermann JE, Schmidt DE. An epidemic of suicide among physicians on probation. *JAMA* 1980;**243**(19):1915–17. doi:10.1001/jama.1980.03300450029016 https:// jamanetwork.com/journals/jama/article-abstract/369845.

28 Horsfall S, General Medical Council. Doctors who commit suicide while under GMC fitness to practise investigation: Internal review [Internet]. 2014. Available from: www.gmc-uk.org/-/media/documents/Internal_review_into_suicide_in_FTP_processes.pdf_59088696.pdf.

29 Bourne T, Wynants L, Peters M, et al. The impact of complaints procedures on the welfare, health and clinical practise of 7926 doctors in the UK: a cross-sectional survey. *BMJ Open* 2015;**5**(1):e006687.

30 Williams S. Multiple jeopardy. *Medical Protection Society: Casebook* 2009;**17**(3):8–10.

31 Office for National Statistics. Suicides in the UK: 2018 registrations [Internet]. 2018. Available from: www.ons.gov.uk/peoplepopulationandcommunity/birthsdeathsandmarriages/deaths/bulletins/suicidesintheunitedkingdom/2018registrations.

32 Camus A. *The Myth of Sisyphus*. 1942. Available from: https://postarchive.files.wordpress.com/2015/03/myth-of-sisyphus-and-other-essays-the-albert-camus.pdf.

33 Gibbons R, Brand F, Carbonnier A, Croft A. Effects of patient suicide on psychiatrists: survey of experiences and support required. *BJPsych Bull* 2019;**43**(5):236–41. Available from: http://bit.ly/2R1TsCE [open access].

34 [Cited in] Campbell D, Hale R. *Working in the Dark*. Abingdon: Routledge, 2017, p. 43.

35 Myers M. *Why Physicians Die by Suicide: Lessons Learned from Their Families and Others Who Cared*, 1st edn. Myers, 2017.

36 Mason G. *Just Carry on Breathing: A Year Surviving Suicide and Widowhood*. Oakamoor: Dark River, 2016.

37 Anderson P. Doctors' suicide rate highest of any profession [Internet]. WebMD. 2018 [cited 10 November 2019]. Available from: www.webmd.com/mental-health/news/20180508/doctors-suicide-rate-highest-of-any-profession#1.

38 Beyond Blue. National Mental Health Survey of Doctors and Medical Students [Internet]. 2013. Available from: www.beyondblue.org.au/docs/default-source/research-project-files/bl1132-report---nmhdmss-full-report_web.

39 Shanafelt T, Balch CM, Dybre L. Special Report: Suicidal ideation among American Surgeons. *Arch Surg* 2011;**146**(1):54.

40 Large M, Ryan C, Carter G, Kapur N. Can we usefully stratify patients according to suicide risk? *BMJ* 2017;**359**:j4627.

41 Carter G, Milner A, McGill K, Pirkis J, Kapur N, Spittal M. Predicting suicidal behaviours using clinical instruments: systematic review and meta-analysis of positive predictive values for risk scales. *Br J Psychiatry* 2017;**210**(6):387–95.

42 Yentis SM, Shinde S, Plunkett E, Mortimore A. Suicide amongst anaesthetists – an Association of Anaesthetists survey. *Anaesthesia* 2019;**74**(11):1365–73. doi: 10.1111/anae.14727. Epub 2019 Jul 2.

43 Feigelman W, Gorman B, Jordan J. Stigmatization and suicide bereavement. *Death Studies* 2009;**33**(7):591–608.

44 Farberow NL. (1991). Adult survivors after suicide: Research problems and needs. In: Leenaars AA (ed). *Life-Span Perspectives of Suicides: Timelines in the Suicide Process*. New York: Plenum Press, 1991, pp. 259–79.

45 Bailley SE, Kral MJ, Dunham K. (1999). Suicide survivors do grieve differently: empirical support for a commonsense proposition. *Suicide and Life-Threatening Behavior* 1999;**29**:256–71.

46 Cvinar J. Do suicide survivors suffer social stigma? A review of the literature. *Perspect Psychiatr Care* 2005;**41**:14–21.

47 Gerada C, Griffiths F. Groups for the dead. *Group Analysis* 2019. Available from: https://doi.org/10.1177/0533316419881609.

48 Brooks S, Gerada C, Chalder T. Review of literature on the mental health of doctors: are specialist services needed? *J Ment Health* 2011;**1**:1–11.

14

Bipolar Disorder and Other Psychotic States

CLARE GERADA

INTRODUCTION

While the majority of doctors presenting to my service have the more common mental health problems (especially anxiety and/or depression), a small number have other mental health conditions such as bipolar, psychotic and personality disorders.

BIPOLAR AFFECTIVE DISORDER (BPAD)

Individuals with bipolar affective disorder have periods of depression (usually feeling very low and lethargic) interspersed with mania, where they feel high and overactive (the less extreme form of mania is known as hypomania).[1] Each episode can last several days, weeks or even longer. The high and low phases of bipolar can be so extreme that they interfere with everyday life. Bipolar is a chronic, lifelong illness. The pattern of remission and relapse is variable. The symptom-free period tends to become shorter as time goes by and depressive episodes become more frequent and longer-lasting. The risk of recurrence is 50% at one year, 75% at four years and 10% thereafter.[2]

There is a high lifetime suicide risk in patients with bipolar disorder; between 25% and 56% have at least one suicide attempt during their lifetime and 15–19% die from the attempt.[3,4] This means that it is important that patients are engaged with good treatment services, sensitive to their needs and that they have support systems to help recognise relapses.

There are no definitive studies regarding the prevalence of bipolar disorder in doctors. It is probably lower than the general population (which is between 0.4% and 2%)[5] given that medicine is so gruelling and as such likely to select out those with severe mental health problems.

Over the last ten years, just over 100 doctors at my service have this illness, which is around 2.5% of all doctors who have registered with us over this time. The gender mix is 50:50 M:F. The average age is just over 40 years old. Of our patients with bipolar disorder, 10% also have alcohol or drug misuse and 6% an additional mental illness (such as severe obsessional disorder, eating disorder or other mental health problems). Of the doctors with BPAD, around 25% are psychiatrists, 33% are general practitioners (GPs) and the remainder are a mix of all specialities.

Before I started working with doctors, I (wrongly) assumed that a diagnosis of bipolar would exclude doctors from being able to work in the medical profession. Of course, I should not have been surprised, as after all, the catalyst for my service being set up in the first place was the death of a psychiatrist with bipolar, Daksha Emson, whom I mention throughout this book. She had a severe recurrent illness, which necessitated several spells of hospital admission. Nevertheless, she was still able to work, and before her death had been a well-respected and highly proficient doctor. Though we will never know, the chances are if she had received treatment for her relapse, it is more than likely she would have been able to continue working when her maternity leave was over.

There are very few personal accounts written by doctors with bipolar disorder, and many are fearful of speaking out about what is seen as a stigmatising condition. One patient told me it would be career suicide if she were to become public about her illness. The GP Wendy Potts did kill herself. She received a complaint from a patient after writing a blog about her experience of living with bipolar disorder.[6] The psychiatrist Ahmed Hankir writes and talks openly about his experience and tweets under the hashtag @WoundedHealer. He conducted a review of first-person narratives of people with severe mental illness and used his experience as the backdrop to his paper.[7] He first became unwell as a medical student. Despite sensing he was very ill he was reluctant to seek help and writes:

> refusing to seek psychiatric treatment out of fear that I was ungrateful for all of what I have been given in life.
>
> A full-blown mania ensued… The aftermath is invariably melancholia… I started to sink into the murky depths of a depressive illness, a depression too dreadful to describe.

He eventually received treatment, gradually recovered (though had to experience homelessness and social isolation *en route*), resumed his studies with renewed vigour and qualified from medical school. He received the Royal College of Psychiatrists Foundation Doctor of the Year in 2013. He now works as a psychiatrist and uses his experience to try to reduce the stigma associated with mental illness in the medical profession.

Throughout this book I have discussed how hard it is for doctors to become patients and often present late for care. This is especially the case for doctors with bipolar disorder. Even where they have tried to seek care, their condition can be misdiagnosed. A retrospective study of doctors with BPAD found it took ten years before the diagnosis was made,[8] similar to other patients where between 3% and 22% are misdiagnosed.[9] The individual is usually told they have recurrent depression, or maybe even borderline personality disorder. For doctors though, such is the stigma surrounding serious mental illness that both the treating doctor and the doctor-patient have a 'vested' interest in giving alternative interpretations rather than the obvious. This collusion is made easier as doctors are able to 'mask' their symptoms, especially through directing their hyperactivity into working harder, staying later and taking on extra shifts, and outwardly appearing normal.

Claire Polkinghorn, a psychiatrist has written about her experience of bipolar disorder.[10] Even when extremely unwell, she tried to deal with her illness by putting on a brave face and working harder. Her colleagues did not notice the change in mood, though it is telling that her patients did. Depressive thoughts can merge into the background negativity that seems to be ever present in the health service. Guilty ruminations can lead doctors to blaming themselves inappropriately for problems at work and for others to accept their explanations as an easy scapegoat. It is not unusual for doctors to use their manic episodes to get more work done, to feel creative and to instil hope into their organisations by their infective optimism. However, these doctors are unwell, often they do not sleep, and they become intensely fatigued. Their 'ideas' when tested, while having a ring of truth, have a delusional feel to them when really examined. A GP wrote anonymously about her experience, 'On madness: a personal account of rapid cycling bipolar disorder'[11] and describes feeling irritable and intensely anxious but attributed these symptoms to the stress of her job. At one stage, she felt so bad that she decided the best action was to crash her car into the central reservation of the motorway (she didn't).

Helping doctors with BPAD has to involve careful history taking, drawing on information from their past, involving significant others in the assessment and carefully piecing together previous episodes to make an accurate diagnosis in any individual. This takes time, something that is often lacking in busy public health services. This might account for the high rate of misdiagnosis. Late presentation is often due to a mixture of internalised stigma, fear and denial. This was the case of the American psychiatrist, Kay Redfield Jamison. She wrote an autobiographical account of her illness in *An Unquiet Mind*. She had years of mood swings, episodes of severe depression with elation, and suicidal thoughts (and made a serious attempt on her own life). She also had manic episodes. It was only when at the end of her mental tether that she reluctantly sought the help from a psychiatrist. She wrote:

> I was not only very ill when I first called for an appointment, I was terrified and deeply embarrassed. I had no choice.[12]

She describes her experience of being assessed as a positive experience and how she was able to relinquish her professional and expert role (she was an expert in bipolar disorder) and become a patient, though still found the process difficult.

> I realised I was on the receiving end of a very thorough psychiatric history and examination: the questions were familiar, I had asked them of others a hundred times, but I found it unnerving to have to answer them, unnerving not to know

where it was all going, and unnerving to realise how confusing it was to be a patient.

Finding it a relief to become a patient was not the case for Claire Polkinghorn. She described it akin to being in a high security prison:

> I found it hard to be a doctor-patient. I was usually in control but now felt a prisoner. I was furious. I even tried ordering a torx key from the internet to unlock my window. Patients shared their stories of past successful escapes. We all enjoyed watching The Shawshank Redemption on DVD.[10]

I mentioned stigma earlier in this chapter and it is a recurrent theme throughout this book, especially where serious mental illness is the issue. Polkinghorn wrote in her personal account how she experienced stigma:

> I had become a psychiatric patient and am embarrassed to say the stigma made me feel physically sick. I felt ashamed of being 'weak' and hated the idea that personal information and 'failings' were going to be kept on an NHS database. It was common knowledge I had been depressed. Most colleagues were kind and supportive, but some avoided me or were visibly uncomfortable in my presence. Covering for a colleague with cancer is definitely seen differently. Tackling stigma against mental illness in doctors is not going to be easy – it is still a taboo subject.[10]

Stigma creates harm and for Wendy and Daksha contributed to their deaths. Stigma also causes delay in seeking help, leads to doctors masking the severity of their symptoms and makes it harder for them to accept they are unwell.

When it comes to treatment and outcomes, this is mixed. Kay Jamison had a treating psychiatrist whom she saw as often as she needed, sometimes two to three times a week, for many years. She was able to develop a close, continuous, professional relationship with this doctor. She writes:

> He saw me through madness, despair, wonderful and terrible love affairs… an almost fatal suicide attempt… and the enormous pleasures and aggravations of my professional life – in short, he saw me through the beginnings and endings of virtually every aspect of my psychological and emotional life. He treated me with respect, a decisive professionalism, wit and an unshakable belief in my ability to get well, compete and make a difference.[12]

This level of continuity and expertise is unusual (certainly in our publicly funded health service). Doctors frequently move address due to training requirements, and in doing so might move to a different catchment area in the process. Even moving across the road may mean the doctor changes their treating team, necessitating a new referral to a new service, which can take a long time to put in place. It is also not unusual for my patients to be deemed 'too well' to be followed up in pressured public health services, instead told to re-present when they feel they are deteriorating, the illusion being that as they are doctors, they will recognise when unwell and in between can self-manage.

Doctors are worried that if it is known they have bipolar disorder they will not be allowed to work. While it can be difficult to hold down regular employment, it is by no means impossible to do so. With treatment, doctors with bipolar can, and most in our service, do work, sometimes requiring reasonable adjustments (for example limits to the amount of on-call duties or working less than full time). While only 38% of doctors with bipolar disorder presenting to us were at work, by the end of treatment this figure increased to 73%. This is much higher than in the general population, where only 21% of people with a long-term mental health condition (including bipolar) are in employment.[13] This means these doctors are back in the workplace, doing what they have been trained to do, and to a high standard. It takes a lot of personal effort for these doctors to return to work as they often come up against intense negativity and stigma.

There are three main reasons why doctors with bipolar might not be able to work. The first is that their illness (or the side-effects from treatment) are too severe, with insufficient periods of respite to allow them to remain in consistent employment. The second is stigma, and that employers assume that they cannot work and find ways of not employing or terminating a pre-existing contract. We know of patients who having told their employers they have BPAD are immediately told to take 'sick leave' as if they have some sort of contagious disease. This is discriminatory. If they instead had admitted to having a new diagnosis of cancer or epilepsy they would be treated differently. If a doctor is receiving and following the advice of their clinicians and, if necessary, reasonable adjustments are made in the workplace, then there is no reason why these doctors cannot work. Finally, the reason a doctor with BPAD cannot work is that the regulator might consider they are not fit to practise. An area of concern for many patients is whether or not they should inform the regulator of their diagnosis. This really depends on the severity of their illness, whether they are engaged with treatment services and whether they require high levels of monitoring that can only be provided by a regulator (or in North America, a Physician Health Service). In our service, while the percentage of those with bipolar disorder having regulatory involvement is high (21%) compared to doctors with other mental illness (15%), the vast majority (79%) with BPAD still do not have any regulatory involvement at all.

All of the accounts included in this chapter have been written by psychiatrists or GPs. This is probably not a coincidence. These two specialities make up nearly 60% of all the doctors with BPAD in our service. It is likely that they are over-represented among doctors with this disorder in the wider medical profession. This might be because doctors in these specialities are more likely to open up about their illness and present for care, or that these specialities are more accommodating of doctors with serious mental illness.

This personal view is from a surgeon. She exemplifies the problems doctors with BPAD can face in the workplace. Some details have been changed, though the essence of her story remains, which she has consented to being told:

Growing up I thought it was normal to want to die all the time. No one would have guessed this is how I felt as I trained myself to be cheerful. I wore this mask throughout medical school and later when qualified. After a particular period of low mood, I began to stockpile tablets bought from various pharmacies, I confided to my husband how I was feeling. I went to see my GP who started me on antidepressants. Four weeks to the day later I experienced a great change in my mood, 'the drugs do work', I thought. I felt I was energetic, clever, beautiful, and full of the best ideas I have ever had. I would wake up early and busily scribble in my diary all my brilliant ideas. I was sociable and very chatty at work. My colleagues commented on the loud laughter in my clinics (laughter in a consultation is quite normal for me but not so loud and incessant). I took over meetings and was extremely disorganised. The antidepressants had triggered mania (I didn't know this of course). My mania was interspersed with days where I could barely crawl out of bed, cried all the way to work and was tempted to drive off a motorway overpass.

Work provided routine and it was there I was at my most stable. During the manic stages I went on spending sprees, fortunately, my natural spendthrift nature meant I spent money on cheap discounted goods, though even with my shopping limited to Amazon, Ikea, Costco, and Aldi special buys I managed to go through £30,000 of savings. My husband was the first person to say, 'I think you have manic depression'. I reacted very badly to this and read the Unquiet Mind and did not recognise myself in the descriptions. But finally, I agreed to go back to my GP who sent me to a psychiatrist who confirmed the diagnosis. I started treatment, took a bit of time off work and when given the all clear by my psychiatrist, returned to work. I told my senior colleague of the new diagnosis and made arrangements to see Occupational Health at the next appointment (four weeks hence as she was on annual leave).

The next day, the surgical director called me into his office. I was told I had to immediately suspend my clinical activities until I had an occupational health appointment and if I disagreed, they would suspend me. I went home absolutely despondent. Until that moment I don't think I had ever realised how much of my identity came from my occupation as a surgeon. The routine of work that kept me stable was removed from my life. I felt humiliated and ashamed. The word bipolar lead to this stigmatisation – as I said to my Director, if I had had a broken leg, they would have found some compromise solution to allow me to work. My mood kept deteriorating despite the psychological support I was paying for privately in order to avoid leaving a trace of my mental health issues in the GP records. One of my overwhelming concerns was that I would never be taken seriously ever again, and my imaginative ideas would be discarded as the ravings of a mad person. I went to see the occupational health physician with my husband, and she agreed I should return to my work.

I had now been off work for six weeks and when I returned, I was given 'the cold shoulder', as if I had a contagious disease. My Director looked at me and said, 'you'd never guess you had a mental illness; you look so normal', another *teased me about my name (which closely resembles the word 'mad'). Looking back now I realise how naive it was for me to trust my workplace with information they were ill equipped to handle. I had never experienced discrimination – here I was an Asian, overseas trained woman (mother as well) who had made it as a consultant surgeon. Yet, here was my mental health causing me problems with my workplace and from my colleagues. I wish my story had a happy ending. It doesn't as I am now leaving the NHS. I cannot trust senior people to hold my information in confidence. There are too many who feel they have a right to know about my health and I feel I am being punished rather than supported for having an illness, which after all, is not of my making. I am not leaving surgery though. I will continue to work in the private sector.*

PARANOID DELUSIONAL STATES

I have been even more surprised that doctors have presented to our service with, as yet, undiagnosed paranoid psychosis. While this is a small number in comparison to the overall cohort of doctors coming for care, it has still been surprising. These doctors are unwell yet have all been working. They present with delusional beliefs centred around their work; the beliefs (as with many delusions) have an air of authenticity about them. For example, they often involve beliefs of being watched, inspected, monitored (usually by the Care Quality Commission or GMC). Almost all have been international medical graduates and the delusions merge with reality; for example, that they are victims of racism, that people are out to get them because they have come from overseas. It is not unusual for the doctor to have raised concerns and whistle blown about events that they have 'uncovered' in their place of work. Almost all of the doctor in our service have been locums, or on short placements. This means that while their odd behaviour might be noticed the doctor has moved on before an action is taken. Even where these doctors are assessed by Occupational Health or seen by their family doctor, the diagnosis is missed. It takes time, trust and expertise to identify a chronic psychotic disorder in highly intelligent and articulate individuals who give plausible explanations for their beliefs.

We have had a small number of doctors in our service present with drug-related psychosis, and this always has to be part of the differential diagnosis of any doctor with psychotic symptoms.

CONCLUSION

Bipolar disorder in doctors is uncommon, but not absent. As with the general population, bipolar disorder is often misdiagnosed or not diagnosed at all. It is often poorly managed (especially in doctors as their training acts against receiving continuity of care). With the correct treatment, doctors with bipolar disorder are able to work, even given the severity of the condition, and do not require any involvement of the regulator.

REFERENCES

1 Fountoulakis K. *Bipolar Disorder*. Springer, 2015.

2 Geddes J, Miklowitz D. Treatment of bipolar disorder. *Lancet.* 2013;**381**(9878):1672–82.

3 Abreu LN, Lafer B, Baca-Garcia E, *et al*. Suicidal ideation and suicide attempts in bipolar disorder type I: an update for the clinician. *Rev Bras Psiquiatr* 2009;**31**(3):271-80. Epub 2009 Aug 7.

4 NHS. Help for suicidal thoughts [Internet]. nhs.uk. 2018 [cited 29 October 2019]. Available from: www.nhs.uk/Conditions/Suicide/Pages/Causes.aspx.

5 Merikangas KR, Jin R, He JP, *et al*. Prevalence and correlates of bipolar spectrum disorder in the world mental health survey initiative. *Arch Gen Psychiatry* 2011;**68**(3):241–51. doi: 10.1001/archgenpsychiatry.2011.12.

6 www.theguardian.com/uk-news/2016/aug/26/gp-found-dead-after-being-suspended-over-bipolar-disorder-blog.

7 Hankir A, Zaman R. Jung's archetype, 'The Wounded Healer', mental illness in the medical profession and the role of the health humanities in psychiatry. *BMJ Case Rep* 2013;2013(jul12 1):bcr2013009990-bcr2013009990. www.ncbi.nlm.nih.gov/pmc/articles/PMC3736293.

8 Albuquerque J, Deshauer D, Fergusson D, Doucette S, MacWilliam C, Kaufmann I. Recurrence rates in Ontario physicians monitored for major depression and bipolar disorder. *Can J Psychiatry* 2009;**54**(11):777–82.

9 Smith DJ, Griffiths E, Kelly M, *et al*. Unrecognised bipolar disorder in primary care patients with depression. *Br J Psychiatry* 2011;**199**(1):49–56. Epub 2011 Feb 3.

10 Polkinghorn C. Doctors Go Mad Too. Available from: www.rcpsych.ac.uk/docs/default-source/about-us/prizes-bursaries/morris-markowe-public-education-prize-2012-doctors-go-mad-too.pdf?sfvrsn=bedd75ee_2.

11 Anonymous. On madness: a personal account of rapid cycling bipolar disorder. *Br J Gen Pract* 2006;56(530):726–8.

12 Redfield Jamison K. *An Unquiet Mind. A Memoir of Moods and Madness*. Picador, 2011.

13 Office for National Statistics. Social and Vital Statistics Division, Northern Ireland Statistics and Research Agency. Central Survey Unit. Quarterly Labour Force Survey, October–December, 2006 [Internet]. UK Data Service; 2014. Available from: http://doi.org/10.5255/UKDA-SN-5609-2.

15

COVID-19 and Mental Illness

CLARE GERADA

I wrote this book before the COVID-19 pandemic turned the world upside down and added this chapter as my country hit the peak of the first wave of infected cases. Pandemic strikes fear in everyone's heart and COVID-19 is no exception. It us the biggest threat in living memory to health and wellbeing, social welfare and the global economy. Within weeks of identification of the first infected person, to one degree or another every country imposed new rules to keep the virus at bay: social distancing, isolation, quarantine, face masks, closure of schools, universities, shops, libraries and so on. Other than essential workers we were all confined to our homes, allowed out only for exercise, food shopping and to receive health care, the aim being to 'flatten the curve', in other words to avoid a peak in those who became seriously unwell and so reduce the pressure on hospital and intensive care services.

I developed COVID-19 in early March 2020, while at a psychiatric conference in New York. I stayed in a large hotel near Times Square and while COVID-19 was an issue (how could it not have been given that at the time Italy and large sways of China were in lockdown?), you would not have known by the lack of precautions in the city. Other than a few bottles of hand sanitiser, New York remained the vibrant, 24-hour place it is famous for. Soon after returning back to London I developed the most violent headache, high temperature, cough and muscle pains. For four days I stayed in bed, rising only to go to the bathroom. Even trying to lift my head to drink was an effort akin to hitting the 'wall' during the marathon. I forced myself to take fluids knowing that developing acute renal failure could lead to a bad outcome. Even once the temperature subsided, the pains in my legs were intolerable. This was followed by fatigue that made the simplest physical effort, such as climbing one short flight of stairs, leaving me exhausted and needing to rest. My illness lasted around three weeks, though by the beginning of the third week I was recovered enough to return to work and get back to helping my colleagues look after patients with COVID and, assuming immunity, even see the most high-risk ones. It is not surprising I wanted to get back to work, it is normal behaviour for doctors (and other healthcare workers) to want to help – especially when caught up in a terrible trauma or tragedy. Doctors, as I have described in this book, can have an exaggerated sense of personal responsibility. So, when their patients are threatened by a fast-spreading and frightening viral illness many want to do everything within their power to help.

However, this altruism can place helpers at increased risk of becoming infected themselves and even of dying.[1] A case of altruism on a global scale was undertaken by one of the first doctors to lose their life to COVID-19, the whistle-blower Li Wenliang. This young Chinese doctor raised concerns about a new illness, which resembled severe acute respiratory syndrome (SARS), now known as COVID-19. Since then hundreds of health workers, including doctors, have died from COVID-19 across the world. In China, it is estimated that around 4% of COVID-19 infections affected healthcare workers, with five deaths,[2] and in Italy the figure was 8%.[3] In the UK by the end of April 2020, 106 NHS health professionals had died from COVID-19, 98 having patient facing roles and in 89 cases, the individual had been working during the pandemic; 25 were doctors.[4] By June 2020 at least 540 health and social care workers had died from COVID-19 in England and Wales.[5]

There is more at risk to health professionals than physical harm. COVID-19 is also affecting their psychological health, with emerging patterns of emotional response to the unfolding situation. This is hardly surprising considering how much grief and anxiety is being brought into the mix due to the death, loss of liberty, sadness and fear as the virus takes its toll on our existence. The levels of trauma, grief, helplessness and to a certain extent hopelessness are high among those presenting to my sick doctor service. One doctor cried as she told me she had seen more deaths of patients in the last month than in the rest of her career put together, these patients dying alone without their loved ones by their side. Unable even to hold the hands of the dying patients, she felt devastated and reminded of the difference between the death of her own grandmother (when all the family were assembled by the bed side) and those, now dying on her ward, alone. What this doctor is experiencing is moral distress, or moral injury.

While not a mental illness *per se*, moral injury is perhaps the most prevalent psychological effect of COVID-19 and other pandemics. Pandemics put health professionals in unchartered territory, which is causing them great distress. For example, having to make impossible life–death decisions, such as having to choose which of two equally sick patients is provided with specific care, one of whom does not survive, because of the non-availability of healthcare equipment; or putting one's own needs ahead of patients' (for example, not providing resuscitation if lacking personal protective equipment [PPE]).

The term 'moral injury' originated in the military and can be transferable to the current situation, more so as for the first time in my 40-year career I am seeing the army in routine healthcare settings, helping address the pandemic.

Moral injury does not just affect individuals who are working in the so called 'front line', but also those who might feel that they are not pulling their weight, not putting themselves at risk or carrying the heavy burden of acute clinical care. Take for example Martin, a general physician who had taken a few years out of clinical care to focus on his research. When the call came for doctors to return to work, instead of his skills being utilised in intensive care he was instead sent to a call centre, speaking to people who had been asked to 'shield themselves'. He felt bereft that as a young doctor he was not taking the place of his older colleagues in accident and emergency departments or urgent care. Or Maria, a radiologist based in a trauma unit, who found her workload had reduced by around 90% as the need for scans due to accidents was reduced considerably. Both approached me with intense feelings of guilt, of not doing enough.

Alongside guilt, another emotion prevalent among doctors (and others) is that of grief. Grief is an emotional response typically associated with a single profound loss, such as the death of a loved one. It is one of the most challenging and universal psychological experiences. The emotions of grief range from shock and denial to anger, bargaining, sadness and, finally (for most of us), acceptance. During this journey, depressive thoughts and even those of suicide are not uncommon. During the COVID-19 pandemic doctors are presenting to my service with grief related to multiple losses: through bereavement, loss of job role or income, friendship networks, work teams, certainty and predictability in life. This grief can be unbearable, leaving doctors without a sense of anchoring or hope. Feelings can come on suddenly, stopping them in their tracks as they try to go about their newly chaotic and constantly changing lives.[6]

During pandemics health staff work under extreme pressure in difficult and often unfamiliar environments. They also have to contend with imperfect systems. For example, safety precautions such as cleaning equipment or surfaces, handling linen and used PPE, adequate handwashing and so on are not always adhered to according to strict infection control guidance. As such health staff might find themselves living in constant fear of becoming infected and experience their working lives as traumatising.

STIGMA

Stigma is often a feature of illness, as I have discussed in many chapters in this book. Stigma sets the individual apart from the rest of society and brings to the bearer shame and isolation. It is more often seen in those suffering from mental illness, although is also present where the illness is a mystery and, as with COVID-19, with no known treatment (as of June 2020). Throughout history, there have been illnesses that stigmatised the infected individual (such as leprosy) or entire populations, such as AIDS, which stigmatised homosexuals, and SARS and COVID-19, which stigmatised Chinese people.

In her book, *Illness as Metaphor*, Susan Sontag, the American writer and philosopher, wrote about how, in an era in which medicine's central premise is that *all* diseases can be cured, those that cannot (TB in the 19th century, AIDS in the 20th century and one could argue, COVID-19 in the 21st century) arouse the most dread. Sontag argues that any disease that is treated as a mystery and intensely feared will be felt to be morally, if not literally, contagious. The individual sufferer is often made to feel that the disease is shameful (and by implication the afflicted individual) and that it is their fault. This is through a process where the disease becomes a metaphor for one's greatest fears. She describes that first the subjects of the deepest dread (corruption, decay, pollution, anomie, weakness), are identified and associated with the disease. The disease then itself becomes a metaphor and in its name (that is using the name of the disease itself as a metaphor), its horrors are imposed onto other things.[7] Infectious diseases are commonly associated with stigma and are more likely to be stigmatised when the disease is considered to be the fault of the individual or the disease is considered to be degenerative.[8] This was certainly the case with AIDS during the 1980s and 1990s, where the person (be they an intravenous drug user or men who have sex with men) was thought to have invited the infection. AIDS was described by Jerry Falwell, a former Republican senator from North Carolina as 'God's judgement' and divine retribution for homosexuals' 'perverted' lifestyle.[9]

While HIV did not specifically affect doctors, nevertheless regulatory guidance was targeted at doctors and served to increase the stigma associated with the disease in this professional group. This was particularly the case around disclosure. While doctors have a right to privacy around their own health, patients also have a right to ensure that their doctors do not pose a risk to them. In some cases, patient's rights versus doctor's privacy are in conflict. Doctors infected with HIV until the late 1990s had a duty to disclose their infection to health services or limit or cease practising. If they failed to seek appropriate counselling or act upon it this could result in restrictions or removal of their licence to practise. The UK was by no means the only country to impose these requirements and not surprisingly led to concealment, secrecy and fear among those in the profession who were either at risk of the infection or had it.

Silence, shame and stigma were all features of the ebola epidemic that affected large areas of west Africa in 2014. Ebola haemorrhagic fever is one of the most virulent diseases known to man and also one of the most terrifying. Death often occurs within days of first infection, with individuals dying from uncontrollable internal bleeding or diarrhoea. The weight of the ebola crisis had a major impact on healthcare workers, with many becoming infected and dying. These were staff working in areas of the world (Liberia, Sierra Leona, Guinea) where there were desperate shortages of health workers at the outset. A factor contributing to the high rate of infection and death of healthcare workers was their commitment to working and 'making their patients their first concern'. With testing and PPE scarce, these professionals would utilise what they had for their patients in the first instance, denying their own needs. Not surprisingly, healthcare workers faced a heavy psychological toll, as they had to deal with large numbers of patients infected with the virus as well the death of their colleagues.

Stigma meant that survivors of ebola, and health professionals working with the sick (or those burying the dead) were rejected by friends and family, and as such had no source of support at their time of emotional need. Those working with ebola-infected patients faced numerous challenges, from the logistical ones such as obtaining enough PPE, to extreme emotional distress from dealing with so much illness and death as well as having to deal with their own fears and grief. Healthcare workers responding to the ebola crisis, became not only the subject of stigma, but also of unwarranted blame for spreading the disease.[10]

While the problems faced by healthcare staff during ebola were compounded by inadequate healthcare systems and infrastructure, nevertheless there have been similar experiences in more well-resourced countries, including the UK. For example, healthcare staff, in particular nurses working during the COVID-19 pandemic, have also been subjected to abuse, violence, stigma and blame. There have been reported incidences of staff being spat at and assaulted and being labelled as 'disease spreaders' amid coronavirus fears.

When Spanish flu hit New York in 1918 there were reports that patients were holding nurses captive in their homes as protection for the frightened inhabitants, as at the time doctors and nurses seemed to be spared from the influenza virus (though not for long).[11]

MENTAL HEALTH

Fortunately, pandemics are rare and as such the literature on their psychological harms on the medical profession is sparse; where it exists, it does suggest that the impact can be profound, with studies suggesting that up to one-half of healthcare workers will experience significant mental health symptoms as a consequence of a pandemic, with more than 10% having on-going problems.[12]

The negative effects experienced by healthcare workers are not just experienced by those who might be putting themselves at physical risk (such as those working in intensive care or critical care) but are also experienced when working in call centres or advice lines and are exposed to the traumatic stories of callers. The negative psychological effects include anxiety, depression, and post-traumatic stress symptomatology (PTSS). To one degree or another all of these are common features of people facing major health epidemics regardless of the specific disease or the time or place where it occurred.[13]

Most recent studies have come from the emotional reactions that emerged following SARS, which broke in China in 2002. In early 2000 a new infection called SARS emerged. Its threat was only recognised when a doctor who was working in a French hospital in Vietnam, Dr Carlo Urbani, first drew attention to a new influenza-like disease. He died of the infection. SARS spread rapidly to countries mainly in south east Asia, though also reaching Toronto, Canada. The psychological impact of SARS was significant, both on the general population and on healthcare professionals. In general, many patients, their families and medical staff were found to suffer from immediate and post-traumatic symptoms, anxiety and depression after the epidemic ended. In China people were reported to have become very anxious, feeling helpless and angry and developed behaviours such as hoarding food or taking their temperature several times per day.

The impact on healthcare workers working in high risk areas during the Toronto SARS outbreak in 2003 found that they experienced a range of psychological disorders, particularly increased levels of anxiety, depression and post-traumatic stress disorder symptomatology (PTSS),[14,15] where up to 12% of health staff developed this disorder.[16] High rates of mental illness were found in Chinese healthcare workers dealing with COVID-19, including symptoms of depression (50%), anxiety (45%), insomnia (34%) and psychological distress (71.5%).[17] The variables identified as placing someone at particular risk included experiencing health fear, social isolation and increased contact with COVID-19-positive patients. Female doctors and nurses, and those closer to the epicentre of the pandemic, had the most severe symptoms.

The effects of the psychological distress can be long lasting.[18] As with grief, the effects of traumatic stress response can be overwhelming, distressing and disruptive for the person experiencing it, but unlike grief it usually subsides quickly within days or weeks. Just a small percentage of traumatised individuals will be left with persistent symptoms and may need specialist psychological support to help them resolve this.

For everyone, social distancing, isolation due to quarantine or 'shielding' are likely to lead to increased cases of anxiety and depression as confined people are detached from their loved ones, deprived of personal liberties and lose structure and even the purpose of their daily lives. This is the same for doctors, many of whom have had their working and professional lives disrupted by the pandemic. There is also the feeling of increasing weariness, or COVID fatigue.[19] The initial eagerness to play a part in this crisis, to get 'stuck in' and to make a difference has been replaced by an intense and overwhelming tiredness and irritability. COVID fatigue is not just felt by those working exhausting shifts in face-to-face clinical practice and directly treating patients, but also (and sometimes more so) by those working behind the scenes, staring at their computer screens all day long. Paradoxically, as the daily commute is reduced to a short walk from bedroom to the new 'office' at home, the amount of work being done and its intensity has increased many-fold as the buffer created by travelling between one meeting and another has disappeared. Gone are the pleasantries at the start of meetings, the sharing of each other's day-to-day experiences or the ritual distraction of asking for coffee or tea orders. COVID-fatigue also affects those who are not working, who are prepared for action, but action is yet to come, such as those newly retired doctors recruited to help yet who are currently largely underused, or those waiting for the virus to appear, all prepared, but the pandemic never reached their area in the numbers initially predicted.

Many of the doctors I see are admitting to drinking more alcohol than they normally do – trying to numb either the pain of their work or the boredom now impacting on their lives. While doctor-specific studies on alcohol consumption during covid are yet to emerge, across the UK there are reports of increasing alcohol use in the general population, especially so in older adults. Alcohol sales increased by 30% just before lockdown started as people stocked up for fear of shortages; 15% of individuals who drink alcohol are drinking more than before lockdown.[20]

It is also important to remember that not all individuals will suffer distress. Doctors can thrive with pressure and challenge and can experience 'post-traumatic growth', which is positive psychological change resulting from adversity. Whether someone develops a psychological injury or experiences psychological growth is likely to be influenced by the way that they are supported before, during and after a challenging incident.

CONCLUSION

A unique feature of COVID-19 is experience of universality, that 'we are all in this together' and it is not just doctors and patients who are bearing the brunt of the infection but the whole world. My life as a doctor, as everyone's, has been changed, maybe for ever. As a health professional caring for doctors I am impressed by how many have coped with their lives, literally, being turned upside down. Despite the predictions that many will develop mental illness, at present doctors have reported feeling re-energised, in control and connected in a way to their colleagues that was absent pre COVID-19. Hospitals have re-created 'doctors messes', decompression or welfare rooms where all staff can go. Some of these are indistinguishable from first class airline lounges (without the flight announcements of course) and are run by air stewards. Staff can have free access to refreshments, reclines to rest, massages and counsellors if needed. In the UK NHS, the need for an annual appraisal, revalidation and inspection have all been paused and systems put in place for fast track reinstatement of doctors to return to clinical practice. Across the world healthcare staff are being applauded (publicly in many areas) and thanked repeatedly for their help and dedication. Calls are for them to be financially rewarded. This is unprecedented in other pandemics – where for example, staff who worked with patients were shunned in case they infected others and there was little recognition of the efforts they had made when working on the front line. All of these might reduce the levels of burnout seen in the medical profession (see Chapter 12)[21] – though only, if on return to normality we learn and retain the positive psychological interventions that have been put in place. Only time will tell.

REFERENCES

1   Choi SH, Chung JW, Jeon MH, Lee MS. Risk factors for pandemic H1N1 2009 infection in healthcare personnel of four general hospitals. *J Infect* 2011;**63**(4):267–73. doi: 10.1016/j.jinf.2011.04.009. Epub 2011 May 1. Available from: www.ncbi.nlm.nih.gov/pubmed/21601925.

2   The Novel Coronavirus Pneumonia Emergency Response Epidemiology Team. The epidemiological characteristics of an outbreak of 2019 novel coronavirus diseases (COVID-19) — China, 2020. *China CDC Weekly* 2020;**2**(8):113–22. http://weekly.chinacdc.cn/en/article/id/e53946e2-c6c4-41e9-9a9b-fea8db1a8f51.

3   COVID-19 Task Force. Integrated surveillance of COVID-19 in Italy. www.epicentro.iss.it/coronavirus/bollettino/Infografica_19marzo%20ENG.pdf.

4   Cook T, Kursumovic E, Lennane S. Exclusive: deaths of NHS staff from covid-19 analysed. Available from: www.hsj.co.uk/exclusive-deaths-of-nhs-staff-from-COVID-19-analysed/7027471.article.

5   Amnesty International. UK amongst highest COVID-19 health worker deaths in the world. www.amnesty.org.uk/press-releases/uk-among-highest-covid-19-health-worker-deaths-world.

6 Walker C, Gerada C. Extraordinary times: coping psychologically through the impact of covid-19. *BMJ* 2020. Available from: https://blogs.bmj.com/bmj/2020/03/31/extraordinary-times-coping-psychologically-through-the-impact-of-covid-19.

7 Sontag S. *Illness as a Metaphor and Aids and its metaphors*. London: Allen Lan, 1989.

8 Green K, Banerjee S. Disease related stigma: comparing predictors of AIDS and cancer stigma. *J Homosexuality* 2006;**50**(4):185–209.

9 Reed C. The Rev Jerry Falwell. 2007. Available from: www.theguardian.com/media/2007/may/17/broadcasting.guardianobituaries.

10 Shah N, Kuriansky J. The impact of trauma for health care workers facing the ebola epidemic. In: Kuriansky J (ed). *The Psychosocial Aspects of a Deadly Epidemic*. What Ebola has taught us about holistic healing. Santa Barbara: Praeger, 2016.

11 Honigsbaum M. *The Pandemic Century*. London: Hurst & Co, 2019.

12 Holmes EA, O'Connor RC, Perry VH, *et al*. Multidisciplinary research priorities for the COVID-19 pandemic: a call for action for mental health science. *Lancet Psychiatry* 2020; published online 15 April 2020. Available from: https://doi.org/10.1016/S2215-0366(20)30168-1.

13 Douglas, PK, Douglas DB, Harrigan DC, Douglas KN. Preparing for pandemic influenza and its aftermath: mental health issues considered. *Int J Emerg Mental Health* 2009;**11**:137–14.

14 Styra R, Hawryluck L, Robinson S, *et al*. Impact on health care workers employed in high-risk areas during the Toronto SARS outbreak. *J Psychosom Res* 2008;**64**:177–83.

15 Boudreau R, Grieco R, Cahoon S, Robertson RC, Wedel RJ. The pandemic from within: two surveys of physician burnout in Canada. *Can J Comm Mental Health* 2006;**25**(2):71–88. Available from: https://doi.org/10.7870/cjcmh-2006-0014.

16 Nortje CR, Moller CB, Andre AT. Judgment of risk in traumatized and nontraumatized emergency medical service personnel. *Psychol Rep* 2004; **95**:1119–28.

17 Lai J, Ma S, Wang Y, et al. Factors associated with mental health outcomes among health care workers exposed to coronavirus disease 2019. *JAMA Netw Open* 2020;**3**(3):e203976. Available from: https://jamanetwork.com/journals/jamanetworkopen/fullarticle/2763229.

18 Maunder RG, Lancee WJ, Balderson KE, *et al*. Long-term psychological and occupational effects of providing hospital healthcare during SARS outbreak. *Emerg Infect Dis* 2006;**12**(12):1924–32.

19 Gerada C, Walker C. Covid fatigue is taking an enormous toll on healthcare workers. *BMJ* 2020. Available from: https://blogs.bmj.com/bmj/2020/05/04/covid-fatigue-is-taking-an-enormous-toll-on-healthcare-workers.

20 Holmes L. Drinking during lockdown: headline findings. Alcohol Change UK. https://alcoholchange.org.uk/blog/2020/covid19-drinking-during-lockdown-headline-findings.

21 Hartzband P, Groopman J. Physician burnout, interrupted. *N Engl J Med* 2020. Available from: www.nejm.org/doi/full/10.1056/NEJMp2003 149?query=RP.

SECTION III

Doctors as Patients

16

Doctors as Patients

CLARE GERADA

It is often said that doctors make the worst patients. Systemic barriers to accessing care as well as cultural and individual factors play their part in keeping doctors away from the consulting room and relying on self-care or 'corridor consultations' instead.[1] Maybe our reluctance to seek help is that we are all too familiar with what it means to be sick, to have vulnerabilities and relinquish authority and trust to another, and we recoil against this. I certainly prefer to manage my own health problems. If I seek help, which I have had to over the course of my life (not even I can deliver my own babies), then it is with a feeling of shame and embarrassment that I am taking up the precious time of another. I have had mental health problems, no-one can go through nearly four decades of caring without some of the emotional impact of our patients sticking to us, and everyone, even the most robust is not immune from the pain of significant life events. But when my depression hit me, when I too became sad, felt worthless, hopeless and even had thoughts of suicide, I found it difficult to seek the help of another doctor, of going to my own general practitioner (GP), someone I knew professionally. I worried she might consider me unworthy and incompetent to care for patients or force me to refer myself to 'the authorities'. I did seek help, but by-passed all 'standard' routes, instead, using a pseudonym I contacted a psychologist, privately. The anonymity did not last long as with the patients in my service who also try to hide behind their mother's maiden name, my email address gave away my real identity. My concerns are shared by many doctors, irrational concerns in the main, but real, nevertheless. Maybe it is because I am older, with my 'stiff upper lip' mentality more ingrained than in the younger, more enlightened generation that I have found it so hard to seek care. Or maybe, as with most doctors I meet, becoming a patient means relinquishing our identity of the powerful, knowledgeable, invincible professional and this is very difficult.

While the problems described in this chapter are not unique to the medical profession, they are amplified in doctors due to the way we are trained, regulated and managed.

RELUCTANCE TO SEEK HELP

In 2008, against a growing concern of suicide among doctors, the report *Mental Health and Ill Health in Doctors* was published; it discussed a broad range of issues relevant to this professional group including stigma, secrecy and shame.[2] The report made the point that these three factors contribute to doctors failing to take on the sick role and instead work when unwell. Doctors average less than three days' sickness per year, while in the general population the figure is eight days and for nurses it is 15. A paper following on from this, published two years later, called *Invisible patients* looked at the barriers to doctors seeking help and the subsequent risks to both patients and doctors due to this failure to seek timely care.[3] That doctors are reluctant to present themselves to services for mental health problems is demonstrated by the findings of a number of surveys. For example, one study published in 2009, found only 13% of doctors would seek help through professional routes, the majority would choose, as I did, alternative paths such as self-medication or informal help from friends or family. Most, when asked why, said they feared their career would be jeopardised if they approached a colleague.[4] This was also the finding of a study that I was involved in, of the barriers and facilitators to seeking care among GPs,[5] and another by Ipsos MORI. Both found doctors would keep their mental illness secret, especially so, as the MORI poll found, if they were suffering from addiction.[6]

A survey sent to all GPs and psychiatrists in Devon and Cornwall found nearly one-half reported that they had suffered an episode of depression, 14% in the last year. Yet, despite these high levels of mental illness (and a knowledge of mental health services given their specialities) they would not seek care, rather prefer to suffer in silence. Reasons given (in order of responses) were: not wanting to let their colleagues down, loss of confidentiality, of letting patients down and worries about their career.[7] Surprisingly, the group most reluctant to seek care for mental health problems are psychiatrists, with one study reporting nearly 90% would be averse to consulting with another mental health professional.[8]

It is not just mental health services that unwell doctors are reluctant to attend. It also extends to occupational health practitioners. Occupational health (OH) is a confidential service for employed staff across the NHS and OH practitioners play an important role in making recommendations and offering advice on placement or return to work after a period of illness or disability. Given their important rôle it might seem reasonable to expect that doctors might wish to engage with this valuable source of help. Yet of those with previous experience of mental illness, only 41% disclosed their illness to OH. Even those doctors who had training in mental illness, who one could assume understood the vital role of OH specialists in helping them back to work, were reluctant. When doctors were asked why, the most frequent response was the same in both subgroups, 'not wanting to be labelled'.[9]

A narrative study of doctors about their problems in seeking help again highlighted the anxieties around disclosure. They were worried they would be seen as failures and this would harm their career. These quotes are from doctors interviewed for the study:[10]

There's some concern that other people see you as weak or not able to cope. I've heard that supervisors have suggested people seek help because they're not really resilient enough or whatever, which is not helpful.

I think that there are still areas where, however much they've got a mental illness policy and all those kinds of things, that actually if you were taking time off with mental health, you probably wouldn't get short-listed for that promotion.

Fear is often at the root of why doctors do not seek care. For some of my own patients this has been so great that it is as if they are trying to conceal a terrible crime. They tell no-one, not even those closest to them, how they are feeling. Others have consulted doctors in the private sector under the mistaken belief that this will buy them anonymity. Even at my own mental health service, patients often mask the full extent of their illness, one patient omitting to tell us that he was drinking two bottles of alcohol and using crack cocaine every day. Needless to say, this was obvious by his malodour, jittery state and dishevelled appearance.

In my experience, what doctors worry about most about falls into two main categories. The first is around loss of confidentiality with others being told about their mental health problems without their consent. The second is that by disclosing mental illness it will mean they will be referred to the regulator or sanctioned in some way. Both of these have some basis in reality. Medicine is a small world and it does not take long for two doctors who have never met each other to find they have mutual friends or colleagues in common. Many doctors also live in the same area they work in (as I do). Their local hospital is often the one in which they work, or their neighbouring practices are within the same clinical network as their own practice. Others have relationships with doctors, are related to them or as with me, are married to one, making our social networks among the profession even more entangled. This makes it very difficult to consult with someone with no personal or professional ties to you or your family. At a pinch, this might be acceptable if the reason for needing a consultation is not sensitive. However, if it is for a mental illness or a personal problem, it can be difficult for medical professionals to discuss it with friends or colleagues. Perhaps the most extreme example I can remember of the inability to obtain a confidential space was a psychiatrist who, having attended his own GP for help with depression, found a few weeks later at his referral management multidisciplinary team meeting that he had been referred to his own team.

The fear of breach of confidentiality also relates to one's personal issues being relayed beyond the privacy of the consulting room to others in their wider educational, professional or employment circles. To be blunt, doctors do not trust the system to keep their problems confidential. This is especially the case once a mental illness has been disclosed in the workplace (for example to a training supervisor) when it is not uncommon to have other individuals, each claiming 'a need to know' also told about the doctor's illness. These can include appraisers, trainers, medical directors, senior managers and human resources and secretarial staff. I once counted 17 individuals being told about a doctor who had recently been diagnosed with attention deficit disorder, all assuming they had a right to know.

Even when a doctor is offered confidentiality at their place of work, this rarely happens. Each staff member tells another 'in good faith' and with the assurance '*I am only telling you in strict confidence but I think you should know, please don't pass on… but… Dr XYZ is off sick with…*'. This then gets passed onto another member of staff, even those who have no direct involvement, and another, with the message slightly altered each time as in the children's game Chinese whispers. In the end, the doctor's problem might as well be posted on the world-wide-web for all to see. Sadly, in my experience, colleagues derive vicarious gratification from the drama that a sick doctor brings to the boredom of their everyday working life, especially if their illness is related to addiction. There is also the issue that once disclosed and placed on work records, it is impossible to remove, and the diagnosis is carried forward for evermore into any new posts. The doctor then has to face with each move of a job (which can be every six months for doctors in training) having to go over their past illness and be interrogated as whether they are fit to practise. This is not I hasten to add just for serious mental illnesses, but for problems such as past history of depression, an eating disorder, dyspraxia or indeed any diagnosis that the doctor has placed on their record.

The second major concern for doctors is that of being referred to the regulator. **This is a largely unfounded fear** (certainly in the UK) as very few doctors with mental illness are investigated by the UK regulator, the General Medical Council (GMC) and fewer still receive sanctions. I discuss this much more in Part 4. However, this does not prevent the anxiety. Even where nothing illegal or unlawful has taken place, the belief that they will be referred for simply having a mental illness is still pervasive. For example, a small study involved interviewing 13 hospital doctors, asking why they would not seek help for mental illness. These were doctors who held senior leadership and/or trainer roles (some had personal experience of being mentally unwell). Given their seniority and by implication understanding of the regulatory system, one would imagine they would be more comfortable with disclosing the need for help. This, however, was not the case. A common thread through their narratives was worry that disclosure would lead to a real possibility of being erased from the medical register.[11]

It is not just in the UK doctors have these concerns. Over the last two decades, increasing numbers of American medical licencing boards ask questions on their initial and renewal application forms whether a doctor has ever received treatment for mental illness. As of 2017, 43 States out of 50 asked questions about mental health conditions, 43 about physical health conditions and 47 about substance use.[12] There is a greater likelihood of being asked for one's history of treatment and prior hospitalisation for mental health and substance use versus physical health disorders, illustrating the lack of parity between physical and mental illness and perpetuating the stigma that mental illness in itself must affect a doctor's ability to practise. This has led to 40% of doctors saying they would not seek help for a mental health problem as by doing so it would impact on their career.[13] For female American doctors with existing mental illness, only 6% had disclosed their condition to their State.[14] There are concerns that these questions may not be legal,[15] and as such Court decisions and the USA Department of Justice have begun to establish that such questions do indeed violate the Americans with Disabilities Act.[16]

In Australia, a new law, The Health Practitioner Regulation National Law and Other Legislation Amendment Bill, was enacted in 2018.[17] This requires doctors to report a doctor-patient if they believe their conduct, health or performance risks placing the public at substantial risk of harm. It also introduced heavy fines or the potential for three years' imprisonment for those who did not comply with the law. The new requirement has created considerable disquiet among practitioners, worried that sick doctors would now be denied access to confidential care. In a poll of Australian doctors, almost 60% of respondents either strongly disagreed or disagreed with the statement that '[they] *can disclose their mental illness to their doctor without fear for their career*', which suggests that many are quietly suffering, increasing the risk of suicide.[18] The law creates the problem it is trying to solve, that is encouraging doctors to disclose their mental illness. Instead it is creating additional barriers such that the treating clinicians feel they must report anyone who presents with anything that could be possibly related to an impairment. By contrast, there are no legal sanctions on doctors in the UK. The requirement is captured in good practice guidance with GMC Good Medical Practice.

Aside from worries around admitting to mental health problems there is also the real concern of not being treated with compassion when they are unwell and wanting care. A doctor, writing anonymously about her own experience, wrote how when she presented to accident and emergency services following an episode of self-harm, nurses would comment 'but you're an intelligent girl, why would you do this to yourself?' or 'you ought to know how to deal with this'.[19] This is not an uncommon view my patients have encountered, where they are made to feel a nuisance rather than unwell. One was told *'you're a doctor you should be able to afford private care'*.

Robert Spooner, the father of a patient of mine, whose daughter died from anorexia nervosa (her weight at the time of her death was under four stone) wrote this about his daughter:

> Our daughter, the late Dr Mel, succumbed to anorexia at the age of 13 when the GP said it was just a normal teenage issue. We knew it wasn't and for most of the next 17 years she suffered a daily mental battle. She left Cambridge as a Senior Scholar and won multiple first prizes at University College before becoming a doctor, training in the London area. During that time a paediatric registrar asking her what was wrong with her, when told 'I have anorexia' replied 'But you're so lovely Mel'. When having to see Occupational Health, on walking in he asked, 'Have you not grown up yet?'. Her last rostered duties were four nights on call. As part of her return to work we understood she would not do such long hours, but she was nevertheless rostered to do them. While the cause of death was cardiac arrhythmia, we found letters showing she had on two occasions found life so bad she had planned to take her life. We have lost our daughter, medicine has lost a brilliant, and a so capable and dedicated paediatrician.

Melanie struggled to seek care as her experience with doctors had made her feel as if she were a child, not an adult desperate to find a way through her eating disorder.

BECOMING A PATIENT

Given the 'rules' of medicine it should be clearer why we find it so difficult to become patients. As I have argued, this is because crossing that invisible divide between health professional and patient is a fundamental challenge to our personal and professional identity. It is patients, on the other side of the consulting room, who become unwell, not doctors. The American neurosurgeon, Paul Kalanithi, has written about his personal experience of being unwell in *When Breath Becomes Air*, published posthumously. He developed a brain tumour. His narrative illustrates how difficult it is for doctors to take on the patient role; he wrote 'Why was I so authoritative in a surgeon's coat, but so meek in a patient's gown?' The answer to his question is because as the complete object, the 'doctor', we create an aura of invincibility around ourselves. Becoming unwell is challenging, even in the short term, as with this comes the loss of the trappings of power, knowledge, status and authority defined by our group norms. In a study of GP attitudes to their own health, one is quoted as saying, 'we think we're superhuman and that we don't get ill, or if we do, we can cope with it'.[20] This quote illustrates the central belief many doctors have, that by virtue of their medical degree, they do not become unwell. As the author, Robert Klitzman wrote in his book *When Doctors Become Patients*, 'We wear magic white coats... we destroy disease all the time: how can it attack us?'[21]

Or as the 'Fatman' says in *The House of God*:

There's a law you've gotta learn… the patient is the one with the disease.[22]

The House of God is a satirical exposition of the work of junior doctors first published in 1978. Adam Kay's *This is Going to Hurt* is the modern-day equivalent. Both a brutally honest, amazingly well-written, painfully funny and extremely sad descriptions of what working as a doctor is about. Both should be essential reading for prospective doctors.

The conviction we are different from our patients is inculcated into us early on in our career, not of course in the formal parts of our education, but as I have mentioned, in the spaces between, the so-called hidden or uncoded curriculum. A study of junior doctors who became ill found they experienced the 'patient role' as alien and shaming. These trainees, even though they were still in the early stages of their career, found it hard to adjust to patienthood. One commented, 'I had this bizarre misconception that like as a doctor you don't get ill...' Although she later came to question this perception as naive, this participant maintained, 'because you're the doctor and they're the patients, and there's some kind of line between you.' The omnipresent finding in this study was that ill health equated to incompetence, and, as such, to seek help is a flaw in the individual.[23] This belief is modelled by teachers and colleagues – who come into work when unwell, and even boast about doing so, as I have done on many occasions throughout my career.

This behaviour of 'working nevertheless' and giving a façade of coping, not just to colleagues and patients but also to ourselves, is hard wired into the medical culture.[24,25] Doctors who take time off are not viewed favourably by those who have to pick up the work left by their absence. This creates the norm that illness equates with weakness, and doctors should be strong and healthy and cope themselves with illness and stress. Colleagues who are absent due to illness tend to create 'sympathy fatigue' and blame rather than compassion and understanding.

When doctors do get into a consulting room, they tend to act differently, as they visibly try to regain control of their medical identity, by for example, 'talking shop' or underplaying their symptoms. I certainly underplayed my symptoms when I had to seek help for a medical condition. Despite my problem being a non-stigmatising issue, I still felt embarrassed at not being able to manage it myself. While in a lot of pain, I did not tell the doctor its extent. The consultation was not helped by myself and the doctor I was seeing choosing to spend a good part of it talking about medical politics and local gossip (a not uncommon scenario when doctors consult with other doctors). The consequences for me were that my condition worsened and the treatment I had to have in the end was more complicated than had I admitted my symptoms in the first place (and had the time to do so). As with Paul Kalanithi's' experience, I literally and metaphorically found it hard, as it is for many doctors, to remove my surgical scrubs and replace them with the patient-gown. This was also the experience of a consultant breast surgeon, who developed breast cancer herself and was being treated in the hospital she worked. She wrote:

> One of the hardest things was to stop being a doctor and learn to become a patient... [but] I don't like bothering people for something I should be able to fix myself.[26]

The move from doctor to patient also involves a challenge to one's self and to '*who am I?*', and '*where do I belong?*' Take this extract from *Doctors Dissected* involving a doctor about to donate a kidney to his wife who was dying of renal failure:

> Well, I was determined not to behave like a patient and to take it all in my stride, but donating a kidney involves a lot of medicalization...You have to go in overnight and they shave off your pubic hair, and it's all quite frightening even for a 42-year-old doctor [my bold]. I was determined not to be one of those extra neurotic doctor patients, so I just looked interested and talked the doctors through the procedures.[27]

Not only did this doctor deny his vulnerability and *not behave like a patient*, but also coped with the trauma of losing a kidney (not a minor undertaking) and having a terminally ill wife by holding on to his medical identity in the hope of neutralising his fears. He is also perpetuating the view that as a doctor, he must put on a brave front, and anything less, would be deemed unacceptable, in his words, neurotic (conjuring up images of a 'flaky' weak individual).

Sick doctors are often embarrassed when consulting with other doctors. A personal account called '*The other side of the sheets: a special case?*' was written by a doctor describing her experience of being admitted to hospital. She writes:

> I recount my experience, not going for sympathy, but to make the point that doctors are special patients. From the start I presented late with a list of

differential diagnoses rather than symptoms. Fear of a laparotomy made the abdominal pain 'not too bad' or 'tolerable', rather than 'awful'. Conscious of the overworked nurses, I ignored the fact that I'd had morphine and was found in a heap on the floor. The night passed in morose tears and indescribable morbid fears. Also, always a doctor I could not ignore my fellow patients.[28]

What this anonymous account and the others I have given illustrate is how sick doctors are different to other patients. They present late, and then with diagnoses rather than saying what is wrong with them. They minimise their symptoms. such as deliberately scoring lower on alcohol screening questionnaires or masking the true extent of their negative thinking.

CONCLUSION

Doctors find it difficult to become patients. This is in part due to the way we are trained (not to show vulnerability) but also to difficulties related to the fear of disclosure. Since caring for thousands of doctors with mental health problems I feel the tide is turning. Once services can offer confidentiality, containment and skill in managing their problems, doctors are willing to present to care, and in so doing reduce their fear of seeking help. Still however, the 'system' is predicated on the assumption that a doctor with mental illness is dangerous and needs monitoring and even restrictions on their practice. This is as far from the truth as assuming that any doctor with cancer needs the same. Of course, unwell doctors, just as those who might have an acute physical illness or broken leg will need time to recover and recuperate, and on return to work they might need reasonable adjustments to be made. But my experience of over 10,000 mentally ill doctors is that the overwhelming majority pose no risk at all to their patients and where they might, this can be identified ahead by the medical team and measures put in place to reduce this risk. Chapter 19 will discuss these mental services.

REFERENCES

1   Kay M, Mitchell G, Clavarina A, Doust J. Doctors as patients: a systematic review of doctors' health access and barriers they experience. *Br J Gen Pract* 2008;**58**(552):501–8.
2   Department of Health. Mental health and ill health in doctors, 2008. Available from: www.em-online.com/download/medical_article/36516_DH_083090%5B1%5D.pdf.
3   Department of Health. Invisible patients: report of the working group on the health of health professionals, 2010. Available from: www.champspublichealth.com/writedir/4344Invisible%20patients%20-%20The%20Working%20Group%20on%20the%20Health%20of%20Health%20Professionals%20-%20Report.pdf.
4   Hassan T, Ahmed S, White A, Galbraith N. A postal survey of doctors' attitudes to becoming mentally ill. *Clin Med* 2009;**9**(4):327-332.

5 Spiers J, Buszewicz M, Chew-Graham C, et al. Barriers, facilitators, and survival strategies for GPs seeking treatment for distress: a qualitative study. Br J Genl Pract 2017;**67**(663): e700–8.

6 Ipsos MORI. Fitness to Practice: The Health of Healthcare Professionals [Internet]. 2009. Available from: https://webarchive.nationalarchives.gov.uk/+/www.dh.gov.uk/prod_consum_dh/groups/dh_digitalassets/@dh/@en/@ps/documents/digitalasset/dh_113549.pdf.

7 Adams EF, Lee AJ, Pritchard CW, White RJ. What stops us from healing the healers: a survey of help-seeking behaviour, stigmatisation and depression within the medical profession. Int J Soc Psychiatry 2010;**56**(4):359–70. doi: 10.1177/0020764008099123. Epub 2009 Jul 17.

8 White A, Shiralkar P, Hassan T, Galbraith N, Callaghan R. Barriers to mental healthcare for psychiatrists. Psychiatric Bull 2006;**30**:382–4.

9 Cohen D, Winstanley S, Greene G. Understanding doctors' attitudes towards self-disclosure of mental ill health. Occup Med 2016;**66**(5):383–9.

10 British Medical Association. Mental health and wellbeing in the medical profession [Internet]. 2019. Available from: www.bma.org.uk/collective-voice/policy-and-research/education-training-and-workforce/supporting-the-mental-health-of-doctors-in-the-workforce#report2 BMA-Mental-Health-and-Wellbeing-Medical-Profession-Oct-19.pdf.

11 Bianchi E, Bhattacharyya M, Meakin R. Exploring senior doctors' beliefs and attitudes regarding mental illness within the medical profession: a qualitative study. BMJ Open 2016;**6**(9):e012598.

12 Gold KJ, Shih ER, Goldman EB, Schwenk TL. Do US Medical Licensing Applications treat mental and physical illness equivalently? Fam Med 2017;**49**(6):464–7.

13 Dyrbye L, West C, Sinsky C, Goeders L, Satele D, Shanafelt T. Medical Licensure questions and physician reluctance to seek care for mental health conditions. Mayo Clin Proc 2017;**92**(10):1486–93.

14 Gold KJ, Andrew LB, Goldman EB, Schwenk TL. "I would never want to have a mental health diagnosis on my record": a survey of female physicians on mental health diagnosis, treatment, and reporting. Gen Hosp Psychiatry 2016;**43**:51–7.

15 Schroeder R, Brazeau CM, Zackin F, et al. Do state medical board applications violate the Americans With Disabilities Act? Acad Med 2009;**84**(6):776–81.

16 Jones J, North C, Vogel-Scibilia S, Myers MF, Owen R. Medical Licensure questions about mental illness and compliance with the Americans With Disabilities Act. J Am Acad Psychiatry Law 2018;**46**(4):458–71.

17 Health Practitioner Regulation National Law and Other Legislation Amendment Bill 2018 [Internet]. Parliamentary Committees; 2019. Available from: www.parliament.qld.gov.au/Documents/TableOffice/TabledPapers/2019/5619T6.pdf.

18 Insight+ Polls - InsightPlus [Internet]. InsightPlus. 2019 [cited 13 September 2019]. Available from: https://insightplus.mja.com.au/polls.

19 Anonymous. Medicine and mental illness: how can the obstacles sick doctors face be overcome? Psychiatrist 2012;**36**:104–7.

20 Thompson W, Cupples M, Sibbett C, Skan D, Bradley T. Challenge of culture, conscience, and contract to general practitioners' care of their own health: qualitative study. *BMJ* 2001;**323**(7315):728–31.

21 Klitzman R. Magic white coats. In: Klitzman R. *When Doctors Become Patients*. Oxford: Oxford University Press, 2008. Available from: https://epdf. pub/when-doctors-become-patients.html.

22 Shem S. *The House of God*. London: Black Swan, 1985.

23 Fox F, Doran N, Rodham K, Taylor G, Harris M, O'Connor M. Junior doctors' experiences of personal illness: a qualitative study. *Med Educ* 2011;**45**(12):1251–61.

24 Harris FM, Taylor G, Rodham K, *et al*. What happens when doctors are patients? Qualitative study of GPs. *Br J Gen Pract* 2009;**59**(568):811–18.

25 McKevitt C, Morgan M. Illness doesn't belong to us. *J Royal Soc Med* 1997;**90**(9):491–5.

26 Ball L. The other side: doctors as patients. Medical Women 2016; Spring: 24–25.

27 Haynes J, Scurr M (eds). *Doctors Dissected*, 1st edn. London: Quartet Books, 2015.

28 Anon. The other side of the sheets: a special case. In: Petra Jones (ed). Oxford: Radcliffe Publishing, 2005, p. 37.

17

Doctors Treating Doctors

CLARE GERADA

INTRODUCTION

It is not just unwell doctors who find it hard to accept that they can be sick, doctors who see and treat other doctors find it difficult as well. Doctors often find it embarrassing to treat their own profession, and that they (the treating doctor) might be less qualified or knowledgeable than the sick one. Consulting with more senior individuals can be especially difficult given the rigid hierarchical practices that exist in medicine. We have all been in this position and it is rarely comfortable, for either party. Having a discussion about the side-effects and mode of action of antidepressants might feel awkward with a professor of psychopharmacology. However, what is important is to try and acknowledge and respect any additional expertise the sick doctor has, but always to allow them, at the same time, to be the vulnerable, ignorant and frightened patient needing simple explanations, reassurance and compassion.

When a doctor becomes a patient, consultations can be difficult, especially where mental health is concerned. In the first instance, both parties prefer 'corridor conversations': snippets of care outside the consulting room. Sitting outside the normal health system can have detrimental effects for the doctor as unorthodox routes risks distorting the delivery of care. At the very least the unwell doctor will not be part of the routine call–recall system and as such not followed-up in the standard manner. They might miss out on medication reviews or necessary tests. For others it can have tragic consequences, as with Daksha Emson and her daughter. In Daksha's case, the boundaries with the health services she interacted with were so blurred that she missed out on many of the safety netting systems designed to manage very sick individuals. I have mentioned Daksha before when talking about suffering and stigma in doctors. She was a young psychiatrist who, following the birth of her first child, developed severe post-natal psychosis and killed herself and her 3-month-old baby, Freya. The subsequent inquiry into their deaths highlighted how Daksha's treatment was different, just because she was a doctor, and this was implicated in causing her to kill herself and her baby. Her previous consultant, who had cared for her for many years retired just before she became pregnant. On his retirement he transferred her back to the care of her general pracitioner (GP), but in his transfer letter diminished the seriousness of her history, concentrating on her 'good' points, creating an unduly optimistic assessment of her health. This despite Daksha, over the years having been so unwell as to require long periods of in-patient care, some under compulsory admission. Daksha did not make her condition and previous history of illness known to her new psychiatrist; she hid this through worries that disclosure would negatively impact on her career. Information was not passed between doctors involved in her care (GP and psychiatrist) to 'respect' her confidentiality. Information sharing was normal practice for other patients. Once unwell, her psychiatrist did not place her on the Care Programme Approach, which would have offered enhanced care, nor discuss her case with colleagues in the team meetings, again in the belief that he should maintain her confidentiality. Finally, only informal arrangements were set up with a community psychiatric nurse, which were not adequate in the circumstances, but made in the belief that as she was a psychiatrist she would know what to do. While singly none of these changes to normal practice contributed to her death, the accumulation of them did. Given the seriousness of her condition she was excluded from the standard of care that would have been provided to any other, non-medically qualified patient with a similar illness and seriousness.

As Daksha illustrates, even once in the consulting room the sick doctor is treated differently and often seen more as a colleague than a patient, sometimes even going as far as to suggest the sick doctor should treat or at the very least know how to manage themselves, even organise their own tests. This has certainly been my experience. The implication being that the only rôle allowed is that of an 'expert-patient'. This is a two-way collusion, as both parties have a vested interest in maintaining the status quo, that is the denial of the wounded healer.

Over the years there have been a number of personal accounts of doctors becoming patients and most of them illustrate how difficult it is for both sick-doctor and treating doctor to deal with. For example, this individual wrote about their experience of being 'the unwilling occupant of a psychiatrist's couch'. This doctor gives advice on how to 'look after one of us' (mentally ill doctors) much of which focuses on the importance of treating the sick doctor as a patient and not as someone in full control.[1] I would echo this advice.

All too often, mentally ill doctors are treated by trainers, employers and regulators, as naughty schoolchildren or wrongdoers at having crossed the boundary from professional to patient.

COLLUSION OF ANONYMITY

Doctors are trained to care for others, not each other. Even if a team member is seen to be struggling, rarely does someone pick this up, or make enquiries. We lack a culture of mutual responsibility for each other, leading to a situation, described by the psychoanalyst Michael Balint, of a collusion of anonymity. This typically was used to describe the collusion that occurs when 'the patient is passed from one specialist to another with nobody taking responsibility for the whole person'.[2] In the case of an unwell doctor at work, while everyone can see that something is wrong, and may even raise concerns with a colleague, no one wants to take any responsibility in the hope that someone else will deal with them or that the problem will disappear. I am not suggesting that we have a 'duty of care' for each other in the sense of needing to provide medical care. Rather that we have a duty of caring for each other as fellow professionals, all working hard towards a common aim of treating patients.

Many years ago, while training in psychiatry at the Maudsley Hospital, one of the psychiatric registrars jumped onto a dining table in the middle of the busy canteen. At the top of his voice he began a tirade about the corruption he had exposed in this hospital, how his consultant (an eminent professor) had tried to cover up a scandal involving the secret service and that only he (John) could save the world from the invasion that was around the corner. It was quite clear he was psychotic, yet no one seemed to know what to do. Here were dozens of psychiatrists, with one of their own clearly in a distressed state and we were paralysed.

Eventually, a member of the kitchen staff gently coaxed him down from the table and took him by the hand to the psychiatric emergency clinic a short way down the corridor. If this doctor, instead of a mental health problem, had had a physical emergency, he would have been overwhelmed with helping hands. John, as I later learnt, had bipolar disorder. He had sought help from his GP in the previous week, who told him that as a psychiatrist he must know the best way to treat his condition or maybe he could ask a colleague for help. Needless to say, he didn't know how to access care, instead he became increasingly unwell, surrounded by his peers blind to his odd behaviour. Sadly, in my experience of working with mentally ill doctors, this scenario is not uncommon.

So good are doctors at not seeing distress in their own kind, they often describe the shock when the sick-doctor's condition is subsequently brought to light. Colleagues perform retrospective trawls through their memory to clues of the doctor's problems; clues that they would have picked up on in their non-medical patients or colleagues. The tell-tale signs of alcohol dependence (no one can fully disguise the stale smell of alcohol on the breath or clothes) or the sudden weight loss of someone not eating through depression, or even the small cuts of a someone self-harming (the 'bare below the elbow' rule makes them even more obvious). It was only after the doctor's condition has come to light that others admit 'they thought something was up' and illustrates how both at the collective and individual level, doctors hold to the notion that they should not be ill.

PATIENTS, THE PUBLIC AND THEIR VIEWS OF SICK DOCTORS

Beyond the obvious of not wanting to wait longer for care, patients do not take kindly to doctors being unwell. This is because it breaks their (the public's) belief that doctors are somehow immune from illness. The sociologist Talcott Parsons described the 'sick role' in terms as having certain roles and responsibilities achieved through maintenance of a paternalistic stance and rigid boundaries between the roles of doctor and patient. These rôles act to maintain the tacit contract between patient and doctor; patients become unwell, not doctors. Both patient and doctors enter unconscious symbiotic processes. The psychiatrist Thomas Main touched on this when he described the defensive interplay of projections between caregivers and patients and the 'fantastic' collusion that occurs between the two:

> The helpful unconsciously require others to be helpless while the helpless will require others to be helpful. Staff and patients are thus inevitably to some extent creatures of each other.[3]

In this process, the nasty, frightening and distasteful aspect of illness can be projected into and contained (held) within health professionals, who given their training and status accept these projections demanded of them by society. If a doctor becomes unwell, how can they hold this pain?

This theme of the collusion between doctor and patient forms the introduction by John Updike of the book the *House of God*:

> We expect the world of doctors. Out of our own need we revere them; we imagine that their training and expertise and saintly dedication have purged them of all the uncertainty, trepidation, and disgust that we would feel in their position, seeing what they see and being asked to cure it. Blood and vomit and pus do not revolt them; senility and dementia have no terror; it does not cause alarm for them to plunge into the slippery tangle of internal organs, or to handle the infected and contacts.[4]

Of course, it makes sense that patients want their doctors to be well, as unwell physicians can impact on patient care.

A study of patients set out to determine how they, based on their own personal experience, perceived doctors' health and its link to care. Three overarching themes emerged. Firstly, patients notice cues in their doctors that they interpret as signs of being well or unwell (so the way doctors dressed, whether they looked tired, ran late, looked stressed, engaged in general dialogue with the patient, and so on). Secondly, patients formed views based on what they noticed, and these judgments directly influenced how they felt about their care. Finally, patients made a direct link between doctor wellness and the care they received.

Unwell doctors were seen in a negative light by the patients in this study. For example, they were seen as less competent and more likely to make errors; less appropriate in their interactions, disorganised; and more likely to place added responsibilities on patients to limit their problem list. Patients also described feeling less comfortable with and less trusting of unwell doctors, even to the point of seeking care elsewhere.[5]

CONCLUSION

In this chapter I have highlighted the difficulties other doctors have when asked to treat their own colleagues. Both the sick doctor and the treating-doctor feel embarrassed and find it difficult to accept the change of role (from professional to patient). Nevertheless, it is important that we all accept when we need help. When doctors do seek help, they have remarkably good outcomes in terms of reduced distress, impairments, abstinence rates and overall improvements in their mental health. This is why it is so important to encourage doctors to make that giant step (for them) from professional to patient. Maybe next time I am unwell, I will be open and honest enough to practise what I preach.

REFERENCES

1   McKall K. An insider's guide to depression. *BMJ* 2001;**323**(7319):1011.
2   Balint E, Courtenay M, Elder A, Hull S, Julian P. *The Doctor, the Patient and the Group: Balint Revisited.* London and New York: Routledge, 1993.
3   Main T. Some psychodynamics of large groups. In: Kreeger L (ed). The Large Group. London: Constable, 1975, pp. 57–86.
4   Shen S. *The House of God.* London: Black Swan, 1985.
5   Lemaire J, Ewashina D, Polachek A, Dixit J, Yiu V. Understanding how patients perceive physician wellness and its links to patient care: a qualitative study. *PLoS One* 2018;**13**(5):e0196888.

18

The Doctors' Doctor

RICHARD DUGGINS

I have enjoyed the privilege of assessing and treating doctors as the mainstay of my clinical work now for 12 years. This chapter allows me the opportunity of sharing my personal reflections and learning from my work with doctors as their psychiatrist and psychotherapist. It is a personal view.

THE IMPORTANCE OF IDENTIFICATION

During the time I have been caring for sick doctors, perhaps the biggest hurdle I have had to deal with is my natural inclination to overidentify with their suffering, to be overly empathic. Of course, empathy is needed, and helps patients feel comfortable. It helps them feel safe enough to open up, and for me to be able to listen to them with compassion (the cornerstone of empathy). It is natural that I identify with my doctor-patients who, after all, may have similar childhood backgrounds, familiar schooling experiences and of course common clinical and personal struggles. However, it is easy to overdo, especially, as I sit and listen to their stories, I feel the anxiety-provoking realisation of 'there but for the grace of God, go I', a sense of survivor guilt. How is it not possible to feel their distress so deeply? Unbridled empathy means that I take on their pain, stress and anxiety. I become angry on their behalf and want to rail against the unfairness of their situation. Taking on their feelings and living through their experience can lead to me feeling hopeless and helpless on their behalf, a form of countertransference as I embody their emotions.

Over-identification can also lead me one of **two ways**. The first is to want to draw closer to them, physically and emotionally so, as if by narrowing the distance between us I can make the pain go away and fix their problem. This form of identification can have the result of me overdoing my help, and even be intrusive, such as offering solutions when none are required or to want to fix things that can remain broken. Identification can have powerful influences on therapeutic boundaries. I might extend the appointment length, offer more sessions than necessary, be too accessible and help with things that I would not normally do.

Alternatively, overidentification can lead me in the opposite direction, to create a greater distance between us, to draw away and put on my inquisitive brakes, being less curious about them. When I reflect why this might be, I suspect somewhere in my unconscious is the fear of contagion, or perhaps not wanting to see myself mirrored in their suffering. This kind of identification might lead me to avoid their pain, and even to discharging my patients too quickly or referring them elsewhere. A balance must be struck.

It is vital for the best outcomes for my patients that I maintain a regular therapeutic stance and distance, and to achieve this it is essential I invest in reflection and supervision to explore the frequent pushes and pulls in my therapeutic relationship with my patients.

THE ACCEPTANCE OF LOVE

An important part of working with patients in general, but in my experience with doctors specifically, is they can induce feelings of love as part of the therapeutic relationship. This is not the romantic love of affairs, but a therapeutic love linked to transference, the predisposition we all have to transfer onto people in the present experiences and related emotions and unmet longings associated with our past. Transference can happen both ways and has to be understood. I have come to accept the powerful transferences induced by my identification with my doctor-patients means that caring for them cannot be a 'nine-to-five' job in my mind. Although I may finish my clinical work, their struggles and pain continue to percolate throughout my mind at home.

MAINTAINING THERAPEUTIC BOUNDARIES

I am a psychotherapist. I understand boundaries and their importance in all therapeutic relationships. Boundaries are linked to safe clinical work and provide a containing space for patient and therapist alike. Given the shared common spaces that all doctors inhabit (such as connections through medical school or later training, or common social networks) it is harder to maintain strict boundaries compared to non-medical patients. However, over the years I have found that doctor-patients yearn for strict boundaries (certainly at the beginning of treatment) as it makes it easier for them to become 'the patient' if I am 'the doctor'. They struggle enough with knowing the correct boundaries they should bring to our relationship and I have learnt to do everything possible to help them with this. They can feel unsure if they should behave as my patient, my colleague or somewhere in between. Their identification with me as a possibly overworked clinician can lead them not to wish to burden me, and perhaps not to open up in a way that is essential for their care. I have learned to be clear with regard to boundaries, including how, when and why, they should contact me between appointments.

Tempted as I am with this 'special group', I have learned that my boundaries need to be the same as for all my other patients; no stricter, but no more flexible, and in that way doctors get the best treatment they can from me. I have learnt to temper my inclination to share my own stories with them, or to divulge personal anecdotes as they map across to theirs.

RESPECTING SHAME

Shame is a powerful force in doctors presenting to me for treatment. Throughout these years I have seen how becoming unwell can feel such a failure for them, maybe similar to how an investment banker must feel if they become bankrupt. I find many of my patients hold a deep fear of physical and mental illness, and a belief that becoming a doctor somehow should magically protect them from ill health. They feel intense shame and personally responsible for becoming unwell in the first place. I have learned that shame colours almost everything in the consultation, and it is important that I am aware of this, and I try to draw it gently into the open for the therapeutic relationship to deepen. The temporary inability to work can cause deep shame, and this shame is often not rational, because it is not relieved by the obvious reality that it is severe symptoms of an illness out of the doctor's control that are currently preventing a return to work.

NOT EXPECTING TOO MUCH

I am impressed with my patients; at the very least they have survived a long and grueling training, and are able to deal with suffering, disability and illness on a daily basis. In common parlance, they are intensely resilient. Yet (or maybe because of) many describe a troubled past, with a childhood where they had to be self-reliant and 'grow-up fast', caring for themselves as one or other of their parents where physically or psychologically absent. One of my key learnings about doctors is that often their intellect develops ahead of other aspects of themselves, such as their emotional intelligence.

In assessing and treating doctors, I frequently find their intellect helps us to come quickly to a rational shared understanding of how past traumas or enduring difficulties with certain emotions, may be influencing their current problems. I am careful, however, not to let their impressive intellectual grasp of their difficulties lead me to expect a similarly rapid emotional processing. I have learned to use at least as much care with doctors around exploring emotionally upsetting topics as I do with all my other patients. A high intellect does not, and should not, guarantee the same level of emotional maturity. I have found it wise to tread carefully, and respectfully build-up the emotional aspects of my consultations. I deeply regret the occasions when I have emotionally 'leapt-in' at the deep end with an intellectually very-able doctor and left them confused and distressed because I have not gone at their pace.

RECOGNISING PERSONALITY STRUCTURES AND DEFENCES

Rationalisation, minimisation and denial are the 'Holy Trinity' of psychological defence mechanisms seen in doctors. They explain why they do not seek care or come late for treatment (and often as a result are more unwell than others). They spend months or years explaining away or ignoring their difficulties. Invariably at our first appointment my patient will explain to me that they feel they are wasting my time, before going on to describe eventually the symptoms of significant psychological distress. In our consultations doctors will play down both their symptoms and their distress. I find the concept of 'compassionate scepticism' to be helpful and leads me to enquire more about their presenting problems. Doctors manage to maintain a brave face, or to put on their mask of coping. They might even lie to themselves (and to me) about the extent of their despair or underscore themselves on routine mental health questionnaires. Asking for objective evidence of illness, such as sleep disturbance or weight loss, is essential. I give special attention to eliciting suicidal thoughts, and take an alcohol and drug history, as these are easily underplayed.

This book has already touched on the common personality structures in doctors, especially perfectionism, obsession and compulsivity. I have found it helpful, and so do many of my patients, thinking about these traits as both a gift as well as a curse. These qualities make us good doctors; they help us work hard, succeed, be persistent and practise safely. They are selected for by medical schools and encouraged in our training. However, many doctors notice as they become more stressed, that these qualities become more pronounced and inflexible. This means that the very qualities that make us good doctors, under stress, make us more likely to become unwell. Doctors' high expectations and associated severe criticism are usually turned inward. I think this often reflects the doctor's experience when growing up, where they learned to be harsh on themselves so as to protect their parents from their anger, criticism and blame. I find I am often protected from criticism in the consultation in a way that mirrors how they protected and still protect others in their life. Their high expectations also lead to overwork, and neglect of replenishing social and pleasurable activities. While doctors are compassionate and kind to their patients, at the same time they can be severe and intolerant towards any personal vulnerability, especially when unwell. This can result in self-destructive suicidal thoughts and plans. Doctors are a high-risk group for suicide, and I work hard in every consultation to keep this thought at the forefront of my mind. I have discovered a potentially dangerous situation can be created if I collude with their wish to minimise, rationalise and deny such risks. I have learned to become more courageous in helping them (and me) gently face the reality of their situation.

IDENTIFYING THE LINK BETWEEN COMPULSIVE CARING AND VICTIMHOOD

The concepts of 'compulsive caring' and the 'wounded healer' are based on the premise that individuals become doctors to try to work through imperfect childhoods. Doctors are trained to put others first even when they are unwell themselves, maybe doing this, not just because it is what is expected in 'make the patient your first concern', but because it deflects from admitting our own vulnerability. Projecting 'weakness' into others, helps bolster our own sense of confidence. Another reason is that many doctors struggle with the emotion of anger.

In my experience, doctors see anger as a negative emotion, and have often, from their childhood, buried it deeply to protect others from it. The problem with repressing anger is that it is then not available to be harnessed in asserting boundaries around personal self-care, and especially in the effective saying of 'no'. I have met many doctors who, on the face of it, appear powerfully competent in their professional demeanour, but who feel they have little control over their workload or relationships. In more extreme cases, this suppression has led my patients to become victims, staying with abusive work arrangements or destructive personal relationships, because they cannot assert their self-care.

A linked theoretical concept is **learned helplessness**. Doctors can often have childhood experiences of parents who are physically or emotionally absent, and as a result learn they are helpless to change their parents, but they can become self-reliant. This self-reliance can lead to a life-long tendency towards passive tolerance of inadequate care from others (be they employers or romantic partners), with no learned experience that they can act to change it.

WORKING, BUT NOT COLLUDING, WITH ATTACHMENT PATTERNS

Everyone has an attachment style, which is our 'go-to' characteristic way of relating. The concept of attachment style comes from attachment theory, one of the leading frameworks for understanding emotional regulation, personality development and interpersonal relationships. Attachment styles are laid down in childhood and persist from cradle to grave.

In my experience, a typical attachment style I observe in doctors is 'dismissive', meaning they play down the importance of emotions and of personal relationships. A dismissive attachment style may be helpful at certain times in a medical career, for example, it may be useful to dismiss our own and others' distress when we are facing significant and prolonged exposure to stress during our training. I find such doctors to be self-reliant, independent, but also 'swan-like', with a cool exterior hiding frantic anxious paddling below the surface. It is important to make allowances for such an attachment style because delving into feelings too quickly will feel unnatural to such doctors and harm engagement. Therefore, with doctors I often make our initial meetings relatively formal and business-like to match their preferred way of relating. I actively structure the session, ask questions and transparently explain why their answers are important. Such doctors can be helped to feel safe in treatment by the use of rational explanations of discussions of their mood, and the defining of an explicit collaborative focus and goals. However, there is a balance to be struck, and it is crucial that I do not collude with their dismissive attachment style for too long by keeping things away from the emotional field. As our treatment progresses and as soon as it feels safe for me to do so, I start to work hard to introduce exploration about their feelings and relationships. This is crucial because it may well be their difficulties with processing emotions, or challenge in managing the softer side of their interpersonal relationships, which has led to their presentation, and is where they need help.

Although less common, the other attachment style I tend to encounter in doctors is 'preoccupied'. In my experience doctors with this attachment style tend to express their emotions freely, and work very hard in maintaining relationships, even if this is at the cost of their self-care. These doctors often report a career with few or no complaints because it is second nature for them to go the extra mile to make sure people are happy. With such doctors it is also important to initially follow their natural attachment style, and in this case this involves facilitating a more open, less-structured approach that allows them to express emotions and fears about relationships. People with a preoccupied attachment style can struggle with slowing down and reflecting rationally on what thoughts and actions are needed. The balance to strike here is to engage such doctors by ensuring they feel emotionally heard and understood, but to slowly work towards helping them to slow down, reflect and plan their recovery.

TAKING CARE OF OMNIPOTENCE

Although most doctors do not recognise it, they enjoy a healthy amount of omnipotence. Omnipotence is helpful and encouraged by our training, for it allows us to take on difficult encounters and have the belief that things will be alright. I certainly needed omnipotence to turn up for my terrifying night shifts as a junior doctor. Our omnipotence also allows us to feel differently from our patients. It allows us to deny the fact that we are as fragile and vulnerable as them.

Omnipotence can be harmful though, as it means we can take on far too much with little sense of our personal limits. We can find we are the person wearing 10 different hats due to our additional roles or working 60 or more hours per week. Omnipotence also encourages independence rather than interdependence, with everyone coming to the doctor for help without the doctor expecting any personal support for themselves.

The most characteristic presentation I see again and again in doctors presenting to me is what I term the 'performance cliff'. This is a sudden crash in work performance associated with an internal switch from omnipotence to impotence, superhero to superzero. In this deeply distressing change, my patients report that they suddenly find they cannot go on, and they need to stop work. I initially felt confused seeing senior doctors with incredible careers presenting to me saying they cannot be a doctor; they are a failure and would be better off dead. I have come to see this as a result of the sudden loss of the defence of omnipotence as these doctors had used this for years to shore-up their self-esteem or mask vulnerability. When omnipotence falters because they finally reach their limit, their unconscious fears of inadequacy break-through. I have learned this presentation needs to be approached with great care, because doctors often feel hopeless and suicidal at this time. However, I find that firm, confident and reassuring holding of the therapeutic relationship can lead to rapid improvement. My work is then to help the doctor recover while not having to return to their previous level of omnipotence, so they can recognise they have a human side that needs to be paid attention to.

In dealing with doctor-patients, I have to be aware that my own omnipotence can be stimulated. This has led me to manage doctors more independently than is helpful, not to involve other professionals or discuss them with my team. To protect myself from this unhelpful behaviour, I maintain a careful watch for such developing omnipotent feelings and make good use of my regular supervision.

ELICITING UNCONSCIOUS CONTRACTS

I have found some doctors have deeply held unconscious contracts with regard to their work and can feel betrayed when they feel these contracts are broken. Examples include, 'if I work hard and do my best then it will be alright', or 'if I treat people fairly then they will treat me fairly'. Another common contract is linked to the psychology of postponement, in which doctors believe if they work hard now their reward will come later. I find it helpful to look out for these beliefs, especially if a doctor is presenting with feelings akin to betrayal. Often, they will not be explicitly aware of these beliefs until we bring them to light.

PSYCHOEDUCATION AND INVOLVING THE FAMILY

My patients find it helpful when I routinely provide psychoeducation around diagnosis, treatment and prognosis, and I make sure not to automatically assume they will already know something because of their training. This does not mean I always go back to basics, but tailored psychoeducation is good practice as part of treatment.

Involving family members has been a more recent addition to my work, and it is a very helpful intervention. Often due to shame and personality factors, doctors minimise their illness and keep themselves isolated in their ill health. I know it is easier to collude with their isolation and shame, but I have learned to be brave and challenge them, especially through encouraging the involvement of a close family member or friend. Early on in getting to know a doctor such a meeting with a family member can be helpful in gathering additional information, mobilising support and sharing my assessment and treatment aims. Towards the end of therapy, these meetings can be helpful in sharing the relapse prevention plan and asking for the family member's support in helping the doctor stay well.

THOUGHTFUL CHOICE OF THERAPY

One of the most rewarding aspects to me of working with doctors, is how quickly they recover when engaged in appropriate treatment. I think this is because doctors are motivated, bright and committed, and these are excellent prognostic factors. I find doctors make excellent use of brief therapy.

In thinking about therapy options for doctors, I increasingly give importance to personality and attachment styles. If they are dismissive and play their emotions down, then they may be attracted to a more cognitive therapy such as cognitive behavioural therapy (CBT). However, often these patients can also benefit from therapy that works explicitly and directly with emotions, even though this may feel counterintuitive. Such therapies include psychodynamic psychotherapy, interpersonal therapy (IPT) and cognitive analytic therapy (CAT). These therapies may be more able to reach the parts that need to be reached. Similarly, if a doctor-patient is full of emotion and finding it difficult to slow down, a psychodynamic approach may feel the obvious fit, but actually a CBT treatment may be more helpful in encouraging structured reflection and change.

I have received fulfilment from running a number of therapeutic groups for doctors, and I am particularly struck by how helpful these can be. Group therapy powerfully helps doctors challenge their feelings of shame, stigma and isolation. Groups also give the opportunity for altruism, which can feel especially helpful for those who currently cannot work due to ill health.

CONCLUSION

Doctors are fascinating people to care for, and to me they are rewarding patients to look after. As with everyone, they also bring their complexities to treatment, and I have learned these complexities demand significant understanding and accommodation if I am to help them engage in timely and effective treatment. I have needed to develop courage and confidence in robustly ensuring good clinical care despite the strong pushes and pulls of identification, boundaries, expectations and collusion. I rely heavily on regular personal reflection, peer reflective practice and supervision in keeping my work on task. One of the joys of my work is that I am always learning, and my patients are the most generous and absorbing of tutors.

19

How to Be a Good Enough Patient

From Sickness to Health

PRACTITIONER HEALTH PATIENT AND VOLUNTEER GROUP
AND CLARE GERADA

> *The physician who doctors himself has a fool for a patient.*
>
> **Sir William Osler, 1849–1919**

The Patient and Volunteer Group is made up of doctors who have all been patients of Practitioner Health. They have helped prepare the contents of this chapter, which provides top tips on being and supporting a doctor as a patient and also:

- How to admit vulnerability and become a patient.
- How we might want to engage with a sick colleague in the workplace, and how do to this **safely** and with **compassion**.

TOP TIPS FOR DOCTORS BECOMING PATIENTS

If you are unwell

- Recognise that it is alright to become unwell – after all, you are human.
- Ask for help in time, don't wait too long. If others, ask if you are OK, don't just give a knee jerk response, think about it – perhaps you are not OK.
- Seek help from another doctor or health practitioner. Now is not the time to be self-diagnosing or self-medicating. Seek advice and listen to it.
- Avoid 'corridor consultations'. Book a date and time to see someone and go with the understanding that in this space you are a patient, not a doctor.

- Remember you can ask for more information about your illness and what happens next. Just because you have medical training doesn't necessarily mean you are an expert in this particular condition, and you also may not be thinking as clearly as you normally would.
- Don't get drawn into organising your own care, arranging tests or examinations. This is the job of the doctor, not the patient.
- Listen to what the health practitioner is telling you, particularly if they are advising time off work. **You don't have to be a hero**. You may feel that you are letting patients or colleagues down if you take time off, but you will get well and be back to work as an effective, healthy clinician far **more quickly** if you follow the advice you are given.
- Make sure you have a good support structure around you. Think about who needs to know about your situation (family, friends, direct line manager) and what level of detail they need. Doctors either overshare or become isolated and hide themselves away when unwell – particularly if they are off work.
- **Think about *why* you became unwell** – is there something in your work life or lifestyle that should/can be changed? Occupational health can be really helpful here in helping to negotiate any changes.

TOP TIPS FOR DOCTORS WHO HAVE COLLEAGUES AS PATIENTS

- Recognise that the sick doctor in front of you is first and foremost a patient, your patient. They may come with some medical knowledge, but don't assume they are in a position to use that knowledge to help themselves.
- Go back to first principles – ask your patient what their concerns, ideas and expectations are. Explore their presenting complaint.
- Understand that the doctor-patient may be feeling emotionally distressed. They may be lacking insight into how unwell they are, or alternatively, catastrophising about how sick they might be (a little knowledge can be a dangerous thing).
- It's important to recognise that they may be knowledgeable about their illness (it's surprising how many doctors get the illness in their own speciality) but remember you are the doctor and they are the patient. Listen to them, answer questions, give information but be clear about what the best treatment or care plan should be.
- Good communication is vital. Make sure the doctor-patient understands what is being said, repeating anything if necessary. Don't assume a level of knowledge they may not have (even if this means explaining the side-effects of antidepressants to a psychiatrist, or the harms of alcohol to a hepatologist).
- Keep good records, write prescriptions and organise tests yourself, don't expect the doctor-patient to do any of this for themselves.
- Doctor-patients are often concerned about the confidentiality of their consultations and records. Think about who might have access to clinical

notes and what you can do to preserve confidentiality. For example, can electronic or paper records be stored so they are not accidentally accessible to all administrators or colleagues of the doctor-patient? Can you place an alert on computer records or restrict access to them?

- Doctor-patients may need support to make decisions, particularly when this involves taking time off to recover. Remember doctor-patients who are away from work can feel guilty at letting patients or colleagues down; they can become isolated and their condition can worsen as a result. Ensure they have support at home, consider their safety net and make sure they are followed-up.
- Don't escalate concerns about whether the doctor-patient should be at work or not **without discussing this with them**. There may be situations when a doctor should not be working in your opinion – remind them that to go against such advice would not be sensible and could put their registration at risk. However, it's also important for them to know that in most cases regulators are not interested in getting involved in health matters if the doctor-patient is seeking and following medical advice. Self-disclosure of a health issue is always preferable to a doctor-patient being 'reported' and you can have a role in supporting them to do this if necessary.
- Do not share information about your doctor-patient outside the consulting room **unless it is absolutely necessary** (and this should mean only where there is a serious risk to self or others). Just because they are a trainee doctor or working in the same hospital does NOT mean you need to inform anyone. You can advise the doctor that they might want to consult with Occupational Health or their clinical director, but you should not be doing this on their behalf without their explicit informed consent.
- Remember, the GMC's own guidance states:

If, with the right support, you are able to manage a health problem so that the care that you give your patients is not affected, then your fitness to practise won't be affected. So, there will be no need for us to be involved or even to know about it.[1]

- Finally, consider if you are OK. Being a doctor to a doctor can be challenging and comes with its own stressors. Consider if you need any support or to discuss how the impact of caring for one of your own has affected you.

TOP TIPS FOR FAMILY AND FRIENDS OF A DOCTOR-PATIENT

- Encourage your friend or family member to be a patient, to listen and take the advice being offered to them.
- Keep an open mind about the level of knowledge they may or may not have about their condition. Remember they may not be able to apply their own learning and knowledge at this time.

- Don't criticise or judge them for not recognising their own illness – doctors are notoriously poor at realising they are unwell or seeking help in a timely manner.
- Stay in touch, particularly if they are off work – they may be feeling isolated or alone.
- Encourage them to attend appointments, to take time off work if needed.
- Be a critical friend. Challenge them if they are pushing back on the medical advice they have been given or refusing to take time off. You may have some medical knowledge of your own but **use this wisely** – don't fall into the trap of becoming a second doctor to them.
- Ensure they have support around them. Encourage them to join a support group or find others in a similar situation. Remember, however, that it can be hard for doctors to access support groups with members of the public. This is not only for reasons of confidentiality, but because group members often may be criticising their own doctors and care, which can put additional strain on the doctor-patient.
- Think about the impact on them of becoming unwell. They may have fears for their future (training or jobs); there may be money worries if they are not currently working; and concerns about other issues they are facing. Ask them and help them identify support.
- **Be kind** – doctors are notoriously tough on themselves when they become ill so having you on their side will be invaluable.

STOPPING AND RETURNING TO WORK

Many of the group have spent long periods of time not working – either due to a restriction on their practise by their employer or the GMC or through illness. Fortunately, a large number have returned to work and this is the advice they give on how to manage both processes (unemployment and return to work).

Time away from work and sick leave

Some do's and don'ts:

- Do ensure you are registered with a general practitioner.
- Do keep a copy of your sick notes when submitted.
- Do ensure managers are notified if you are going to be away from home or uncontactable for more than a few days, to avoid missed emails or appointments. If you are on paid sick leave you can still take holidays and be paid for it.

If you are attending your workplace for a review, try to make the appointment soon after, rather than just before, an occupational health appointment and allow time for any correspondence to be sent and seen. Most occupational health reports do not go into clinical details but are restricted to issues relating to fitness to work, adjustments that might be needed and a time frame for returning to work. You are not under obligation to discuss details of your illness with your colleagues or managers. If necessary, seek advice from your Trade Union if there are issues relating to your contract or where your employer is making it difficult for you to return to work.

Regular contact with your clinical director or manager is vital. It allows for general progress reports to be given to a single person rather than for everyone to know your personal issues. This makes it easier for planning for returning to work (or not) and allows for a coordinated approach to your case. A link with colleagues and the workplace is maintained, which helps avoid the feeling of isolation and being totally estranged from work. Any restrictions or conditions on employment can be accommodated and integrated into the return to work plan. Importantly, any possible changes in pattern of work on return can be planned well ahead.

If the workplace and its stresses are a significant factor in your illness, this can be discussed in order to minimise recurrent illness. Continuing reviews after return should allow for any new difficulties to be discussed. You do not need to be 100% well before returning to work (in fact no one is ever 100% physically or mentally well) but remember it is difficult to take more time off once you have returned, so equally don't feel pressurised to return too soon.

Things to do before returning to work

- Rehearse returning to work – especially important if you have been off work for a while. Practise getting up early for at least a week before and take the route to work, in rush hour for a few days beforehand.
- Try to find a colleague who will allow you to sit in with them for a few days before returning to work.
- Acclimatise yourself if there have been any changes in the workplace or if you will be starting in a new environment.
- A prolonged period away from work may result in accumulation of annual leave. Sick leave of more than six months will result in half pay but taking annual leave after being signed off sick leave and before return to work is at full pay rates. This may be regarded in a negative way by some colleagues, but two weeks holiday and rest are very different to being on sick leave.
- Each employer will have rules about carrying over annual leave not taken in the previous year, frequently five days. This should be confirmed by agreement with the appropriate manager and documented. More than this can sometimes be negotiated.
- It is important that your clinical director and the rota master know of any conditions or voluntary undertakings from the GMC, as these should be built into and considered in the return plan; for example, requirements around supervision, on-call or not working alone.
- If you have an associated depressive illness, night-time medication may initially cause some morning drowsiness and it is important you are stable on these treatments. It may, for instance, require postponing starting night-time duties. Similarly, if you can't drive following a drink-driving offence, allowances may have to be made.

Return to work

A date for return to work should be reached after discussion with relevant staff. Do not rush back or try to bring the return date forward – the specialists looking after you know what time frames are reasonable far **better than we ourselves may perceive**. Nothing is to be gained from doing what you think would go down well with the department – you may be quite emotionally vulnerable for a while. Often there is a feeling of being 'tested' and under criticism from colleagues. It is important to bring up any problems during your phased return and maybe accept that your previous sessions require some alterations. When you first return to the department, **don't be a 'people-pleaser' and take on too much**. You may feel isolated to start with, and that colleagues are a bit wary of you.

Remember that colleagues probably had to cover for you and put up with some difficult behaviour before you went on sick leave; some may still feel resentful, so trust has to be rebuilt slowly. Don't feel the need to tell everyone everything. Going to 12-steps meetings or counselling encourages you to be honest and involves sharing some deeply personal information. That is appropriate in a safe place, but those not familiar with the 12-steps recovery programmes often find this honesty a little threatening and are not expecting it and don't know how to react. People will talk about you, that's human nature, but this won't go on for very long. Everyone is busy and preoccupied with their own lives. Even if your case has made the local or national papers, it will be 'tomorrow's fish and chip paper' – i.e. things will die down, people will become bored and will get on with other things.

In those first few weeks back at work:

- Go to bed early.
- Don't be surprised if it feels like a bit of a culture shock – **it is**!
- Don't worry if, for a while, all you do is get up, go to work and get a good night's sleep.
- Don't feel obliged to organise or take on new ventures – it is easy to feel a bit guilty after a while away and tempting to make up for it by volunteering for new things. Your personal welfare must come first at this stage.
- Try to be positive and appropriately enthusiastic, but don't do things because you feel you ought to.
- Make sure any outpatient and other follow-up appointments are allowed for in your initial work plan.

It can be daunting to return to work after a period of sick leave, but be reassured, it is not difficult, and many do make this transition very safely.

REFERENCES

1 General Medical Council. Your health matters Practical tips and sources of support [Internet]. 2014. Available from: www.gmc-uk.org/-/media/documents/dc7210---your-health-matters-1215_pdf-56661104.pdf.

20

Services for Mentally Ill Doctors

CLARE GERADA

Jo felt terrible. He had tried to ring the help number on the card left at the end of a lecture on burnout he'd attended last month. Each time he tried to ring he put the phone down before anyone answered. Every day now he wanted to die and had even begun to dream about dying. He had begun to stockpile drugs that he was buying from different pharmacies. He felt as if he was wearing dark glasses all the time, his life seemed so grey and empty. Work was his only distraction and the alcohol that numbed his thoughts at the end of the day. He was depressed. It had been triggered after the death of a baby from sepsis a few months ago. He knew he wasn't to blame, but somewhere deep down he felt he was. If he had been more experienced things might have worked out differently. Now he was checking everything he did, twice over. He was even beginning to go into work on his days off just to check up on his decisions. He felt useless as a doctor. All his training didn't save the baby. He couldn't get the look of anguish on the mother's face from his mind. He was terrified about seeking help. What if 'they' made him refer himself to the Regulator. He didn't want to give all his details in case 'they' told someone. He wasn't even sure himself who the 'they' were. He tried the number again. This time he let it ring and after four rings a friendly voice the other end answered 'hello, this is Nadia, how can I help you'. Jo started to cry and told Nadia that he was desperate and needed help. Within the next few minutes he had been given an appointment to see a doctor the following week.

Doctors' health problems are not unique, nor is the environment in which they work. Jo does not have a special illness; he has depression. Nor does he require different medicines or interventions than any other patient. Doctors' mental illnesses respond just as well, or for some conditions better, than their non-medical counterparts. Where doctors do differ is how they go about seeking help, and how those who care for them, treat them (see Chapters 15 and 16). It still surprises me the lengths mentally ill doctors will go not to access care. Maybe I too am guilty of this.

This chapter discusses what services are available, how they differ across the world and what makes a good service (good with respect to improving access for care).

PHYSICIAN HEALTH SERVICES

Advantages of doctor-specific services include:

- They encourage early presentation.
- They provide expert management of mentally unwell doctors.
- They help doctors in different inter-related areas, including dealing with mental illness, complaints, return to work and support in disciplinary action.
- They can respond and begin treatment quickly.
- They provide value for money.
- They ensure better protection for the public in having potentially impaired doctors in treatment.

The first specific programmes for doctors were established in North America with the aim of preventing malpractice, mainly related to drug and alcohol misuse. Other programmes have now been developed across the world. Some of these are probation-like (monitoring, supervision, coordination), others are more akin to community mental health treatment services. There are some general features that improve the chances of doctors using physician health services.

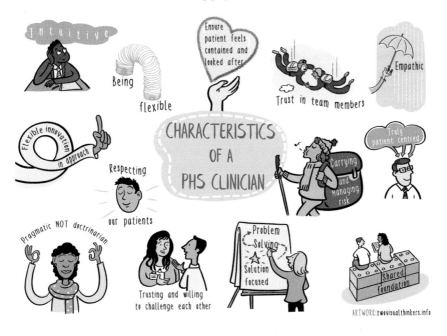

Assessment

Jo was seen for his first assessment. He sat back in the chair facing the doctor he was seeing. The doctor had already told him that everything he said would be kept confidential unless there were serious concerns about him or his patients. He felt reassured. He had never seen anyone for a mental illness, but here he was. Despite his anxiety about being there he began to tell his story. He told about his guilt following the death of the baby. The doctor asked him some questions. He wasn't expecting them, but they made him think. He was asked why he chose to study medicine. He hesitated. It sounded such a cliché – but the reason was because he was inspired by a local GP when he was younger. He had been a very sick child and was having to see his GP on many occasions. The man had always been so kind and given him a small packet of sweets every time he went. He wanted to do the same as his GP and 'stop children dying'. The doctor asked him about other issues and helped him think through what else might be underlying his catastrophic response to the death of the child. Just talking about his mood helped. At the end of the consultation he couldn't understand why had had been so worried about seeking help.

Doctors who treat their colleagues must, as with any other doctor–patient interaction, be able to take a proper history. This might be the first time the doctor has been able to tell their story, and it is important to listen with compassion but also to ask pertinent questions along the way. Questions such as why they chose to study medicine, who influenced this decision, why they chose their medical school and particular speciality. These give a sense of how secure their medical identity is and the influences behind their decision to study medicine. We ask about complaints or difficulties at work or gaps in service. For some patients it is important to seek, with consent, corroboration from a third party, such as a family member or close colleague, especially in the management of addiction, patients with bipolar disorder or other complex mental health problems.

Assessment might include a physical examination and, where necessary, routine haematological or drug and/or alcohol testing (urine, blood or hair).

Our assessment covers:

- Personal and family history (including other doctors in the family).
- Past medical and psychiatric history, including any addictive behaviours.
- School, postgraduate and medical school, training and work history.
- Breaks in training or service and why these have occurred.
- Current work (including private practice, academic work).
- Academic achievements, including prizes, distinctions, failures or deferments.
- Involvement with complaints, significant events, referral to regulator.
- Any financial problem.

History taking helps formulate the doctor's problem. I find the 5-P framework helpful with developing a formulation.[1]

Predisposing factors – for example, early traumatic events, family history of mental illness, childhood trauma, disabilities.

Precipitating factors – triggers leading to someone asking for help, and why now.

Presenting problem – which the person describes as the issue they want help with and why they feel the problem as arisen.

Perpetuating factors – unhelpful behaviours and thoughts that are maintaining the problem or on-going problems secondary to the presenting issue, such as financial or health issues.

Protective factors – including healthy coping strategies, support networks, sustaining and enjoyable employment.

Multidisciplinary teams

Physician health services that operate in a multidisciplinary way bring added benefits to the patient from the different expertise clinicians bring. It also allows for decisions and risks to be shared, important when caring for patients who themselves work in a high risk and difficult environment.

At my service we meet weekly, and all new patients are discussed and anyone we are concerned about. Usually the case is straightforward, but sometimes we mull over issues such as who else needs to be involved, whether they are safe to work or whether they need to stop and what other risk factors might be present.

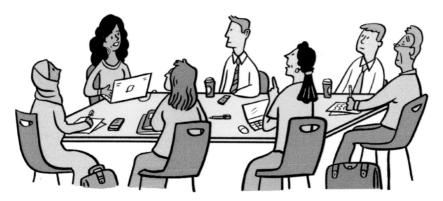

Assessing risk

Most physician health services have a means of assessing, addressing and minimising risk. This is important when caring for mentally ill doctors, as we have to be mindful that there are two sets of patients in the mix: the patient in front of us (the doctor) who might pose a risk to themselves (including professional self-harm) and secondly the patients who these doctors manage and who might be harmed if a doctor is unfit to practise. There is also the potential damage a sick doctor might pose to their organisation. At our service, we carry out a risk assessment on every patient.

Depending on the problem and severity, patients are risk-rated as either green (lowest), amber or red (greatest). The risk category determines how often the patient is seen and how proactive we are at following them up. Green for example, means that the patient attends on an as-necessary basis. Red, that we have serious concerns about the patient and would want to review them (either face-to-face or telephone) at least weekly. The process of ascribing a risk status to patients ensures we look in depth at their issues and how these might impact on their behaviour (e.g. suicide risk or risk of breaking down at work). An important aspect of any assessment is to make sure that the doctor if unwell, is safe to continue working.

> *Arif lived in hospital accommodation. He recently started working as a locum. His family live in Libya and he came to work in England a few years ago. It is hard now for him to return. Arif had recently been suspended after a complaint from a patient who said he had been rude to her and shouted. He denies this, saying he had been upset as the patient had been racist to him and had said she didn't want to see a foreign doctor. Even before this, he had noticed how irritable he had become and had lost interest in most things. All he seemed to do was work. He had no friends, no family in England and no real social network. He started to cry. He said he would be better off dead.*

Arif was rated as the highest risk, red. He lives alone, in hospital accommodation and is socially isolated. He undertook his primary medical qualification overseas, which means he has additional cultural, professional and social issues to contend with. He is depressed, has a complaint and is suspended from work. We would make sure that we kept close contact with him (at least weekly) and offered treatment, most likely including antidepressants, talking therapy and a place at our group for doctors who are excluded from work. We would also offer support around the complaint and hopefully de-personalise the issue and help him see it in perspective.

Risk Assessment Group (RAG) rating	Examples
RAG Risk Green Reviewed 'as and when'	Mild to moderate symptoms Good social and/or family network Other factors (for example, no major financial issues, partner supportive) Work colleagues involved and supportive
RAG Risk Amber Reviewed monthly	Bipolar affective disorder, in contact with other services but still acutely unwell Mental illness with other issues that might cause problems (e.g. waiting on the outcome of a regulatory determination) Few social supports Financial issues, but still able to pay bills

RAG Risk Red Reviewed weekly or more often	Bipolar affective disorder and not in contact with any other service Severe depressed mood BMI <16 Intravenous drug use Anaesthetist who uses any drugs Anaesthetists with depression Serious complaint or referral to the regulator Lives alone, especially if in hospital accommodation Previous suicide attempt International medical graduate

Confidentiality

CONFIDENTIALITY

One feature, which might seem obvious, is for staff to understand the regulatory framework in which doctors work. It is crucial that the treating clinicians are competent in recognising when and to what extent it is appropriate to maintain patient confidentiality. This can be a fine line, best decided in the context of team working where issues are discussed, risks assessed and a treatment plan formulated. Those not familiar with treating mentally ill doctors might feel they have to escalate issues unnecessarily. I can remember one patient who sought help for depression, finding that unbeknown to him, his own psychiatrist had made a referral to the regulator; sadly, this psychiatrist wrongly assumed that all mental illness needs to be disclosed.

Doctors must trust the service they present to and really believe they will be treated in confidence. Fear of breach of confidentiality is probably the single most common reason given for doctors not accessing care for mental health problems.

Our service has a series of measures to ensure confidentiality is secure, including:

- All electronic correspondence uses a unique confidential number.
- We avoid paper correspondence wherever possible.
- Doctors can register using a pseudonym.
- All staff, including external contractors, have to adhere to our confidentiality policy.
- A patient has a right to bar any clinician from seeing their records or being present at discussions about them.
- We are mindful of, and mark the notes accordingly, where we might have members of the same family or close friends/colleagues also attending the service (which often happens).

- We do not disclose records to any third party except where required by law.
- We work on the principle that there is 'nothing about me without me'. This means that, bar exceptional circumstances, what is said in the service stays in the service and the doctor's confidentiality is paramount.

Even given all of these reassurances, there are situations where unavoidably, confidentiality needs to be breached. This is the same for all of our patients, irrespective of their professional groups. For example, in the UK, we have to notify certain infectious diseases, certain criminal behaviours and child and adult safeguarding issues. For doctors, given our additional roles with patients, there are times when a treating doctor has a duty to disclose them to the regulator (or the doctor has to self-disclose). This is where there is evidence that the doctor might be putting patients at risk or continues to engage in criminal activity.

Ancillary services

Good physician services offer structured after-care, including group and individual options. They also offer a range of other services, such as access to in-patient rehabilitation treatment, return to work support and prescribing.

EXAMPLES OF PHYSICIAN HEALTH SERVICES

North American Physician Health Programmes (USA PHPs)

The North American physician health services have been in operation for over 50 years.[2] They were established as a response to high number of suicides and increasing rates of addiction among doctors, and in an effort to replace disciplinary action with a more empathic, treatment-like approach. They have since become a billion-dollar industry providing support to and monitoring of doctors in almost all States. They have evolved under the authority of the medical licencing boards with support from the American Medical Association. They have the dual role of helping addicted physicians attain sobriety while also providing assurance to colleagues, hospital insurers, licencing boards and the general public that these physicians can practise safe care.[3] They are essentially probation services, though they do have other functions with respect to education, training and prevention activities. The underlying assumption is that early detection and active management of substance misuse protects patients and the public and can help prevent legal, regulatory and employment problems for the doctor, such that their career and life can be protected.

PHPs provide monitoring and supervision of doctors who have signed formal, binding contracts for participation (generally extending for five years). State medical licencing boards often accept the care of the PHP in lieu of imposing disciplinary action, as long as any failure to stick to the recommendations and/or return to the use of alcohol or other drugs is reported back to them. Contracts typically stipulate attending accredited treatment providers, regular random drug testing (typically five out of seven days a week for at least five years) as well as unscheduled work site visits for extended periods. While American PHPs do not directly provide treatment, nevertheless they recommend treatment pathways doctors have to adhere to. For the most part, this would include abstinence-orientated residential care with a 12-step-orientated outpatient treatment, most espousing the principles of Alcoholics Anonymous, Narcotics Anonymous and other 12-step programmes. The doctor is responsible for the costs of treatment, drug monitoring and costs of seeing a therapist or psychiatrist.

Physicians who engage and comply with treatment, and provide negative tests receive support and advocacy from the PHP with their licencing boards and others. On the other hand, those who refuse the terms of the contract and/or are found to continue substance use risk reporting to their boards, which may result in loss of their licences.

American PHPs claim to be non-disciplinary in nature. For example, they are not empowered to subpoena, require participation, impose sanctions or take punitive or disciplinary action. However, as part of a monitoring contract signed by participants, most require reporting of non-compliance or relapse, and other specified situations including reporting by approved clinicians treating the doctor. So, though they have no direct authority to restrict or remove a doctor's licence to practise, they have considerable indirect power to do so via these reporting mechanisms. Therefore, even though they offer 'strict confidentiality' they do not in fact have a traditional doctor–patient relationship. Saying this, PHPs help doctors avoid formal complaints along with any punitive measures that could be imposed by the Medical Boards. They create structure and accountability and offer support, long-term monitoring and management, advocacy and other assistance to doctors. Over the years these interventions have led to high success in terms of abstinence, return to work rates and saving doctors' lives. For those who engage in the programme they achieve excellent outcomes, with reported five-year abstinence rates for substance use disorders of 81%, return to work rates of 86% and little or no evidence of serious risk or harm to patients.[3]

However, despite their success they have their critics, in particular that conflicts of interest of the service to make money can lead to some doctors being coerced into unnecessary treatment programmes leading to significant financial debt.[4] Fees can run into several hundreds of thousands of dollars over the course of engagement. There have been accusations that some PHPs contribute to suicide of doctors.[5] Some programmes are accused of being punitive and unmonitored, depriving doctors of their rights and preventing them from challenging or objecting to diagnoses they disagree with.[6] Treatments and interventions are almost always self-funded, such that doctors with less favourable prognostic outcomes or with financial problems may not engage in the first place and not be included in any outcome figures.

General Medical Council (GMC)

The GMC is the UK medical regulator. As with North American PHPs, the GMC does not treat doctors, rather it provides case management, through undertakings ('promises') or conditions (mandatory requirements) placed on a doctor's licence to practise.[7,8] Within the suite of requirements will be to:

- Attend regular recovery meetings (12 steps).
- Attend therapy.
- Agree to remain under the care of a psychiatrist.
- Allow for any sharing of information between those involved in the care/management of the doctor.
- Limit the number of hours worked.
- Agree to testing (if the concerns involve alcohol or substance misuse).

For those with other mental health problems requirements could include seeking the help of and adhering to the treatment suggested by their treating psychiatrist, workplace monitoring and restricting time or places of work. As with North American PHPs, doctors will be expected to attend for treatment and adhere to the recommendations of their treating doctor. They will also be allocated a GMC approved medical supervisor (a psychiatrist) who will oversee progress and provide reports to the GMC case manager based on information from the doctor's workplace supervisors and other medical practitioners.

NHS Practitioner Health (PH [formally PHP])

The service I lead exemplifies the truism, 'if you build it, they will come'. Our doors opened in November 2008, and I remember with great anxiety wondering whether any doctor would present themselves for care. I need not have worried. Our first patient made contact within minutes and a decade later thousands have registered. The service was the first of its kind in the UK (nationally funded, free at point of use) and has now become one of the largest physician health services in the world. Doctors cannot be forced to attend as part of a disciplinary or performance process – though some are encouraged to attend by their supervisors or employers. Since October 2019 it has been available to all doctors and dentists on the medical register across England.

We provide interventions that would normally be found in a standard outpatient mental health department, with the addition of in-patient treatment for addiction. Where needed we can prescribe medicines and a range of psychological interventions, including group, remote, face-to-face and web-based therapy. If a doctor requires monitoring as part of a disciplinary or regulatory requirement, then this is not undertaken by us but by other bodies such as the GMC, employer or occupational health department. This was a deliberate action to ensure that we maintained our core function as a treatment rather than a probation-like service.

The service provides the following interventions:

- Telephone advice.
- First contact assessment, formulation and treatment planning with a multi-professional approach to care.

- Brief intervention, cognitive behaviour therapy, relapse prevention, brief psychotherapy, case management.
- Prescribing for mental health conditions.
- Community-based detoxification and access to in-patient drug and alcohol detoxification and rehabilitation.
- Substitute medication for opiate addiction.
- Therapeutic blood, urine and hair testing as part of treatment.
- Report writing.
- Attendance at employment tribunals or other work-related hearings.
- Specific interventions, such as behaviour therapy for repeated exam failure.
- Direct liaison with defence organisations/barristers.
- Liaison with educational supervisors/training programme directors where necessary.
- Theraputic Groups.
- Expert help for doctors out of work for long periods (e.g. due to illness or erasure from work).
- Expert patient forum.

Over the first ten years, more than 6,200 doctors have attended our service for help.[9] Around 80% of the patients who come suffer from mental health problems; 10% have a substance misuse problem and the rest a mix of other diagnoses. Of those with mental health problems, around 80% have problems with anxiety, depression, obsessive-compulsive disorder or adjustment disorder; the remaining 20% have serious mental health problems, mostly eating disorders or bipolar affective disorder, and a few have personality disorder or psychosis. For substance misuse disorder, around 75% are related to predominantly alcohol misuse, 10% drug use and the remainder behavioural addictions or mixed drug and alcohol. Over the ten years, the problems doctors present with have stayed more or less the same: anxiety, depression, obsessive-compulsive disorder, alcohol and drug addiction. What has changed is the proportions of each. During the first year more than one-third of all doctors (36%) presented with problems related to either drug or alcohol misuse (mostly alcohol). This figure for the ten-year period (2008–2018) has dropped to 10.1%; for 2017–2018 only around 7% of doctors are presenting with addiction issues.

In actual numbers, and across all specialities, general practitioners (GPs) are most likely to present with problems related to addiction (35% of the total), but this is related to the GPs proportionately being the biggest speciality. However, when weighted according to the numbers presenting from each speciality, anaesthetists, emergency department doctors and dentists have the highest percentages presenting with problems related to addiction. Another change over the years has been a significant drop in those involved with the regulator, from 33% (2008/9) to 5.1% (2017/18). The mean over the years 2008–2018 is 11%. Over the ten years the patients have become younger, and more are female. At the start, more men presented than women (M53% vs. W47%) but by the end of the first decade women far outnumbered men (M32.5% vs. W67.5%). The average age has dropped from 51.6 years (2008/9) to 38.9 years (2017/18); across the ten-year period, the average age is around 41 years (with a range from 24 years old those in their early 70s). Consultants and GPs are more likely to present with complex mental illnesses. Addiction is a feature of all ages.

CONCLUSION

Jo was referred for CBT, which he chose to do as a mix of online and face-to-face with the therapist. By the time he went for his follow-up appointment with the psychiatrist he was feeling a lot better. Once he felt better, he thought it would be useful for his future mental health to join a peer reflective practice support group, which he did.

With the right support doctors not only make good patients, but excellent ones and are able to return safely to work. They follow advice and respond to treatment. They are invested in their recovery and many thousands of those attending my service and similar ones across the world, get better. All of these factors illustrate the importance of having an accessible and confidential service available for doctors, run by staff who understand the special needs of this hard-to-reach group.

REFERENCES

1   Friendly Formulation – Psychology Tools [Internet]. Psychology Tools. 2020 [cited 23 January 2020]. Available from: www.psychologytools.com/resource/friendly-formulation.
2   Federation of State Health Physician Programs [Internet]. Fsphp.org. 2018 [cited 28 September 2019]. Available from: www.fsphp.org/state-programs.
3   McLellan A, Skipper G, Campbell M, DuPont R. Five-year outcomes in a cohort study of physicians treated for substance use disorders in the United States. *BMJ* 2008;**337**(1):a2038.
4   Tjia J, Givens J, Shea J. Factors associated with undertreatment of medical student depression. *J Am Coll Health* 2005;**53**(5):219–24.
5   Lenzer J. Physician health programs under fire. *BMJ* 2016;**353**:i3568.
6   Anderson P. Physician Health Programs: More Harm Than Good? [Internet]. Medscape. 2015 [cited 28 September 2019]. Available from: www.medscape.com/viewarticle/849772#vp_5 and https://disruptedphysician.blog/2015/09/12/physician-health-programs-more-harm-than-good-state-based-programs-under-fire-pauline-anderson.
7   General Medical Council. How we work with doctors with health concerns [Internet]. Improving medical education and practice across the UK. 2017 [cited 23 January 2020]. Available from: https://gmcuk.wordpress.com/2017/09/12/how-we-work-with-doctors-with-health-concerns.

8   General Medical Council. Your health matters. Practical tips and sources of support [Internet]. Available from: www.gmc-uk.org/-/media/documents/dc7210---your-health-matters-1215_pdf-56661104.pdf.

9   Gerada C, Ashworth M, Warner L, Willis J, Keen J. Mental health outcomes for doctors treated at UK Practitioner Health Service: a pilot study. *Res Adv Psychiatry* 2019;**6**(1):7–14.

21

The Migrant Doctor

CLARE GERADA

The term International Medical Graduate (IMG) is used for doctors who have completed their primary medical qualification overseas.

A Staff and Associate Specialist doctor (SAS) is a doctor who works in a subconsultant (leadership) or non-training grade role.

Black Asian Minority Ethnic group – BAME.

There is unequivocal evidence that doctors whose primary medical qualification was not obtained in their host country suffer from additional challenges and discrimination. Compared to doctors who were not trained overseas, these doctors are:[1]

- More likely to experience problems with bullying and harassment.
- More likely to feel less included in their workplace.
- Almost twice as likely to say that they would not feel confident in raising concerns about patient care.
- More likely to say they feared being blamed or suffering adverse consequences.

A vicious cycle ensues, where the inequalities impact on mental well-being, which in turn can affect clinical performance leading to difficulties at work and in turn to more psychological distress. Migrant doctors' problems are compounded as they need to adjust to a new country, a different organisational environment, professional culture and juggling with practical realities of moving to a new country: securing accommodation, setting up bank accounts and so forth. These doctors are under-represented in treatment services and over-represented in disciplinary processes.

INTERNATIONAL MEDICAL GRADUATES AND MENTAL ILLNESS

Some doctors with mental health problems are more invisible than others. Only 15% of the patient population in my service are international medical graduates

(IMGs), despite making up around 40% of UK medical registrants, rising to 25% during COVID-19.[2] This under-representation may be due to IMGs having lower rates of mental illness than those trained in the UK. I do not think this is the case; instead I believe they find it even harder to attend for care. There is evidence that the health of those forced to migrate tends to be better than the general population in both the sending and receiving country. This 'healthy immigrant' effect reflects that those who cross continents have to pass through several ordeals to reach their host country, and only the fittest will survive. However, doctors tend to be drawn from a highly mobile, educated and privileged group, irrespective of the country where they have undertaken their primary medical qualification, and there seems no reason why the health of those who choose to leave might be any different from that of those who stay behind. Until detailed and systematic research is conducted in this area, this can only be conjecture. Those IMGs we see in our service have often struggled alone not knowing where to seek help, and they arrive in an emotionally labile state. Due to language and cultural difficulties they are more likely to have their mental illness misdiagnosed as a performance issue, and instead of being signposted to occupational health or their GP they find themselves embroiled in disciplinary processes. These doctors attend as they have become depressed following a complaint at work, usually because they have been accused of 'not acting as a team player' or being aggressive to staff. I have known doctors, who have come from war-torn areas of the world, having undiagnosed post-traumatic stress disorder 'misdiagnosed' as being a poor communicator.

There may be additional barriers to seeking help, even to accepting that the problem might be psychological at all. Doctors may come from cultures where mental illness as such is not recognised and instead 'disguised' or sublimated into a physical health (somatic) disorder. It is also not uncommon for these doctors to fear that their licence to practise will be removed if they admit to having a mental illness, or worse, that they and any dependents might face deportation. This fear is exacerbated where family members, in the same country or abroad, are dependent on the IMG doctor being in work.

SPECIFIC PROBLEMS THAT IMGS FACE

IMGs face additional pressures that do not apply to UK-born doctors. Leaving one's home country is difficult for anyone, not just for doctors. Migrants face isolation and loneliness, they have to cope with loss and often face discrimination in a variety of forms. My father, who qualified overseas, came to England from Malta in the middle of the 1960s. To secure work he had to accept any job. As such, he took on a series of locum posts across England, dragging with him his wife and four small children, soon to be five. We eventually settled in the east of England, where he accepted a vacant single-handed general practice in a deprived part of Peterborough. While he succeeded in his career, he never belonged to the more established, home-grown general practice community and felt, for his entire life, an outsider to the emerging Royal College of General Practitioners. I wonder what he would have made of his daughter eventually leading the College, which was a role I was honoured to do, and was only the second woman in their 50-year history to hold this post. My father's story is not unique. The 1960s saw the arrival of huge numbers of doctors from south east Asia recruited to fill gaps in deprived communities, or hard-to-fill clinical areas. The reasons why these areas found it difficult to recruit doctors are much the same as today: remote and rural areas (such as north Wales); inner city areas with high levels of immigrants (such as the midlands or the north east of England); and specialities such as psychiatry, general practice and emergency medicine. Often, these individuals were unable to continue in their original specialities and some became trapped in non-consultant, non-training grade positions for the rest of their careers. As with my father, they made an invaluable contribution to the NHS and to their communities. A past President of the Royal College of General Practitioners, Mayur Lakhani, in celebration of south Asian doctors commented:

> General practice in the UK would not be what it is today without the hard work, innovation, and courage of our predecessors, and their dedication to delivering high-quality patient care. Indeed, without them, our profession and the NHS might not even exist at all.[3]

Despite their contribution, these doctors and every migrant doctor since faces problems that make them more at risk of mental illness.

Moving to another country means becoming separated from social, cultural, financial and other supports. From the moment they decide to leave home, migrant doctors face logistical difficulties: strict visa requirements, complex medical registration processes and language tests. The challenges continue when they arrive in their new country as they have to work through complex employment and training requirements.[4] Even if fluent in their new country's language, then idioms, linguistic subtleties and accents still need to be mastered, let alone the non-verbal aspects of communication. They need to learn how to notice and understand facial expressions, gestures, posture, tone of voice and body movements – when to move closer for greater intimacy in the consultation when breaking bad news, for example. Difficulties can also arise when patients might also misinterpret non-verbal communications; or if the doctor does not recognise the patient's signals, they might be seen as unempathic or even rude.[5]

Financial insecurity is a common concern among migrant doctors. Even once through the preliminary administrative hurdles (which can take months or even years), finding a foothold in work is hard. Invariably, overseas graduates have to take on unpaid clinical attachments before being able to apply for paid employment, which in turn is more likely to be a non-training position, a series of temporary contracts (locum or short-term) or in a subconsultant grade.[6] Not surprising therefore that white UK trained doctors dominate the consultant and training grades and Black, Asian and Minority Ethnic (BAME) groups, especially IMGs, have a greater representation in non-consultant (such as, SAS) posts.[7]

People have a fundamental need to form social connections with others. It is what sustains us in difficult times. These connections are harder to make for those in a constant state of transition, moving across different locum posts, or working in areas where the workforce is constantly changing (such as in urgent care and out-of-hours). These are the areas of medicine in which migrant doctors are most likely to work. This personal perspective written by a migrant doctor describes this sense of non-belonging:

> Two years ago, I arrived in Britain on the overseas doctors' training scheme in psychiatry. This was my first trip to a foreign country. I came with little money and no friends or relatives in Britain. For someone who has always been one of us, it is impossible to imagine the feeling of being the other that engulfs you soon after arrival in a new country. The deafening silence of the countryside; the palpable discomfort at meeting a stranger's gaze; astonishment at everyone's attempts to hide behind a newspaper in the London tube; inability to react to the smile of a stranger that never quite reaches the eyes; and the early awareness of racial stereotypes are all disconcerting experiences. You are torn between the need to make human contact and a greater need to hide. For most people a summation of discrete experiences crystallises into this feeling of otherness.[8]

A widely-read report by the academics Doyin Atewologyn and Roger Kline entitled *Failure to Refer; Reducing Disproportionality in Fitness to Practise Concerns Reported to the GMC* found doctors who trained overseas faced strong 'out-group' bias and exclusion, being seen as 'workhorses', 'invisible labour', 'second class citizens' and 'nameless and faceless'.[9] He described insider and outsider group dynamics in the medical establishment relating to broad social processes that many might be familiar with in the playground groupings of their childhood. These dictate access to privileges and are linked to the position of doctors from different ethnic, cultural and employment groups along a pecking order. IMGs are typically seen as the bottom of this hierarchy and having '*not as good medical qualifications*'; locum doctors are deemed by managers as '*not one of our employees*', and SAS doctors perceive their peers see them as '*not good enough to be consultants*'. Furthermore, during the research for the report, the authors heard from doctors about the different 'tribes' that they witnessed in health services. These tribes were mainly demarcated by the colour of one's skin: non-Caucasian, non-British educated (seen as the 'outsiders') versus Caucasian British educated (the 'insiders'). Interaction between the two tribes is extremely difficult as both groups, for different reasons, become entrenched in their beliefs, expectations, working patterns and social networks. The insider group is characterised by having strong cohesive and non-diverse working teams and supporting and coaching each other during difficulties.

Perhaps the biggest (and least spoken about) problem IMG doctors face is discrimination. This can be from patients, colleagues, managers or members of the public. Three-quarters of GPs from BAME groups (many of whom were trained overseas) have faced racial discrimination from patients.[10] The racism experienced by a Scottish doctor, Punam Krishan and a senior surgeon in the north west of England, Radhakrishna Shanbhag, has thrown into sharp focus how this discrimination affects doctors who are the victim of such behaviours.[11,12] Both examples involve UK doctors with Indian heritage. Punam, a GP in Glasgow was told that a patient did not want an appointment with 'an Asian' doctor. When the receptionist responded 'She's Scottish' the patient replied 'She doesn't look Scottish', to which the receptionist asked 'What do Scottish people look like?' Radhakrishna Shanbhag was reduced to tears and made to feel worthless when relaying how a patient had demanded they were treated by a white doctor.

Punam and Radhakrishna were brave to speak out; many do not. Two successful overseas-trained doctors, Kailash Chand and JS Bamrah, have also spoken out. They describe how they have experienced discrimination in exams, interviews and selection for jobs. They comment that though both of them are successful in their respective careers (one is a senior consultant psychiatrist and the other a GP leader) it has not always been plain sailing for them. They wrote 'seemingly well-meaning colleagues who have made remarks that would be considered discriminatory today. The stress of this, on top of everything else, is unimaginable.'[13]

When I was Chair of the Royal College of General Practitioners, I had to face a Judicial Review for alleged discrimination of ethnic minority doctors with respect to the College's professional examination (MRCGP), the compulsory professional examination for all GPs in the UK. For most exams, whether computer-marked, written, simulation or oral, there is differential achievement by different demographic groups undertaking the same assessment. It is due to a complex range of personal, cultural, institutional and structural factors impacting on parity. The gap in achievement between different demographic groups undertaking the same assessment applies across all medical specialities and to all non-white ethnic groups, with the odds of failure of BAME doctors being two and a half times higher than that of white doctors.[14] For the MRCGP examination BAME UK graduates were nearly four times more likely to fail the examination at their first attempt compared to their white UK counterparts, with BAME IMGs almost 15 times more likely to fail.[15,16] This pattern of attainment is the same across different speciality examinations.[17] The challenge to the College's examination was a deeply painful time in my leadership. By implication, I felt accused of discrimination against BAME and IMG doctors by denying them the right to become GPs. Given my background as the daughter of an immigrant, it seemed ironic that this accusation came on my watch. The legal challenge was eventually dismissed but it led to significant soul searching by other Royal Colleges, not just my own, as to why there was such a difference in pass rate between the groups and why our hardworking colleagues were being let down by a system we had created. The GMC report suggests the disparity in pass rate reflects learning styles rather than academic ability or the examination itself.[8] Learning is a social activity and therefore it is not surprising that in medicine strong peer support and learning networks significantly affect performance. Given what I said about 'tribes' it is likely that non-white doctors are excluded from learning and revision groups that might help them prepare and they lose the advantage of modelling answers on those who have previous experience of UK examinations. There is a suggestion that trainers might also be uneasy giving feedback to those from a different background, meaning that bad habits or poor practice cannot easily be changed. However, what cannot be denied is that examinations are set according to the socio-cultural norms of the host country and as such, in the UK, are likely to prioritise dominant white culture over other manners of learning and examination, which would explain the higher failure rate of UK-born, BAME doctors.

There are other areas where non-white and non-UK trained doctors are over-represented other than those who fail examinations. These doctors are much more likely to have complaints lodged against them and be subjected to disciplinary action and receive harsher sanctions than non-IMGs. Between 2012 and 2016 just under 25% of IMG BAME GPs were subject to complaints, compared to 17% of their UK BAME counterparts. IMGs have 2.5 times higher rate of being subject of serious disciplinary action and referred to the GMC compared to UK graduate doctors.[9] There are reasons put forward for this, including entrenched biases in the system that unfairly affect IMGs. It is also likely that IMGs doctors (as with my father) are likely to work in more deprived areas, areas that have fewer resources in terms of manpower or money and have more work-related pressures due to unfilled posts and greater burden of disease among their patients. Graduates trained abroad also disproportionately treat migrant and minority populations, where neither the GP nor the patient share the same common language.[18]

Individuals who have been separated from their family and network will have reduced financial, practical and emotional supports, all of which are vital to maintaining mental well-being. Bamrah and Chand write that the emotional burden of migration is the main contributor to health problems of immigrant doctors:

> It is well within the gift of employing authorities and statutory organisations to make a better effort in ensuring that these factors are earnestly tackled. Not doing so comes at a considerable cost not just to the NHS but to the individual doctor and their families as the consequences of stress and depression are substantial, from loss of income, re-employment issues, visa restrictions, stigma of mental health and at its worst, suicide of the affected doctor.[13]

CONCLUSION

For IMGs, having to navigate the complex medical regulatory and healthcare system is, to put it lightly, tough. Add to this the additional hurdles facing migrants generally – including learning the nuances of language; adjusting to cultural norms; and finding a way through the strict hierarchies of medical practice – it is no surprise that for IMGs the road to a successful career has many added challenges that put them at increased risk of mental illness.

Mohammad's experience illustrates the complex problems faced by IMGs:

Mohammad arrived for his first appointment 2 hours and 2 minutes early. It is not unusual for doctors to be early for their first appointment, but 2 hours and 2 minutes may be a record. Even before this first appointment Mohammad had made himself known to our office. He'd called the previous week asking for help, saying that it was urgent – 'You must help me!', he shouted down the telephone, and continued, 'If you don't help me, I will lose my job'. His accent and rapid speech made it difficult to understand him fully, but the urgency of his distress came over and the first available appointment was given to him (17.15 4 days later) and a confirmatory email sent. He rang the following day to confirm the time, place and who he was going to see. He rang the day before the appointment to check it was still happening and he rang on the day to say that he was on his way but might be a little late as the traffic was so bad. He arrived for his appointment at 15.17, having misunderstood the 24-hour clock in his anxiety.

Mohammad told his story. He had qualified in Egypt and had to move to England when his political beliefs became known to the authorities. He initially arrived as an asylum seeker. He had left a post as a senior surgeon but had to start again in very junior grades when he arrived in the UK. He told me that back in Egypt he had been a high flyer, had come top in his finals and got very good jobs, 'not like this place', he interjected, 'where they treat you like shit and make you do all the terrible jobs'. He had come alone, leaving his wife and two young sons with his parents; he sent money home to them every month. He had hoped his family would join him once he was settled, but he was never settled, and they never did. He rarely saw his two sons, who were now adults, but still sent money home to his wife.

After passing the necessary language examinations he had to find an unpaid attachment, then worked in endless locum jobs and finally managed to get a position working in accident and emergency (he tried surgery but never got shortlisted for jobs). In recent months he had worked as a locum wherever he could find work. In one three-month period he had worked in ten different hospitals across England and Wales, from far north to extreme south. When not provided with accommodation he would check into a bed and breakfast if needed, but mostly he lived in his car, parked in the hospital carpark; after all, this was a lot cheaper than spending money on a few hours in a hotel bed.

He found that he had lost his appetite and was beginning to lose weight. Though he didn't notice at the time, he realised now that he was getting increasingly tired and demoralised. He told me he felt sad all the time and would often have fleeting thoughts of killing himself. After another night shift, a nurse complained about his care of a patient. He disagreed with her view. He accepted that maybe because he was tired and angry that his voice might have become raised. Over the next few days he worried that the nurse was watching him, even recording him when he did his shifts. He noticed her in the staff room and was sure she had been laughing at him. A few days later, he was asked to see the Clinical Director. He was told that his services were no longer needed and that he had to leave. He felt desperate and thought of killing himself. Instead, he contacted our service, having seen a leaflet in one of his hospital on-call rooms.

Mohammad illustrates the multiple problems doctors who have trained overseas face. This doctor is clearly depressed – with hypervigilance, paranoid ideation, feelings of worthlessness and hopelessness. He was unable to sleep, not surprising given his condition. He, as with others, faced barriers to seeking care and these were exacerbated by his isolation. He feared disclosing his of mental illness in case (as he thought) he would be deported. In general, he also lacked the vocabulary and emotional language to describe his feelings. My service helped him to formulate the problems he was facing. We acted as his advocate, provided reports to his workplace and treatment for him. This included antidepressants, a brief course of cognitive behaviour therapy as well as enrolling him into a doctor-only therapy group where he could safely share his experiences.

In times of stress those who are the weakest, most vulnerable are at greatest risk. Many of our IMGs, who have come to support our struggling health service, fall into this category. It is important that we acknowledge the difficulties these doctors face and their increased risk of mental illness. These doctors are the lifeblood of the NHS. They do the jobs many UK trained doctors do not wish to do, including the back-breaking, long red-eye shifts. Without these doctors our health system would collapse. We must ensure that they are cared for in the same way they care for us.

REFERENCES

1 Harris S. Are BAME doctors treated unfairly? Available from: www.medscape.com/viewarticle/924049?nlid=133703_5170&src=WNL_ukmdpls_200129_mscpedit_gen&uac=288666AV&impID=2260058&faf=1.

2 The medical register [Internet]. Gmc-uk.org. [cited 18 January 2020]. Available from: www.gmc-uk.org/registration-and-licensing/the-medical-register.

3 RCGP. Migrants who made the NHS. Available from: www.rcgp.org.uk/about-us/news/2018/april/migrants-who-made-the-nhs-college-pays-tribute-to-gps.aspx.

4 Ratcliff C. Integrating international medical graduates. *Future Healthc J* 2019. DOI: https://doi.org/10.7861/futurehosp.6-1-s176.

5 Coelho K, Galan C. Physician cross-cultural nonverbal communication skills, patient satisfaction and health outcomes in the physician-patient relationship. *Int J Fam Med* 2012;376907.

6 Fazel S, Ebmeier K. Specialty choice in UK junior doctors: is psychiatry the least popular specialty for UK and international medical graduates? *BMC Med Edu* 2009;**9**(1):77.

7 GMC. Survey of specialty and associate specialist (SAS) and locally employed (LE) doctors. Available from: www.gmc-uk.org/education/standards-guidance-and-curricula/projects/survey-of-specialty-and-associate-specialist-and-locally-employed-DOCTORS.

8 Singh S. Cultural adjustment and the overseas trainee. *BMJ* 1994;**308**(6937):1169.

9 Doyin Atewologyn D, Kline R. *Failure to Refer; Reducing Disproportionality in Fitness to Practise Concerns Reported to the GMC 2019.* Available from: www.gmc-uk.org/news/news-archive/fair-to-refer.

10 Mahase E. Quarter of BME GPs experience patient discrimination at least once a month [Internet]. *Pulse Today.* 2018 [cited 18 January 2020]. Available from: www.pulsetoday.co.uk/news/quarter-of-bme-gps-experience-patient-discrimination-at-least-once-a-month/20036640.article.

11 Johnson S. My patient made racist remarks about me. I decided to do something about it [Internet]. *The Guardian*. 2019 [cited 18 January 2020]. Available from: www.theguardian.com/society/2019/jan/22/patient-racist-remarks-nhs.

12 'Can I have a white doctor for the operation?': Racist abuse against NHS staff almost triples, ITV News finds [Internet]. ITV News. 2019 [cited 18 January 2020]. Available from: www.itv.com/news/2019-10-31/can-i-have-a-white-doctor-for-the-operation-racist-abuse-against-nhs-staff-almost-triples-itv-news-finds.

13 Bamrah JS, Chand K. Medics, migration and mental illness. *Sushruta* 2020;**13**(1). Available from: www.sushruta.net/March-2020.

14 Shah R, Ahluwalia S. The challenges of understanding differential attainment in postgraduate medical education. *Br J Gen Pract* 2019;**69**(686):426427. DOI: https://doi.org/10.3399/bjgp19X705161.

15 GMC. Relationship between general practice selection scores and MRCGP examination performance. Available from: www.gmc-uk.org/about/what-we-do-and-why/data-and-research/research-and-insight-archive/relationship-between-general-practice-selection-scores-and-mrcgp-examination-performance.

16 Patterson F, Tiffin P, Lopes S, Zibarras L. Unpacking the dark variance of differential attainment on examinations in overseas graduates. *Med Educ* 2018;**52**(7):736–46.

17 Regan de Bere S, Nunn S, Nasser M, Plymouth University Peninsula Schools of Medicine and Dentistry. Understanding differential attainment across medical training pathways: a rapid review of the literature Final report prepared for The General Medical Council [Internet]. Available from: www.gmc-uk.org/-/media/documents/GMC_Understanding_Differential_Attainment.pdf_63533431.pdf.

18 Atri A, Matorin A, Ruiz P. Integration of international medical graduates in US psychiatry: the role of acculturation and social support. *Acad Psychiatry* 2011;**35**(1):21–6.

22

Medical Students

CLARE GERADA

I can remember the day, just after Christmas in 1977, when I received the letter telling me I'd been accepted into medical school. It was, at that point, the happiest day of my life.

At last, I was on my way to do what I'd wanted to do ever since I was a little girl. In the weeks before I started, my father took me to Lewis' book shop, on the corner of Gower Street, next door to University College Hospital, **my** medical school. He bought me *Gray's Anatomy* and *Price's Textbook of Medicine*, which are still treasured possessions. I made my closest friends over the dissecting table (we spent many a formative hour there). I learnt to love the theatre, good food and London. There were bad times, of course. I spent the first few months struggling with loneliness, as it took time to make friends; the realisation of the vast knowledge I had to acquire and the anxiety that went with it; and the ups and downs of broken relationships. After all, what does one expect when you arrive at medical school barely out of adolescence? Over the five years, I learnt not just the lines needed to become a doctor, but also how to take my place on the medical stage.

I wonder if the young men and women starting out today, as I did nearly 50 years ago, know what they are in for. Though everyone has a concept of what it is to be a 'doctor' (if only from the 'fly on the wall', or fictional accounts on television), not even I (who spent my childhood surrounded by the trappings of medicine) could have imagined the depth, breadth and volume of information I needed to accumulate – much learnt today and gone tomorrow (I still can't fathom why I needed to memorise the Krebs cycle).

Each year of training the gap between the lay person who starts medical school, and the professional who ends as the doctor years later, widens. Between the time of making the commitment to study medicine and ending as the final product of 'the doctor', we must pass through rites of passage that ease this transition, and which I introduced in Chapter 1. The first sight of a cadaver in year one; the time I placed my hands on a real (live) patient in the second pre-clinical year; proudly donning the short white coat in the third year, taking blood in the fourth year and carrying the bleep as a student locum in the final year, are all memorable milestones. Perhaps the most memorable is ringing my father from the payphone soon after finding the results of my final examinations and saying, 'hi Dad, its Dr Gerada here'. Even today, I shudder with pride remembering this experience. As a result of our training, we learn to think and talk about patients and diseases in a different way, to look upon death and disability, not with horror as a lay person might, but with compassion and sufficient detachment. We learn along the way to retain our idealism (hopefully) but add a good measure of realism alongside. Idealism now shaped by knowledge (which might be the definition of scepticism). Looking back, if asked and knowing what I know now, I would certainly choose medicine again and again and again. I hope this is the same for young people starting this journey today.

This chapter will explore mental illness in medical students and the impact it has for individuals through their training. As with many studies involving the medical profession, there are very few that allow for comparisons across different years, and it is still unclear whether the rate is increasing.

MENTAL HEALTH OF STUDENTS

The mental health of medical students has been a topic of research for several decades. There have been books following them up through their years of training – examining, as if animals in the wild, their natural habits, relationships and development.[1] My favourite is Simon Sinclair's book, *Making Doctors, an Institutional Apprenticeship*.[2] Simon Wessely, past President of the Royal College of Psychiatrists (and my husband) has been cited as saying that all doctors should read this book.[3] I agree with him. Sinclair trained as a psychiatrist and then as a medical anthropologist. His book is an anthropological analysis of medical students (from their first year pre-clinical to registration year). He spent a year at University College Hospital Medical School (where I trained) watching students as part of his 'field work' as they went about their work, rest and play. He studied them in the dissection room, tutorials, ward rounds, in the student's common room, the rugby club and of course their bar. What he referred to as the 'backstage "stuff" of training' and in so doing, how students acquired what he referred to as 'Dispositions' (or cognitive categories). These are other ways of knowing other than purely based on factual knowledge. Dispositions, in areas such knowledge, experience, status, economics and responsibility, are silently absorbed during the medical training, which while unspoken, determine the behaviour of students as they move towards making their final transition to becoming a doctor. During their training students move from 'that of the audience in lectures, through combined audience and actors on ward rounds, to full time actors as housemen' and in so doing, learn to look at the world through a different lens, as Simon describes, 'first through scientising then through pathalogising'. Most students make this transition but along the way they have to adapt to their changing habitus, and some become more disillusioned, cynical and mentally unwell.

The academic Jenny Firth-Cozens has studied the mental health of medical students since the early 1980s. All students face pressures due to their academic requirements and social adjustments. Medical students, in particular, have additional challenges due to their long training, large workload, number of assessments and learning to deal with the clinical environment. Firth-Cozens has attempted to evaluate what impact these have on students' mental health. I have always been interested in her studies, not just because of their academic prowess, but because the timing of her research exactly matched by my own career progression. The first study was of second-clinical year students in 1980 (I was also a second-year student in 1980). She found that the prevalence of 'emotional disturbance' was 31%, compared to 10% in young unemployed men, with no difference between men and women.[4] There was no evidence that these high rates were associated with similar numbers of these students going on to become patients. Most didn't seek out help, rather 'coped' alone (a pattern that would continue once qualified). When asked to rate causes of their distress, the most frequent reasons were 'not being valued', 'feeling useless'. The second study was two years later, apparently the catalyst was the suicide of two junior house officers.[5] The students, now first year housemen (the first year post qualification), were tested in the same way, though a measure for depression was now included. The rate of emotional disturbance was now 50% (compared this time to civil servants, where it was 36%) and of depression, severe enough to warrant treatment, was nearly 28%. This rate of depression is high and even now I am shocked by this figure, which was at a time when mental illness was not discussed, let alone addressed. So much mental pain at a time when young people were just finding their 'doctoring-feet'. This time the most cited reason individuals gave for their distress was '*overwork*'. At the time, the average number of hours worked by house officers was around 80 hours per week, but it was not unusual for this to increase to 120 hours per week, for example when on-call over an entire weekend. However, and surprisingly, though the house officers self-reported overwork as the major cause of their distress, when mapped to scores for depression, there was no correlation between the two variables. In fact, the opposite was found in her later study[6] and mirrored by other researchers,[7] that the doctors who coped best worked longer hours.

MENTAL ILLNESS TODAY

Since Jenny Firth-Cozens' studies (and there were others earlier carried out largely in North America), there have been hundreds of others involving medical students from across the world. The vast majority find rates of mental illness among doctors at least as high, if not higher than age-matched background populations. There have been a number of systematic reviews. For example, one published in 2016 involved studies from 43 different countries;[8] the overall prevalence of depression or depressive symptoms was 27% ranging from 9% to 56%. Suicidal ideation ranged from 5% to 36%.[9,10] In the studies that assessed depressive symptoms before and during medical school, the increase in symptoms was 14% (range 0.6% to 35.3%). As with the early Firth-Cozens study, students preferred to 'go it alone' and only 16% of those who screened positive for depression had sought psychiatric treatment.

The academics Valerie Hope and Max Henderson carried out a systematic review of publications looking at the mental illness of medical students. The papers were all published in the UK, Europe and English-speaking world outside of North America between 1948 and 2013.[11] The overall prevalence was 8% to 66% for anxiety, 6% to 67% for depression and 12% to 97% for psychological distress. Most studies found depression, anxiety and psychological distress reduced the closer the student was to qualification, maybe because there is 'light at the end of the tunnel'. This was the finding of a study involving Portuguese medical students.[12] The prevalence of depression changed from 22% to 13% over two years (against an overall rate of depression in Portugal ranging from 6% to 22%). While depression scores decreased as they progressed through training, for one-fifth of the students they were sustained at high levels over the whole time. Other studies have found that mental health deteriorates during medical school and continues to decline as the individuals starts work.[13]

The extremely wide prevalence range reflects the variable quality of the studies, with better quality ones tending to find lower prevalence rates. As with studies on mental illness in doctors, differences in rates reflect the robustness of the study, sample size, instruments used, cut-off points and so on. Students are not blinded to the purpose of the study, that is they know it is designed to measure mental distress and therefore risks conflating rates. Most studies use self-report instruments with no independent validation of mood state or ability to function.

As with qualified doctors, psychological distress impacts on the individual, and also affects their interaction with patients, ability to empathise,[14] and causes a decline in academic performance[15] and impairment of professionalism.[16]

A personal account of depression by the medical student Karyn Joss illustrates the factors that can lead to mental illness:

> I had recently commenced my second semester and I had come to realise that everything had begun to seem a bit darker, a lot darker in fact. The intense pace of medical school, the striving for excellence, incredibly high stakes, and the fierce competition can, perhaps unsurprisingly, pit an individual's mental well-being against a perfect storm.[17]

Medical school is the 'perfect' environment to create the distress we see. We place individuals who have excelled in their school life, achieved outstanding scores in whole areas of their personal and academic life and place them in an environment where, by definition, one-half will now be below average. Given their identity is already bound up with academic success, they work harder to achieve more and become 'above average'. We then give them the opportunity to try and 'overachieve'. We bombard them with immense volumes of work, intense scrutiny, assessments and the need to constantly compete with their peers. We also place them in an environment where failure is not allowed and any transgression, academic or personal, is punished. Added to this, the culture around mental illness being 'a weakness' or character flaw persists, meaning that those who might have mental illness are frightened of seeking help. Echoing the words of Karyn, in the medical student with depression, we create a perfect storm.

HOW TO ADDRESS MENTAL ILLNESS IN STUDENTS

Despite mental illness of medical students being the subject of study for nearly 70 years little seems to have been done to reduce the high levels, other than perhaps putting in place 'resilience training' which has little efficacy (as discussed in Chapter 6). Interventions such as advising self-care, engaging in mindfulness, sport, yoga or other self-help interventions or participation in group work do little to address the underlying systemic cause – namely the burden of what is expected of students, intense competition, assessments, financial pressures and bullying. These and the culture that training has to be demanding in the effort of 'toughening up' students and removing those who cannot cope, in essence, 'survival of the fittest' have not changed significantly since I started training nearly 50 years ago. Medicine is a broad church and we need all sorts to work in it, not just those who are outwardly 'the toughest'.

It is the culture of medical training that has to change, and a study conducted at St Louis medical school has attempted to do this. It adapted the pre-clinical curriculum in a deliberate attempt to reduce levels of depression and anxiety in their medical students.[18] Over a four-year period, the changes included introducing a pass/fail grading rather than scores, a 10% reduction in curricular time, efforts to reduce the amount of detail taught, longer electives, theme-based community learning and spaces for peer group reflection. As well as all of these changes, they implemented a confidential option to track depression and anxiety. Those students who screened positive were contacted by a mental health provider and offered treatment. The effects of these interventions were different as the students progressed through their training. The impact of the changes was greatest for the first-year students. Objectively (as compared to a questionnaire administered to all American medical students) and subjectively (on free text comments) these individuals had lower rates of mental illness and better 'satisfaction' with their training. However, as they progressed through medical school, the interventions appeared to have less of an impact and it became harder to control the negative effects of external stressors, such as the first part of the National Medical School exam. Once students entered their clinical training, the impact of interventions, including peer group support, did not create any effect. The authors attributed this inability to reduce rates of mental illness as being due to **four main factors**:

1 The learning environment involved multiple posts making it very difficult to provide a consistently supportive offering.
2 The pre-existing poor mental health of residents and physicians that the students encountered might have had a contagious effect on their mental health.
3 The competition for future residency posts, which acted as a significant source of stress.
4 Despite the efforts to provide 'resilience' training, this did little to counteract the psychologically stressful conditions students were exposed to in their clinical posts.

Most commentators and much of the work I have reviewed for this book make the same point, that is **medical education** must change, with more effort and resources directed to the study of different teaching methods or new content. Yet, almost without exception, interventions focus only on addressing the well-being of students. While advising students and even perhaps funding resilience-building interventions might make educators feel and possibly look good, it merely shifts the locus of disturbance to the individual rather than where it should sit: their learning environment. Until a way is found of reducing these psychological stressors, high rates of mental illness in students will remain. We cannot resilience train our way out of this issue. It requires medical schools to commit to addressing their processes and implementing changes throughout their students' training. This is not about mollycoddling students; it is about removing extraneous pain from an already difficult training regimen and ensuring they have the space, time and energy to successfully make the transition from student to doctor.

CONCLUSION

It goes without saying that medical school is stressful. The workload is intense, the exams are frequent, individual excellence is demanded and one is surrounded by high-achieving individuals that provide fierce competition. This is one of the unspoken rules of medicine that many are aware of when choosing to enter the profession. Despite knowing this, how individuals respond and adapt to the challenges and the stressors they face is only realised when they arrive at medical school, most of them adolescents fresh from their A-levels. The literature included in this chapter paints a picture of psychological distress, emotional disturbance and depression. From a personal perspective, the cited incidence and prevalence rates of mental illness almost defy belief. Clearly many medical students are not coping or faring as well as they had hoped. This chapter highlights the struggles that plague medical students throughout their training. A critical point to reinforce is the difficulty students face of finding themselves to be 'average' following 13 years of academic excellence. This false sense of mediocrity can be a powerful driving force for making students work longer, graft harder, achieve more and strive for excellence. The fierce competition only fuels this mentality; friends and peers are engaged in a silent battle to publish papers, attend conferences, perform charity work and more, to boost their credentials and fill their CV with evidence of their achievements. While this pursuit of perfectionism is admirable, it can create a vicious cycle of stress and overwork, eroding individual resolve and leaving them susceptible to mental health illness. For the current generation of medical students, awareness of mental health issues has never been more prominent. Students are talking, sharing and directly addressing the issue at hand, rather than repressing and bottling their emotions due to fear and shame. Despite the challenges, the stresses and the trials and tribulations, the resounding response is that most students wouldn't want to be anywhere else.

Contribution by Michael Owen, a first-year graduate medical student.

REFERENCES

1 Becker H, Geer B, Hughes EC, Strauss A. *Boys in White. Student Culture in Medical School.* New Brunswick (USA) and London (UK): Transaction Publishers, 2007.

2 Sinclair S. *Making Doctors. An Institutional Apprenticeship.* Oxford: Berg, 1997, p. 297.

3 Wessely S. Making doctors: an institutional apprenticeship. *BMJ Clin Res* 1998;**316**(7132).

4 Firth J. Levels and sources of stress in medical students. *BMJ* 1986;**310**:1177–80.

5 Firth-Cozens J. Emotional distress in junior house offices. *BMJ* 1987;**295**:533–5.

6 Firth-Cozens J. The role of early family experiences in the perception of organizational stress; fusing clinical and organisational perspectives. *J Occup Organ Psychol* 1992;**65**:61–75.

7 Hale R, Hudson L. The Tavistock study of young doctors: report of the pilot phase. *Br J Hosp Med* 1992;**47**:452–64.

8 Rotenstein LS, Marco BA, Ramos A, *et al.* Prevalence of depression, depressive symptoms, and suicidal ideation among medical students: a systematic review and meta-analysis. *JAMA* 2016;**316**(21):2214–36. doi:10.1001/jama.2016.17324.

9 Wan YH, Gao R, Tao XY, Tao FB, Hu CL. Relationship between deliberate self-harm and suicidal behaviors in college students [in Chinese, Abstract in English]. *Zhonghua Liu Xing Bing Xue Za Zhi* 2012;**33**(5):474–7.

10 Osama M, Islam MY, Hussain SA, *et al.* Suicidal ideation among medical students of Pakistan: a cross-sectional study. *J Forensic Leg Med* 2014;**27**:65–8.

11 Hope V, Henderson M. Medical student depression, anxiety and distress outside North America: a systematic review. *Med Educ* 2014;**48**:963–79.

12 Silva V, Costa P, Pereira I, *et al.* Depression in medical students: insights from a longitudinal study. *BMC Med Educ* 2017;**17**:184. PMCID: PMC5633876. Published online 2017 Oct 10. doi: 10.1186/s12909-017-1006-0 PMID: 29017594.

13 Dyrbye LN, Thomas MR, Shanafelt TD. Medical student distress: causes, consequences, and proposed solutions. *Mayo Clin Proc* 2005;**80**(12):1613–22.

14 Thomas MR, Dyrbye LN, Huntington JL, *et al.* How do distress and well-being relate to medical student empathy? A multicenter study. *J Gen Intern Med* 2007;**22**:177–83.

15 Dyrbye L, Shanafelt T. A narrative review on burnout experienced by medical students and residents. *Med Educ* 2016;**50**:132–49.

16 Dyrbye LN, Thomas MR, Shanafelt TD. Systematic review of depression, anxiety, and other indicators of psychological distress among US and Canadian medical students. *Acad Med* 2006;**81**(4):354–73.

17 BMA. Darkness or blankness, a medical student's experience of depression. Available from: www.bma.org.uk/connecting-doctors/b/work/posts/darkness-or-blankness-a-medical-student-s-experience-of-depression.

18 Slavin SJ, Schindler DL, Chibnall JT. Medical student mental health 3.0: Improving student wellness through curricular changes. *Acad Med* 2014;**89**:573–7.

23

Different Specialities and Risk of Mental Illness

CLARE GERADA

GENERAL ISSUES

The choice of speciality is the second most important decision a doctor makes in their career, the first was to study medicine at all. For some, they come with a pre-existing idea of what they want to be. I knew for example that I wanted to be a general practitioner (GP) and did so via general medicine and psychiatry, as I felt it was all too easy to be 'like my father' and wanted to put distance (time and geography) between us. However, it was clear that I was a generalist at heart. Every rotation I did I enjoyed and what I missed most was the variety of caring for people from cradle to grave and when well and sick. In the end, the other jobs were only a means to an end, to be a GP. For others their choice is a more gradual process as they are exposed to the variety that medicine can offer, or a process of elimination as they cannot get into their career choice and have to choose second, third or even more least-best options. Finally, for some it is luck, as it was for me when I had 10 months 'spare' after the birth of my first child and worked in substance misuse, only to spend the rest of my career working in the interface between addiction and general practice.

Whether a particular speciality creates more or less risk in terms of mental illness is related to the character of the doctor as well as the area of medicine and other factors that are independent of both the speciality and the individual. It is very difficult making comparisons between different areas and there are few studies to draw on.

Headlines from my service
GPs are over-represented in the service
Anaesthetists are most likely to present with addiction

| Anaesthetists have the highest rate of death through suicide |
| Surgeons are a hidden group |
| Paediatricians have the lowest rate of addiction (less than 1%) but are over-represented in the service |

GENERAL PRACTITIONERS

By way of background, GPs in UK have the shortest of training of all medical specialities, at only three years. One of these is spent in general practice (as a GP registrar) and two in hospital practice (ST1, ST2). GPs, once qualified, can work as GP partners/principals (having full responsibility for their practice with no limit on workload and a requirement to deliver against a contract set by NHS England; this includes the number of patients seen vs. list size. GPs can also be salaried doctors (paid according to work done and contracted by the practice partners) or work as a locum (essentially set their own working hours, place of work and working pattern). Unlike qualified GPs, GP registrars have some of the most protected working conditions, with their working hours strictly capped, longer appointment time with patients, limited responsibilities and usually a one-to-one relationship with a trainer for the time spent in practice as well as a half day release for education and training with peers. Most GP practices would not have a GP trainee (and even those that do, it is unlikely to be more than one or two trainees), unlike hospitals where training grade doctors are its workforce backbone.

Given their position at the 'front door' of the health system, GPs are probably bearing a disproportionate burden of workload against diminishing resources. Workload has increased by 16% over recent years without a corresponding rise in the work force.[1-3] It is hardly surprising, therefore, GPs often top of the list for mental distress and burnout in the medical profession.[4-7] This is translating into increasing levels of dissatisfaction, anxiety, chronic stress, depression and suicidal thoughts,[8] not just in the UK, as European and American GPs are also struggling with high rates of burnout.[9,10]

I have been working in the same general practice for 30 years. The same room, same community of patients and the same starting time (8 am). Over these years I have seen improvements in the use of technology, for example, our medical records became paperless more than 15 years ago; we offer a higher quality of care and a better skill mix as we now have an army of allied medical professionals to help us in our work. Yet, given all of these, my daily work has become immensely harder. While 30 years ago I finished my morning surgery by 11 am, did home visits till midday, collected my small children from nursery, fed them and spent some time with them. I would then invariably have an afternoon meeting, then return for my evening surgery at 4 pm, and be home by 6.30 pm. Unless I was on call – which was one in five nights – the working day would end then. A generation before me, my father who was for many years a single and then a dual-handed GP would start his surgery at 8 am, return home for a large lunch usually with a glass of wine, have an afternoon siesta (calls from patients would be taken by his receptionist at the surgery), waking in time to do house calls before returning to do evening surgery at 4 pm and returning home by 7 pm. He was on call one night in two, and though he was invariably called (as I was) at least once every night, it was still manageable. Today, a GP is barely able to finish their morning surgery before the evening one has started. Eleven hour working days, with no break, are now the norm and while few GPs do out of hours anymore, it is not unusual for paperwork and tasks not completed at the surgery to be finished at home, with the GP easily working into the late evening. Clinics at the start of my career would be largely full of patients with minor self-limiting illnesses, requests for repeat prescriptions or sick certificates or women for antenatal care or contraception. Now all of these have been removed from my consulting room and I am left with complexity: patients with five or six issues, complicated medication regimes to sort out, serious mental health problems and patients who not long ago would have been the domain of the hospital specialist. My experience is borne out by the literature.[11]

Headlines
Only 27% of trainees intend to work full time in general practice one year after qualifying and only 5% after ten years; the intensity of the working day remains the leading factor in GP trainees not wishing to undertake full-time GP work, with 69% of respondents citing this. Many referred to the risk to their own health.[12]
The volume and intensity of GP workloads is driving many to either reduce their hours or leave the profession altogether. While more GPs than ever are being trained, today's figures show that GP numbers continue to decrease, with a 2% drop in the number of permanent, full-time equivalent GPs in the past year and 6.2% fewer in September 2019 than in 2015.[13]
Four in ten GPs intend to quit general practice in the next five years amid growing workload pressures.[14] Nearly 90% of GP partners are at high or very high risk of burnout, 30% of GP partners and 40% of sessional GPs had received a formal mental health diagnosis at some point in their career.[15]

PSYCHIATRISTS

Psychiatrists are reported to have higher rates of mental illness than most other doctors, with high levels of stress, job dissatisfaction, depression and burnout.[16,17] Psychiatrists might be at increased risk for a number of reasons. Perhaps as a group they are vulnerable to experiencing burnout, more so than other physicians and surgeons. In this paper, various definitions of burnout are reviewed and the tools available for quantifying burnout are compared. The factors that make psychiatry a stressful profession are also examined. These include factors such as patient violence and suicide, limited resources, crowded inpatient wards, changing culture in mental health services, high work demands, poorly defined roles of consultants, responsibility without authority, inability to effect systemic change, conflict between responsibility toward employers vs. toward the patient, and isolation. In order to investigate how exposure to such stressors results in burnout, two theoretical models are examined. Recommendations are also made, on the basis of anecdotal reports, for addressing burnout in psychiatrists. They, more than most doctors, they use themselves as the tools of their trade, as they listen, interpret and reflect back to the patients. The courageous actions of psychiatrists are largely invisible. It takes enormous mental strength to remain focused when having to listen to the psychic pain of patients, day in and day out. This intense doctor–patient relationship is difficult and unpredictable. Patients evoke emotions such as the need to rescue them, and a sense of failure and frustration when the illness does not respond to treatment.[18] This forms part of the emotional work that all doctors have to confront (discussed in Chapter 3). However, for psychiatrists, the chronicity and fluctuating nature of their patients' illnesses can be particularly challenging. Tom Main, a psychoanalysis who for many years was in charge of the therapeutic community, The Cassell, described these difficulties. When a patient gets better it is a

> most reassuring event for his doctor or nurse . . . cured patients do great service to their attendants. However, the sufferer who frustrates a keen therapist by failing to improve is always in danger of meeting primitive human behaviours disguised as treatment.[19]

Other ther factors such as violence from patients,[20] overcrowded in-patient wards and an increasing culture of blame, increases the risk of burnout.[21] While blame seems to be inherent in the whole health system, for psychiatrists this is particularly acute as they are held responsible when a patient with mental illness takes their own life or kills or harms another. Psychiatrists have to undertake a difficult, if not impossible task of assigning risk status to a patient ahead of discharge, of essentially predicting future behaviour. The majority of psychiatrists experience the death of a patient by suicide at least once in their career[22] and this can have profound and long-term effects on their personal, psychological and professional life.[23]

It might be that those who go into the mental health field (counsellors, psychiatrists, psychotherapists) are more likely to have a history of mental health problems themselves, entering the field as a vicarious desire to understand their own difficulties or in the hope of repairing past traumas. I talked of this in Chapter 3, when looking at the concept of the wounded healer. A 2015 survey of Canadian psychiatrists found that of 487 psychiatrists who responded to a questionnaire, nearly one-third said they had experienced mental illness.[24] This suggests that those who enter the field of psychiatry might be influenced by their own history of mental illness.

There is evidence that despite higher rates of mental illness, psychiatrists are more reluctant to attend for treatment, even when these services offer confidential care.[25] Stigma to mental illness is not an abstract issue for this group. They see their own patients exposed to it on a daily basis. When mentally unwell themselves, they are on the receiving end leading to deep-seated shame and guilt.[26] Self-stigmatisation is not uncommon. It is also very difficult for a psychiatrist to receive confidential help; as with GPs, if they work and live in the same area it is not unusual for them to know those who work in mental health services, personally or professionally.

Psychiatrists find enormous purpose and meaning in their job as well as high levels of personal accomplishment and job satisfaction. They are also experts at using a host of coping strategies, which include staff support groups, confidential counselling and staff sensitivity sessions.[27]

Psychiatrists as a group are vulnerable to experiencing burnout, more so than other physicians and surgeons. In this paper, various definitions of burnout are reviewed and the tools available for quantifying burnout are compared. The factors that make psychiatry a stressful profession are also examined. These include factors such as patient violence and suicide, limited resources, crowded inpatient wards, changing culture in mental health services, high work demands, poorly defined roles of consultants, responsibility without authority, inability to effect systemic change, conflict between responsibility toward employers vs. toward the patient, and isolation. In order to investigate how exposure to such stressors results in burnout, two theoretical models are examined. Recommendations are also made, on the basis of anecdotal reports, for addressing burnout in psychiatrists.

Keywords: Burnout, psychiatrists, stress management, workforce

SURGEONS

An aura of authority surrounds surgeons and it is generally unquestioned. They confront acute life and death situations more commonly than any other group of doctors and they are seen as more confident individuals. This might be why compared to numbers on the medical register, surgeons are under-represented at treatment services,[28] including at my own service. Over the decade we have seen around 150 surgeons; 90% had mental health problems and 9% presented with addiction problems (which is less than the average across all specialities).

Surgeons' lower rates of presentation could be due to having more protective factors (e.g. better resilience to cope with occupational stress). There might be some validity in this, as those who cannot cope with the pressure and competitiveness of a surgical career may fall along the way, leaving only the fittest to survive. Surgeons might be protected by their close working relationships with others, allowing for sharing of distress, successes and general support.

Perhaps then, surgeons genuinely have a lower rate of mental illness than other doctors. However, an alternative explanation is that they are a hidden group, with even greater reluctance to seek help. There is some evidence for this. Different surveys show high levels of suicidal ideation (especially in older surgeons) and significant levels of distress, anxiety and/or burnout.[29,30] A systematic review in 2017 looked at burnout in American surgeons.[31] Based on the review, the levels of surgeons meeting the criteria for burnout ranged from 32% to 40% depending on surgical subspeciality. Shanafelt and colleagues[32] carried out one of the earliest and largest studies of burnout in American surgeons in 2009. These authors surveyed nearly 25,000 members of the American College of Surgeons; 40% met the criteria for burnout and 30% screened positive for depression.

A study looked at burnout and alcoholism of surgeons employed in a single institution over a 25-year period.[33] Amazingly, 97% of all present and past employees were ultimately included in the study (100 males and 14 females). There had been two deaths (one through an accident and one from suicide). Four doctors were no longer practising due to alcohol/substance dependency. The divorce rate was 21.4%. Overall, major health issues occurred in 32%, and in 50% of those aged over 50 years old. Of the 110 surgeons available for interview, eight were recorded as having a significant dependency history; six were primarily alcohol related with the other two having opiate dependency. This gives a rate of 7.3%, in line with estimated alcohol dependency rates reported in the literature and lower than in the general population.

It should not be surprising that surgeons suffer from mental illness given the long, unpredictable hours and high stress work they undertake. All doctors have their own unwritten group norms, developed over generations. For surgeons, these include working long hours (sometimes when not even rostered to do so); meeting multiple deadlines; rarely complaining; keeping emotions or personal problems away from the workspace. They also have some of the longest training in medicine and make substantial personal sacrifices to achieve their chosen profession. Surgeons have to perform well, at all times, under the spotlight of others (at the very least, scrub nurses, anaesthetists). They also need to appear competent irrespective of their internal demons. In the operating theatre, when the going gets tough, it is the surgeon who has to take control and rescue the situation. Even when off duty surgeons may ruminate over the difficult operation or worry about the patient in intensive care.

There are other contributing factors in the development of mental illness among surgeons. Patients are at their most vulnerable when they see a surgeon, whether unconscious on the operating table or lying on their hospital bed in anticipation of reassurances, pre- or post-operatively. Patients trust surgeons, totally. They relinquish all authority and power to them. They become helpless. The surgeon's job requires that they constantly contain others' fears of death. This places a heavy toll on the individual doctor. The expectations placed on surgeons might make it harder for them to accept vulnerability and present for care when needed; instead they have to project the image of being tough and resilient.

With respect to substance misuse, the low rate of dependence has face validity. Close working relationships, with every move witnessed, as well as long and unpredictable hours of work, frequent on-call shifts and out of hours work, would make it difficult to disguise an alcohol or drug problem.

In my experience, surgeons generally struggle more than other doctors to see themselves as patients. They find it hard to accept they might be ill, or when they do, they seek a quick fix. Almost every surgeon who presents talks about the fear they have of other colleagues finding out about their mental health problems. They report that colleagues don't 'believe in' mental illness, and they fear that they will be excluded by their peers if their illness is discovered.

ANAESTHETISTS

Easy access to intravenous opioids and opiates and anaesthetic agents, including inhalation gases, places anaesthetists at particular risk of addiction and death due to drug overdose. Estimating the true prevalence of substance misuse disorder is difficult as even in surveys promising confidentiality there is a reluctance to admit to having a problem that could result in criminal and professional sanctions. Where studies have been done, the risk for anaesthetists is reported to be 2.7 times that of other doctors.[34] At my service, anaesthetists present with substance misuse disorder at around twice the rate of all doctors.

A retrospective study of North American trainee anaesthetists 1975–2009 found the overall incidence was 2.16 per 1000 resident-years for men and 0.65 per 1000 resident years for women.[35] The most common substance was intravenous opioids, followed by alcohol. The time from the beginning of training to first use was around 30 months and from first use to detection four months. Of these doctors, 28 had died during residency, all as a result of their drug use. Estimated relapse rates over a 30-year career were above 40%; less than 50% achieved specialist certification. These are very poor outcomes. It is unclear from this study whether these doctors were enrolled in Physician Health Programmes (PHPs) or treatment services. More recent studies of doctors with addiction in PHP programmes show much more favourable outcomes: 95% who remained engaged with PHP monitoring and supervision were still licenced and less than 1% had died after five years. In contrast, of those who did not remain engaged, only 21% were still licenced and 17% had died.[36] No patient harm was detected.[37]

Unfortunately, the first indication that an anaesthetist has a problem might be death from accidental or deliberate overdose. Suicide is reported to be the cause of death in approximately 6–10% of anaesthetists,[38] and the risk of a drug-related death to be nearly three times that of a general physician.[39] A matched cohort analysis found anaesthetists with a substance use disorder found a 14.1% mortality rate vs. 1.3% in matched controls.[35]

Nearly 40% of anaesthetists working in the UK and Ireland have had first-hand experience of an anaesthetic colleague who has died by their own hand (either accidental or deliberate).[38] This shows the impact and reach that a death has on those in the same speciality. Most of these deaths involved anaesthetic agents.

With respect to overall levels of mental illness, a sample of Australian anaesthetists were sent a survey about their mental illness and use of services. Around one-quarter had visited their GP or health professional for a mental health-related issue. Of all the respondents, 13% reported that they had been diagnosed with a mental illness. Overall, 25% had previously self-prescribed anxiolytics, antidepressants or sedatives and 17% admitted to using alcohol to deal with stress, anxiety or depression; 3% reported they had used drugs such as marijuana, cocaine, opioids or amphetamines to deal with stress or depression, rather than as a purely recreational activity; and 16% of respondents reported sustained suicidal thoughts, although less than 1% reported having attempted suicide.[40]

OBSTETRICIANS AND GYNAECOLOGISTS

As with other specialities, obstetricians and gynaecologists (O&G) doctors are reported to have high levels of burnout, depression and other forms of mental illness.[41] This may be related to the 'high stakes' nature of their work and the high propensity for medico-legal issues to surface when things go wrong. However, there are lower levels of presentation at my service and it might be due to specific protective factors. These include the following:[42]

- It is a speciality that allows a mixture of medical (including primary care), psychological and surgical skills.
- It is a team activity where doctors work side by side with other practitioners from different specialities.
- Perhaps more than any other speciality, doctors really do change the lives of their patients and are by their side at the most significant and momentous moments of a woman's life, across all ages.
- It is a speciality that has in-built 'victories' – delivering healthy babies. This provides constant positive reinforcement.

However, these doctors appear to be at higher risk of post-traumatic stress disorder (PTSD). A study published in 2020 looked at the problem of post-traumatic stress in obstetricians and gynaecologists.[43] The main findings were that two-thirds reported exposure to traumatic work-related events. Of these, 18% of the doctors reported clinically significant PTSD symptoms. Staff of black or minority ethnicity were at increased risk of PTSD. Clinically significant PTSD symptoms were associated with lower job satisfaction, emotional exhaustion and depersonalisation. The culture in O&G was identified as a barrier to trauma support.

PAEDIATRICIANS

There is much paediatricians love about their job, yet increasing numbers are presenting to my service with mental illness (they now represent over 6% of our patient population). Neonatologists and intensive care specialists form a significant subset of this group. Almost all paediatricians presenting have mental illness as opposed to addiction. Safeguarding apart (where the wishes of parents might not always be aligned to those of children and doctors), paediatricians have traditionally enjoyed a close working relationship with children and families, and this has been a positively reinforcing factor for those working in the field. A further attraction has been the almost transformative act of improving children's health, at speed. Even when seriously unwell we have the romantic image in Luke Fildes' iconic painting (1891, Royal Academy London) where a doctor sits in a labourer's cottage beside a sick child, watched by his parents. The doctor stares pensively at the child willing him to survive. The painting is based on Fildes' experience following the death of his first son. The idealised doctor immortalised on canvas is the archetypical paediatrician. However, advances in technology and medicine means that this is changing. As more children are surviving with medically complex conditions, paediatric wards are no longer filled with patients who bounce back to health within 24 hours; instead, beds are occupied by children with multiple healthcare needs, disability and/or life limiting illnesses. The fragmented health, education and social care systems often fail to serve these children and their families well. Inadequate resources, difficulty managing complexity and uncertainty and a mismatch between expectations and what is deliverable adds to this inability to deliver best care. As a result, parents are often distressed, frustrated and exhausted. Paediatricians report high stress levels just doing a routine ward round in the face of this tension. I also discuss in Chapter 3 how all doctors have to 'contain' as in hold patients' fears of death. Until now of course, children rarely had chronic illness. Now this is becoming the norm, and it is paediatricians who have to become used to holding onto these fears of chronic ill health and their attendant anxieties.

OTHER SPECIALITIES

Space, but more importantly lack of evidence precludes me from discussing all the other areas of medicine. It is important though to say, that wherever one looks, surveys show the distress of different groups. For example, doctors working in intensive care,[44] palliative care, clinical oncology[45] and accident and emergency[46] are all reported to have high rates of depression, anxiety and burnout. In some areas the speciality is important, for example, substance misuse in anaesthetists, burnout in GPs, but in the main it is not the area of work that makes the difference, but the environment in which the doctor works.

REFERENCES

1 Hobbs F, Bankhead C, Mukhtar T, *et al*. Clinical workload in UK primary care: a retrospective analysis of 100 million consultations in England, 2007–14. *Lancet* 2016;**387**(10035):2323–30.

2 British Medical Association. Quarterly tracker survey: Current views from across the medical profession Quarter 2, June 2017. BMA 2017. Available from: www.bma.org.uk/collective-voice/policy-and-research/education-training-and-workforce/quarterly-survey.

3 Gibson J, Checkland K, Coleman A, *et al*. Eighth National GP Worklife Survey. 2015. Available from: www.research.manchester.ac.uk/portal/files/39031810/FULL_TEXT.PDF (accessed 16 April 2019).

4 McCain R, McKinley N, Dempster M, Campbell W, Kirk S. A study of the relationship between resilience, burnout and coping strategies in doctors. *Postgrad Med J* 2017;**94**(1107):43–7.

5 Imo U. Burnout and psychiatric morbidity among doctors in the UK: a systematic literature review of prevalence and associated factors. *BJPsych Bull* 2017;**41**(4):197–204.

6 Halliday L, Walker A, Vig S, Hines J, Brecknell J. Grit and burnout in UK doctors: a cross-sectional study across specialties and stages of training. *Postgrad Med J* 2016;**93**(1101):389–94.

7 Orton P, Orton C, Pereira Gray D. Depersonalised doctors: a cross-sectional study of 564 doctors, 760 consultations and 1876 patient reports in UK general practice. *BMJ Open* 2012;**2**(1):e000274.

8 Spiers J, Buszewicz M, Chew-Graham C, *et al*. Barriers, facilitators, and survival strategies for GPs seeking treatment for distress: a qualitative study. *Br J Gen Pract* 2017;**67**(663):e700–8.

9 Soler JK, Yaman H, Esteva M, et al. Burnout in European family doctors: the EGPRN study. *Fam Pract* 2008;**25**(4):245–65.

10 Peckham C. Medscape Lifestyle Report 2017: race and ethnicity, bias and burnout. Available from: www.medscape.com/features/slideshow/lifestyle/2017/overview. Accessed 15 December 2018.

11 Baird B, Charles A, Honeyman M, Maguire D, Das P. Understanding pressures in general practice [Internet]. The King's Fund; 2016. Available from: www.kingsfund.org.uk/sites/default/files/field/field_publication_file/Understanding-GP-pressures-Kings-Fund-May-2016.pdf.

12 The King's Fund. Through the eyes of GP trainees: workforce of the future. 2018. Available from: www.kingsfund.org.uk/blog/2018/08/gp-trainees-workforce-future.

13 The King's Fund. Comments on new GP workforce figures and NHS vacancy data. www.kingsfund.org.uk/press/press-releases/gp-workforce-figures-nhs-vacancy-data.

14 Iacobucci G. Two fifths of GPs want to quit in the next five years, poll finds. *BMJ* 2019;**364**:l960. https://doi.org/10.1136/bmj.l960.

15 British Medical Journal. Mental health and wellbeing in the medical profession. 21 November 2019. Available from: www.bma.org.uk/collective-voice/policy-and-research/education-training-and-workforce/supporting-the-mental-health-of-doctors-in-the-workforce.

16 Kumar S. Burnout in psychiatrists. *World Psychiatry* 2007;**6**(3):186–9.

17 Howard R, Kirkley C, Baylis N. Personal resilience in psychiatrists: systematic review. *BJPsych Bull* 2019;**43**:2009–15.

18 Meier D. The inner life of physicians and care of the seriously ill. *JAMA* 2001;**286**(23):3007.

19 Main T. The ailment. *Br J Med Psychol* 1957;**30**:129–45. [Republished in *The Ailment and Other Psychoanalytic Essays*. London: Free Association Books, 1989, p. 129.]

20 Rathod S, Roy L, Ramsay M, Das M, Birtwistle J, Kingdon D. A survey of stress in psychiatrists working in the Wessex Region. *Psychiatr Bull* 2000;**24**(4):133–6.

21 Deahl M, Turner T. General psychiatry in no-man's land. *Br J Psychiatry* 1997;**171**(1):6–8.

22 Alexander D. Suicide by patients: questionnaire study of its effect on consultant psychiatrists. *BMJ* 2000;**320**(7249):1571–4.

23 Guthrie E, Tattan T, Williams E, Black D, Bacliocotti H. Sources of stress, psychological distress and burnout in psychiatrists. *Psychiatr Bull* 1999;**23**(4):207–12.

24 Hassan TM, Sikander S, Mazhar N, Munshi T, Galbraith N, Groll D. Canadian psychiatrists' attitudes to becoming mentally ill. *BJMP* 2013;**6**(3):a619.

25 Bel M, Lusilla P, Valero S, et al. Psychiatrists admitted to a physicians' health programme. *Occup Med* 2015;**65**(6):499–501.

26 Tagore A. Personal experience: coming out – the psychotic psychiatrist – an account of the stigmatising experience of psychiatric illness. *Psychiatr Bull* 2014;**38**(4):185–8.

27 Fothergill A, Edwards D, Burnard P. Stress, burnout, coping and stress management in psychiatrists: findings from a systematic review. *Int J Soc Psychiatry* 2004;**50**(1):54–65. http://dx.doi.org/10.1177/0020764004040953.

28 Balch C, Freischlag J, Shanafelt T. Stress and burnout among surgeons. *Arch Surgery* 2009;**144**(4):371.

29 Benson S, Truskett P, Findlay B. The relationship between burnout and emotional intelligence in Australian surgeons and surgical trainees. *ANZ J Surgery* 2007;**77**(s1):A79.

30 Sharma A, Sharp D, Walker L, Monson J. Stress and burnout in colorectal and vascular surgical consultants working in the UK National Health Service. *Psycho-Oncology* 2008;**17**(6):570–6.

31 Dimou F, Eckelbarger D, Riall T. Surgeon burnout: a systematic review. *J Am Coll Surg* 2016;**222**(6):1230–9.

32 Shanafelt TD, Balch CM, Bechamps GJ, *et al.* Burnout and career satisfaction among American surgeons. *Ann Surg* 2009;**250**(3):463–71.

33 Harms B, Heise C, Gould J, Starling J. A 25-year single institution analysis of health, practice, and fate of general surgeons. *Ann Surg* 2005;**242**(4):520–9.

34 Lefebvre LG, Kaufmann M. The identification and management of substance use disorders in anesthesiologists. *Can J Anesth/J Can Anesth* 2017;**64**:211–18. DOI 10.1007/s12630-016-0775-y.

35 Warner D, Berge K, Sun H, Harman A, Hanson A, Schroeder D. Substance use disorder among anesthesiology residents, 1975–2009. *JAMA* 2013;**310**(21):2289–96. Available from: https://jamanetwork.com/journals/jama/fullarticle/1787405.

36 McLellan AT, Skipper GS, Campbell M, DuPont RL. Five-year outcomes in a cohort study of physicians treated for substance use disorders in the United States. *BMJ* 2008;**337**:a2038.

37 Skipper GE, DuPont RL. Anesthesiologists returning to work after substance abuse treatment. *Anesthesiology* 2009;**110**:1422–3; author reply 1426–8.

38 Yentis S, Shinde S, Plunkett E, Mortimore A. Suicide amongst anaesthetists – an Association of Anaesthetists survey. *Anaesthesia* 2019;**74**(11):1365–73.

39 Alexander BH, Checkoway H, Nagahama SI, Domino KB. Cause-specific mortality risks of anesthesiologists. *Anesthesiology* 2000;**93**:922–30.

40 McDonnell N, Kaye R, Hood S, Shrivaslava P, Khursandi D. Mental health and welfare in Australian anaesthetists. *Anaesth Intens Care* 2013;**41**(5):641–7. Available from: www.ncbi.nlm.nih.gov/pubmed/23977916.

41 Smith R. Burnout in obstetricians and gynecologists. *Obstet Gynecol Clin N Am* 2017;**44**(2):297–310.

42 Gibson H. Why Obs and Gynae? [Internet]. Royal College of Obstetricians & Gynaecologists. 2018 [cited 22 September 2019]. Available from: www.rcog.org.uk/en/careers-training/considering-a-career-in-og/why-choose-og/harry-gibson.

43 Slade P, Balling K, Sheen K, *et al.* Work-related posttraumatic stress symptoms in obstetricians and gynaecologists: findings from INDIGO a mixed methods study with a cross-sectional survey and in-depth interviews. *BJOG* 2020. Available from: https://doi.org/10.1111/1471-0528.16076.

44 Coomber S, Todd C, Park G, Baxter P, Firth-Cozens J, Shore S. Stress in UK intensive care unit doctors. *Br J Anaesthesia* 2002;**89**(6):873–81.

45 Berman R, Campbell M, Makin W, Todd C. Occupational stress in palliative medicine, medical oncology and clinical oncology specialist registrars. *Clin Med* 2007;**7**(3):235–42.

46 Burbeck R. Occupational stress in consultants in accident and emergency medicine: a national survey of levels of stress at work. *Emerg Med J* 2002;**19**(3):234–8.

24

Talking Helps

CLARE GERADA, CAROLINE WALKER AND RICHARD JONES

Doctors respond well to talking therapies. This is hardly surprising seeing that they use listening and talking so extensively in their own clinical practice with patients. The most common form of talking treatment, cognitive behaviour therapy (CBT) involves correcting abnormal thinking and behaviours. Other therapies such as psychoanalysis, examine the psychological processes linked to one's upbringing and parental attachments to bring about long-lasting change. Different types of treatment are effective depending on the presenting issue.

This chapter will explore the therapies used and which are the most effective for different conditions.

DOCTORS ABNORMAL THINKING PROCESSES

In our service we see some specific unhelpful ways of thinking (*cognitive distortions*) that doctors engage with. These can become entrenched and lead to mental illness.

Worrying

It is not uncommon for doctors to have automatic negative thoughts and ruminations centred on being a bad doctor. They doubt their work, feel guilty for something they have done (or not done) and often feel overly responsible for things out of their control. They are self-critical and paradoxically this gives them the illusion of control, for example, 'If it's my fault then I can do something about it'. However, this just fuels the anxiety and self-doubt and leads to a constant fear of failure. If unchecked it can lead to anxiety, depression or other mental illness.

Fatima had just started her third year after qualification. She was working in a very busy medical job. One day her consultant said that she had failed to mention an abnormal blood result on her hospital discharge paperwork to the general practitioner. This led to a delay in treatment by the patient's family doctor. Fatima felt devastated that she had made this mistake and started to check her discharge letters repeatedly. She began by checking them all twice through, but before long she was checking every letter between 10 and 20 times over. She began to stay later at work to keep on top of her workload. Her boyfriend was becoming so frustrated at never seeing her that he was making murmurings that they should split up. She stopped going to the gym and seeing friends and was finding it increasingly hard to sleep at night, worrying about having made another mistake. She convinced herself that she was a bad doctor, someone who shouldn't be trusted with patients and that she should leave medicine completely.

Fatima's abnormal thinking was triggered by a minor complaint. She then entered a cycle of obsessive worrying, a negative spiral where worrying becomes excessive, unproductive and difficult to control. The longer one spends worrying the harder it gets to stop the worrying thoughts.

In therapy Fatima started to understand the catastrophic thinking driving her cycle of anxiety and worrying. She was able to start challenging these 'worst-case scenario' thoughts and disrupt the vicious cycle of checking and reassurance seeking. She learnt these behaviours made her anxiety worse not better. In time she was able to do them less, eventually just checking her letters through once briefly before signing them off. She was encouraged to re-engage with her running and to go out at least once a week with friends.

Doctors might believe that they are the only ones who worry, that their peers are more competent and 'always know what to do'. In reality all doctors have doubts about their competence and mastery of their job. The lack of safe, confidential spaces to talk about this anxiety means that these worries are never shared or normalised.

The myth of certainty

There is a myth that modern medicine can provide clear and certain answers. Doctors have to discover very early on in their career that this is not the case. Dealing with uncertainty is fraught with anxiety but a key skill to learn.

In our experience the second year after qualification (in the UK called Foundation Year 2 [FY2]) is the time when most newly qualified doctors have to accept responsibility for their decisions and actions. Until now, the job is mainly around following instructions, clerking patients, ensuring a patient is 'worked-up' for theatre and tests, discharge summaries and take-home medicines are prepared. It is at the move to FY2 where more responsibility starts and where doctors begin to experience anxiety as they have to learn to accept not just uncertainty but also fallibility. For some, this anxiety can become overwhelming and lead to constant checking behaviour.

As with Fatima, doctors might ask for repeated reassurance from senior colleagues about their treatment plans and return to the hospital to review patients even when off duty – not trusting their own handover instructions to others.

Considerable time can pass with the doctor in a heightened state of anxiety while other areas of their lives are neglected and relationships suffer, hobbies wane and self-care deteriorates. In this state there is a tendency to overestimate the problem and underestimate personal coping strategies.

Medicine is fraught with situations where one can fret over decisions made. In therapy doctors who find it difficult to accept uncertainty (and all doctors must accept it if they are to survive a career in medicine) are encouraged to reframe their fears. For example:

> Hugh was finishing his Friday emergency clinic at his GP practice. He saw Jane, a 3-year-old with a mild temperature, rash and generally unwell. He examined the child, reassured the parents and gave advice about using paracetamol and keeping the child well hydrated.

This is a common consultation, repeated many thousands of times every day by GPs across the country. Hugh had to address his fears of 'what if?' (the 'if' being a serious illness such as meningitis), based on his experience, knowledge and skills. If Hugh is not able to accept uncertainty (and assuming he cannot send every patient to hospital 'just in case'), then he might fret and engage in unhelpful behaviours and thinking. Instead, his training should have taught him to use a number of cognitive and behavioural processes, for example, asking himself, 'How likely is it that this child has meningitis?' or 'If there is a very small chance, can I live with this?' Finally, he might ask himself, 'What have I done to reassure myself that I have handled this case well?' All of these are examples of **cognitive re-framing**. This is discussed more in Chapter 5 when we look at specific coping strategies doctors might find helpful.

'Imposter syndrome'

No matter how many accolades a doctor receives, or positions of authority they hold, they can still feel that it is undeserved and that sooner or later someone will discover 'the real them' – someone not good enough, a failure and an individual who has just got to where they are through luck rather than their own making. The 'imposter syndrome' was first described in 1974 to define high-powered women who fear they are not as good as their peers. It is common among doctors attending for treatment in our service, especially so in female doctors. The clinical symptoms most frequently reported are generalised anxiety, lack of self- confidence, depression and frustration related to inability to meet self-imposed standards of achievement. The impostor phenomenon is difficult to overcome as there are many reinforcers that maintain the syndrome – especially diligence and hard work. Hard work and study pay off in excellent performance and approval from authorities. Instead of bringing cessation to fears about not being good enough, it fuels the individual to work harder to achieve higher grades, achievements and performance. Each achievement leads to elation, but this is short lived, and the cycle continues. The individual develops an unstated and paradoxical belief that if she (and it is usually a she) were to think she could succeed she would actually fail. Her belief takes on the quality of a magical ritual, which will guarantee at least an overt success. However, the success is an empty one, and the good feelings are short lived because the underlying sense of phoniness remains untouched.

When working with doctors we challenge their ingrained sense of needing to succeed. In therapy we ask them to work less, accept failure or to do things in what they initially perceive as a 'half-hearted' fashion. For example, when we ask a doctor to deliberately leave a spelling mistake in a letter, they look at us as if we had landed from the planet Mars. However, if they can learn to challenge their own rigid standards and tolerate a less perfect way of practising (within the guidelines of safe practise of course), they often find their day-to-day working lives become much easier and more manageable over time and they begin to accept themselves for what they are – high achievers.

TRIGGERS FOR ABNORMAL THINKING

Guilt

The feel of guilt is common in doctors.[1] Doctors' sensitivity to guilt is heightened as if they hold themselves to a higher standard of behaviour and judge themselves harshly if they fall short of this. Guilt is especially seen in burnt-out doctors who blame themselves for dwindling empathy towards their patients. Guilt is also a common feature of doctors when they need to take time off from work due to sickness.[2]

Competition

> If you compare yourself with others, you may become vain and bitter; for always there will be greater and lesser persons than yourself.
>
> **From *Desiderata* by Max Ehrmann**

Competition is a quintessential part of medical life. From the earliest days of trying to gain a place at medical school to the constant assessments and jostling for ranking and jobs, it is part of the daily fabric of a doctor's life. Competition rather than cooperation appears to be the norm in medicine (certainly in the modern era). At school, prospective medical students stood out as the best of their class, yet once at medical school they are just one more A* student among many and excellence is the norm. To achieve the highest ranks means working harder and denying oneself extracurricular activities. Not achieving despite (or in spite) of enormous efforts (efforts that in the past would have been rewarded with accolades) can lead to a gradual erosion of self-esteem. Expectations are either raised to unrealistic heights and never met or lowered to levels that leave the doctor feeling ashamed and lacking.

Fatigue

Doctors often work gruelling shift patterns and are left feeling tired at work due to lack of sleep. Sleep deprivation may be a crucial factor in the vulnerability of doctors in making errors and developing post-traumatic stress-like symptoms.

Constant change

Doctors undergo a large number of changes throughout their training and later working lives. Rotations might be short and involve moving distances between attachments. Frequent changes of addresses mean constant uprooting of components of support networks – including social, professional and medical supports. While change can be exciting, it also creates anxiety and can add to their psychological burden. It also makes it harder to form and sustain long-term life partnerships.

Grief and shock

It is not uncommon for a doctor in their first clinical year, after working years towards that goal, to find themselves realising that the job is far from what they expected or hoped. In adjusting to their new roles, young doctors often go through a grief-like process akin to bereavement. They frequently express themes of:

- Confusion, disillusionment and shock ('This isn't what I expected', 'How did I get here?').
- Anger ('This isn't fair! I never see my family!').
- Denial and rationalisation ('It's just a bad week, the next job will be better.').
- Bargaining ('If I just work a bit harder it will get easier.').
- Depression ('What's the point of carrying on if it's this hard?').
- Acceptance ('This is hard but I'm doing the best I can.').

Each step on a doctor's career path involves relinquishing one rôle to take on another – meaning needing to start again at the bottom of a steep learning curve. This can create joy and excitement, but also loss and sadness for what has been left behind. Add to this the constant actual or threatened loss of patients' lives, cuts to beds and services and saying goodbye to colleagues, and we can see that grief is ever present in the everyday experiences of doctors. And yet it is rarely spoken of (except perhaps in the palliative care environment or those lucky enough to be part of a peer-support group). It is the missing emotion within healthcare, conspicuous by its absence. Without external supports or a space to ventilate the emotional burden of these, losses can become internalised and lead to depression or anxiety. Discussions about loss and grief are commonplace in the therapy rooms of our service.

TREATMENT

What follows is a brief run-through of different talking modalities that can help doctors suffering from mental illness.

Cognitive behavioural therapy (CBT)

CBT has become one of the most common forms of talking therapy. It is based on the concept that one's thoughts, feelings, physical sensations and actions are interconnected, and that negative thoughts and feelings can trap the individual in a vicious cycle of unhelpful symptoms and behaviours. For example, if you interpret a situation negatively then you might experience negative emotions as a result, and those bad feelings might then lead you to behave in a certain way, such as withdrawing from social interactions. CBT uses a problem-focused approach aiming to reframe unhelpful thoughts (cognitive distortions) and encourage more helpful behavioural reactions.

There are a number of common cognitive distortions people use. These include:

Cognitive distortion	What happens	Example
Mental filtering	Focusing only on the negative and screening out the wider context	This commonly happens when a doctor receives multi-source feedback and spots the only negative comment among the sea of positive ones
Over-generalisation	If it happens once, it will happen again	'I made a mistake over a drug dose; I will always make the same mistake'
Jumping to conclusions	Thinking that you can read other people's mind (mind-reading) and in so doing predict the worst possible scenario (fortune telling)	'They didn't answer my email about wanting to drop down a session They think I am useless and not worth speaking to They are going to force me to move to another job'
Polarised thinking (or 'black and white' thinking)	This is all or nothing thinking	'If I fail an exam module, I must be useless, therefore I must give up medicine as I will make a terrible doctor'
Catastrophising, maximising, minimising	Expecting disaster to strike, no matter what Bad news is a disaster, good news is 'no big deal'	'I received a complaint; I am going to be struck of the medical register' Or 'I won a prize… so what?'

(continued)

Cognitive distortion	What happens	Example
'Shoulds', 'musts' and 'oughts'	Imposing rules on oneself; the emotional consequence is guilt Experiencing negative emotions such as guilt, anxiety, low mood and shame	'I should pass this exam the first time around' When a person directs should statements toward others, they often feel anger, frustration and resentment
Personalising	Blaming oneself if something goes wrong	'The clinic ran over time; it must be my fault' (not that it was because three extra patients were slotted in)
Emotional reasoning	Taking one's emotions as facts	'I feel like a failure, so I must be one'

Practically speaking CBT is an ideal therapy for doctors as it is relatively short (usually six to 20 sessions), cost-effective and can be fitted flexibly around their shifting work patterns (especially when provided remotely). It also lends itself to work in couples and groups. Doctors respond well to CBT, enabling them to return to the workplace with a new set of tools to support them in daily practise. It is a highly-structured therapy and doctors like it – maybe because it mirrors the structured approach to medicine. Homework is part of the treatment. The therapist needs to be mindful that the doctor might embrace homework too readily – as their competitive nature kicks in and they want to demonstrate how good they are as patients.

Mindfulness-based interventions (MBI)

Mindfulness is the state in which one becomes more aware of one's physical, mental and emotional condition in the present moment, without becoming judgmental. A 'mindful' person becomes more aware of their experiences, such as their bodily sensations, thoughts and feelings and learns to accept them without being influenced by them. There appears to be an appetite for mindfulness-based interventions on a more organisational level in the prevention of doctors becoming unwell and maintaining well-being once treated.[3,4]

MBIs include a range of interventions, based on using mindfulness and include mindfulness-based stress reduction (MBSR) and mindfulness-based cognitive behaviour therapy (MBCT). MBSR can help people address stress, pain, anxiety and depression. MBCT combines CBT techniques with mindfulness strategies in order to help individuals better understand and manage their thoughts and emotions to achieve relief from distress.

The best evidence base for MBCT is in relapse prevention for those suffering from recurrent depressive disorder.[5-7] The therapy is normally delivered as weekly groups over a course of eight weeks, with each session lasting two hours.

Schema therapy

Schema therapy combines aspects of cognitive-behavioural, experiential, interpersonal and psychoanalytic therapies into one unified model. It shows good results in helping people to change long-standing negative, self-defeating patterns of thinking and behaving. These schemas might include, 'I'm a failure', 'I will never be good enough'. Schemas tend to be laid down in childhood and reinforced in later life. Working as a doctor is a good breeding ground for negative schemas given the unachievably high levels of perfectionism, altruism and self-sacrifice that are demanded from them.

Individual psychotherapy

Psychotherapy helps doctors understand unconscious experiences, linked to their past, and how these affect their current behaviour. Several approaches are described under the general heading of 'individual psychotherapy'. While there may be subtle differences between them, they almost all are longer-term therapies, lasting six or more months, where the agenda for each session is purposefully left open, and the client/patients leads the discussion, with reflections and gentle guidance from the therapist. The focus is on early life experiences and how these may be affecting current life, the relationships we form, the situations we find ourselves involved in and common patterns of behaviours in similar situations.

Compassion and compassion-focused therapy (CFT)

CFT is a form of psychotherapy developed by the British clinical psychologist, Paul Gilbert. It incorporates techniques from CBT, Buddhist psychology and neuroscience and aims to transform problematic patterns of thinking and feeling related to anxiety, anger, shame and self-criticism.[8] Given its focus on shame and self-criticism it is particularly helpful among doctors. CFT highlights how important it is to be 'held in mind' even if this is by an imaginary caregiver, as in the case of the perfect nurturer.[1] Being held in the mind of others is one of the most powerful mechanisms for change when doctors heal together in groups.

Group therapy

Given the choice, most patients, including doctors, would prefer individual- to group-based therapies. Yet group therapy is an extremely useful therapeutic intervention. It allows patients to learn, not just from the therapist, but from each other. Problems and ways of addressing them can be shared among the group members. Interpersonal learning through modelling of behaviour by other patients or giving or receiving feedback in a safe environment can be invaluable in helping with maladaptive ways of thinking or behaving. For individuals who have had problems with their primary family group, the therapy group can help them explore childhood experiences and learn not to repeat destructive or unhelpful behaviours.

In our experience, and irrespective of the type of group (for example, suspended doctors, addiction, bereavement), an overwhelming theme is that group members are reassured in knowing they are not alone. The group provides an antidote to shame – the doctor no longer is an outcast from the larger group of 'medicine', and in fact feels included, accepted, 'normal' and even loved. Given the shadow side of medicine where shameful projections are thrown at sick doctors, it is not surprising that before joining a group, prospective members express anxiety about being humiliated or judged by colleagues. These fears are allayed once members identify with shared struggles. Groups are successful in breaking the isolation doctors feel at all levels or specialities in medicine, normalising the most basic human need for support.[9]

TREATMENT OF SPECIFIC PROBLEMS IN GROUPS

Managing exam stress

I have managed to succeed in passing my exam, which was a huge hurdle, having failed it twice, which was one of the contributing factors to the initial deterioration in my mental health. I am progressing well at work and my confidence and self-esteem has flourished.

A junior doctor

One specific workshop run over the years is aimed at managing exam stress. This workshop is targeted at doctors who have failed examinations on repeated occasions and introduces how their emotions impact on their ability to pass. Through the use of cognitive and behavioural techniques, the workshops give trainees the skills and strategies to manage their stress and anxiety. The underpinning principle of these workshops is to help the doctor understand that the exam itself does not have the power to make them feel anxious (or to feel anything for that matter). Instead, it is the doctor who holds the power to control the emotion they feel about the threat of the exam. Doctors are not blamed for the anxiety that they are feeling, but instead empowered to change this into a more functional and adaptive emotional response. The feedback from this course, and the number who go on to pass their examinations, is very good.

Groups for doctors with drug/alcohol or other addictions

Group work in addictions can make a huge contribution to recovery. For addicted doctors the experience of being included in a group reduces isolation and stigma. Members share their experiences of recovery and, those in established recovery, model success for people just starting out. Most therapy groups for doctors with addiction adopt an alcoholic or narcotics anonymous (AA/NA) philosophy and engagement in the 12 steps.

Groups for doctors who have had their practising rights suspended or have been erased from the medical register

Doctors who have had their licence to practise removed (either permanently through erasure or temporarily through suspension) probably carry the greatest shame and are the most isolated of all mentally ill doctors. A therapy group for these doctors allows containment of their grief, anger, resentment, shame and guilt. The space gives doctors room to express themselves. New doctors can gain support from returning doctors, as well as allowing the sharing of experiences while unable to work; to think about how best to manage the unwanted feelings affecting them and to reflect how they came to be in their current situation.

The following is a description of the group held at our service for suspended, excluded and erased doctors.

The suspended doctors group meets once a month for 90 minutes. Attendance is voluntary and doctors come to get peer support. The setting is a room to which public access is denied. Clear boundaries of confidentiality and respect for each other are important requirements in the group. New members are invited to say briefly what has brought them to the group. Older ones update on their progress since the last group. The focus is to try and understand the thoughts and feelings underlying the experiences they are going through while unable to work; to think about how best to manage unwanted feelings affecting them. Initial feelings of shame lead to depression as their suspension makes them face the reality of their actions. It is common for the doctors' feelings to turn into negativity against the 'system' that they feel has led to them becoming involved with the regulator. They rail against the GMC and their long, drawn out and punitive processes. This can become a distraction preventing doctors from being able to look more deeply at the part they have played in events leading to their suspension. A sense of despair quickly takes hold, leading to a deepening of depressed feelings; anger, frustration and resentment then build up. Meeting in a group helps the doctors regain hope, seeing light at the end of their dark tunnel.

Groups for those bereaved following the death by suicide or sudden accidental death of a doctor

One of the authors (CG) has been running a group for those bereaved following the death by suicide or sudden accidental death of a doctor. Sadly, commonplace among the bereaved is loneliness and the fear of being judged by others, and the experience of those who have attended non-medical support groups is reported as mixed. Doctors (general practitioners and psychiatrists in particular) are frequently held responsible in the aftermath of a suicide for failing to prevent the death of their patient. When attending support groups for the general public, this fault can be transmitted back to the medically bereaved who are vicariously held responsible for failures in their loved ones' care. The bereaved can also become the container for the shame of the medical profession in failing to keep their own kind alive.

The bereavement group allows for 'healthy' mourning and a space where the wall of silence can be broken; where denial and inconsolable preoccupation with the lost loved one can be transformed from monologue to dialogue and then discourse.[10]

CONCLUSION

Doctors respond remarkably well to talking therapies. They respond to being able to reframe and normalise their emotions. What we have found especially helpful is group work, something that at first doctors find difficult to contemplate (their first thought might be 'how can we share what we feel with others?') yet find the support, learning and attachment to a group, transformational.

REFERENCES

1 Lee DA. (2005). The perfect nurturer: a model to develop a compassionate mind within the context of cognitive therapy. In: *Compassion: Conceptualisations, Research and Use in Psychotherapy*. London: Routledge, 2005.

2 Henderson M, Brooks SK, del Busso L, *et al*. Shame! Self-stigmatisation as an obstacle to sick doctors returning to work: a qualitative study. *BMJ Open* 2012;**2**(5):e001776.

3 Mindfulness All-Party Parliamentary Group (MAPPG). Mindful nation UK report. 2015. Available from: www.themindfulnessinitiative.org/mindful-nation-report.

4 Kabit-Zinn J. *Coming to Our Senses: Healing Ourselves and the World Through Mindfulness*. New York: Piatkus, 2005.

5 Segal ZV, Walsh KM. Mindfulness based cognitive therapy for residual depressive symptoms and relapse prophylaxis. *Curr Opin Psychiatry* 2016;**29**(1):7–12.

6 Williams M, Penman D. *Mindfulness: A Practical Guide to Finding Peace in a Frantic World*. London: Piatkus, 2011.

7 Kuyken W, Hayes R, Barrett B, *et al*. (2015). Effectiveness and cost-effectiveness of mindfulness-based cognitive therapy compared with maintenance anti-depressant treatment in the prevention of depressive relapse or recurrence (PREVENT): a randomised controlled trial. *Lancet* 2015;**386**:63–73.

8 Gilbert Paul (2009). Introducing compassion-focused therapy. *Adv Psychiatr Treat* 2009;**15**(3):199–208. doi:10.1192/apt.bp.107.005264.

9 Gerada C. Healing doctors through groups: creating time to reflect together. *Br J Gen Pract* 2016;**66**(651):e776–8. DOI: 10.3399/bjgp16X687469.

10 Gerada C, Griffiths F. Groups for the dead [Internet]. https://doi.org/10.1177/0533316419881609.

SECTION IV

When Things Go Wrong

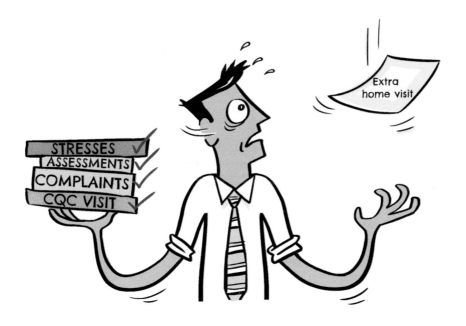

25

Sticking to the Rules
Professional and Unprofessional Behaviour

CLARE GERADA

When I qualified in 1983, it was assumed that in accepting my medical degree I was also agreeing to abide by the values of the profession. I understood these to include a set of behaviours that reflected the trust patients and the public had in me. The definition of a profession varies, but it is generally thought of as having a vocational calling, with distinct ethical codes. It also involves a lengthy, elitist training, specialised knowledge and autonomy in how that knowledge is put into practice, as well as the final say on whether that knowledge is 'valid'. Professionalism generally means self-regulation. What I did, and how I did it was largely determined by the prevailing culture of the medical community and, bar the most grossly incompetent or negligent behaviour, I would be free to practise my trade for the rest of my career with little external scrutiny. I paid a relatively small amount of money to the General Medical Council (GMC) to place my name on their register, and in return received a small pamphlet that contained their expectations of me. These were basically about being open and honest, putting patients first and not engaging in sexual relationships with them.

That was then.

In the UK, there are now over thirty different sets of guidance for doctors to adhere to in areas relating to clinical, managerial, leadership, medico-legal, research, communication and other areas of our daily professional and even personal lives. This chapter will discuss what is expected of us, our professionalism and areas where we fail.

PROFESSIONALISM

The foundations of an ethical code for medicine were laid down over 2,000 years ago in Greece by the Hippocratic school and enshrined by the Hippocratic Oath. These include the principles of medical confidentiality and the requirement to 'at first do no harm'. This has since been modernised into the Geneva Declaration. The original version of this Declaration was conceived just after the Second World War by the World Medical Association. It was felt necessary to have a new ethical code following one of the most troubled periods of modern history, where doctors participated in atrocities during the Nazi era. The Declaration essentially was a modern replacement of the Hippocratic Oath, and since has been modified. Until recently, the first line was 'I solemnly pledge to dedicate my life to the service of humanity'. The most recent Geneva Declaration (October 2017) was amended by the World Medical Federation, such that the following has been included, 'I will attend to my own health, well-being, and abilities in order to provide care of the highest standard'.[1] This amendment was added to reflect the growing number of doctors who were becoming mentally unwell. While the code of conduct under-pinning medical professionalism still exists, it has essentially been superseded by detailed mandatory requirements laid down by the regulator.

GENERAL MEDICAL COUNCIL (GMC)

The GMC has been regulating doctors in the UK since the Medical Act of 1858. The Medical Act 1978 extended its functions, particularly in relation to medical education, and separated the disciplinary processes from those that deal with doctors whose performance is impaired by ill-health. In 1995, the GMC published *Good Medical Practice* (GMP). GMP told every doctor, in plain English, what exactly was expected of them, that is, their professional obligations. It was the first national code of practice for the medical profession in the world, though it was rapidly replicated in many different countries. GMP provides an overview of what is expected in terms of professional behaviour.[2] If we violate these codes, there is a legitimate expectation we could be subjected to formal disciplinary proceedings, including the loss of our licence to practise medicine. What is expected of us now encompasses areas not just in our professional but also in our private lives, as we are expected to uphold certain standards from living room to consulting room. This extends to behaviour that does not involve us working as doctors *per se*, for example, behaviour on a reality TV show or the use of social media. There have even been suggestions that obese doctors should be struck off the register for setting a bad example to their patients.[3]

The most far reaching changes to the way doctors are regulated followed Dame Janet Smith's Public Inquiry, which was called following the actions of the general practitioner (GP), Harold Shipman.[4] Shipman was the most prolific serial killer of modern times. He murdered his patients using lethal injections of morphine and diamorphine. Although 'only' 15 cases were heard at his trial (he was found guilty of murder on all counts and also one of forgery), it was estimated that he had killed between 200 and 400 of his patients, mostly elderly women. As many would later comment, the most striking feature of his murders was that they were being carried out in plain sight of his colleagues, the community and the professional establishment. Up to the time of the discovery of his misfeasance, by most public-held accounts he had been considered to be an 'upstanding member' of his medical community, a GP leader of the local medical trade union, a reliable colleague who other than being thought of as arrogant was liked and respected by his peers and patients. The local undertaker noticed that Shipman's patients seemed to be dying at an unusually high rate and exhibited similar poses in death: most were fully clothed, and usually sitting up or reclining on a settee. It wasn't until much later, when Shipman forged the Will of one of his patients (whom he murdered) that his nefarious actions came to light and the subsequent police investigation uncovered his spree of killing. A Public Inquiry delved deeply into motives, methods, omissions and commissions that allowed Shipman to commit these crimes for so long undetected. The Inquiry even speculated that he might have been 'addicted to killing', (as he had been to pethidine years before). The actions of Shipman sent shock waves throughout the medical community, especially my speciality, general practice. He was 'one of us' and yet instead of healing he was killing his patients. Many of us felt ashamed by association and frightened that a death of our patients from now onwards would suggest that we too were murderers. His actions changed how terminally ill patients were managed in the community. We became fearful of initiating strong opiates, even for severe pain in terminal cancer. This persists even today. It also changed how the GMC functioned; the Inquiry was critical of them,[4] and the final report, which is over 1,000 pages long, made 109 recommendations, involving more robust procedures for disciplining doctors, revalidation, separation of the judge and jury functions of the GMC and brought in the Medical Practitioners Tribunal service (MPTS). It also removed the separation between how doctors with mental illness and those referred for other issues were dealt with. Health is now considered alongside performance and conduct.

Reasons to be referred to the GMC

Before the Smith Inquiry, it was unusual for doctors to be sanctioned by the GMC, let alone removed from the medical register. One study, conducted through laborious examination of the GMC's minutes and reports in the medical press, classified the sometimes tragic, often salacious, and occasionally scarcely credible reasons for disciplining the 584 doctors who were erased in the first 133 years of the GMC's existence from 1858 to 1991.[5] The most common reason for the erasure of doctors who qualified in England was adultery with patients and for those who qualified in Ireland the reason was often alcohol related. Before 1970 procuring an illegal abortion was also a common reason for erasure.[5] During this period, erasure from the register would not necessarily terminate a career: 16 doctors had been erased twice, and two, three times.

This is very different today. Around 8,000 doctors each year are referred to the GMC and about 200 receive a serious sanction, most commonly suspension, and between 60 and 80 doctors have their licence to practise removed. Because human behaviour itself is complex, it is hardly surprising that the ways in which it can become deviant from normal mores are so diverse. Of the 119 cases in 2015 that resulted in suspension or erasure, 103 cases related to transgressions involving the doctor's professional life (most often related to dishonesty, clinical issues or inappropriate relationship with patients) vs. 16 cases that involved their personal life (drink driving, sexual issues).[6] Dishonesty and inappropriate sexual relationships made up nearly one-third receiving these sanctions. Most complaints leading to erasure or suspension arose from employers, not members of the public. Cases referred by members of the public were more likely to relate to clinical issues and inappropriate patient relationships.

DOCTORS AND CRIMINAL BEHAVIOUR

Academic excellence has always been a pre-requisite for admission into medical school, but so too is an unblemished criminal record and, as such, doctors who commit and are charged with crimes are rare. Given the competition, even getting a foothold into medical school is very difficult, if not impossible, if someone has committed a crime. For example, Ahmed was 16 years old when he got a conviction for burglary and given a community service order. He then went on to turn his life around, studied hard and obtained top grades in his A levels, did voluntary work and worked in a GP surgery to gain experience. He then applied to study medicine but was rejected from Manchester, Cambridge, Leeds, Sheffield, and Imperial on the basis of his previous conviction. He did eventually get in, after appeal (helped by the publicity relating to his particular mitigating factors related to his personal upbringing). Ahmed's case sparked a debate about how difficult it is for any potential applicant to be 'flawed' in any way.

Once qualified, strict professional codes of conduct and public expectations means that the vast majority of doctors follow the rules, honour the trust given to them by virtue of their status and never break the law for their entire career. However, occasionally they do transgress and fall short of these standards, some so seriously that they receive a criminal charge and, on rare occasions, the harshest of all sanctions, a custodial sentence. Criminal sanctions against doctors are rare. Data from the GMC for the period between 2005 and 2019 show just over 2,000 doctors in the UK had criminal records (against more than 200,000 on the register). More than 50% of crimes were for vehicle-related offences such as dangerous driving (speeding, drink- or drug-driving) and motoring offences (driving without insurance or tax). While it is only speculation, it is likely that many of these are related to alcohol and/or drug use – this means for treatable mental health problems if the individual had sought help before the criminal incident.

There are other offences (occurring much less often) that involve forgery, fraud, possessing indecent images of children and sexual offences. Fortunately, there have been no more doctors since Shipman who have been charged with murder.

Doctors are surprised that an offence committed quite unrelated to work (for example, being found guilty of offences against health and safety regulations) can impact on their career. Most regulators expect that doctors conduct is of a certain standard, even if they are not at work. The UK regulator says that 'you must make sure that your conduct justifies your patients' trust in you and the public's trust in the profession'. Any conviction or caution received anywhere in the world needs to be disclosed and doctors must follow the GMC guidance in this respect.[7]

Possession of a criminal conviction does not automatically disbar a doctor from working, though the more serious crimes, such as possession of indecent images of children and sexual offences, will almost always lead to erasure. This seems reasonable given public confidence has been breached when a doctor transgresses so seriously. Also, the most robust predictor of future serious offence (such as violence or sexual assault) is a history of past offence.[8,9] For less serious crimes the chances of being able to work are mixed. Many, but not all, minor criminal convictions give reason to doubt a person's honesty, which is a vital requirement expected from a doctor. Cheating in exams is one of the most powerful predictors of future dishonest behaviour.[10] Some offences, however, such as using illegal drugs or motoring offences, do not necessarily imply that a person is dishonest though suggest they are willing to engage in behaviour that is illegal and harmful to themselves or others. Clearly such offences raise serious questions about possible risks to patients, the possibility of more serious crimes being committed or other unprofessional behaviours.[11] All of these issues are taken into account by a regulator and a proportionate balance made on an individual case-by-case basis.

For a doctor to receive a custodial sentence is very rare. At my service, around five doctors have served some time in prison and around ten more have received suspended sentences. Most are for drink- or drug-related offences. This doctor described his experience of a prison sentence (I have changed his name and some details though he has given consent for his case to be told):

Diyan, an accident and emergency doctor, began drinking after a traumatic break up of a relationship. His drinking rapidly rose to two bottles of whisky per day. At work he masked the smell of alcohol by chewing mint-flavoured gum and eating onions. To offset withdrawal shakes towards the end of 12-hour shifts, he persuaded his GP, who was also a friend, to prescribe him benzodiazepines (telling the GP it was for anxiety). He then used drugs and prescriptions stolen from work to augment these. Despite smelling of alcohol and looking increasingly dishevelled, no-one challenged him or suggested he sought help.

After a series of drink-drive offences (including driving while disqualified) Diyan appeared in court and following his trial received a custodial sentence (three years' imprisonment). The trial judge said at sentencing:

This is the most tragic of cases where someone who has taken a profession to care for others has, on the face of it, failed to care for themselves and allowed themselves to fall into the state where dishonesty became a routine way of life for a period of the offending.[12]

Diyan describes his bewilderment, as he stood in the dock, when the judge read out his sentence and that he was receiving a custodial sentence. This is what he recalls of those first few days:

> I didn't know what it meant, being sent into custody. I thought I was going to a detention camp. I thought it was like the refugee camps back home (he had spent part of his childhood in one). Open access, healthcare, schools, food served in canteens, sleeping in barracks. Once the judge left the court, the prison guards put me in handcuffs and took me downstairs to a small cell. I had to take my suit and then all my clothes off, including my underwear. I was naked in this room. They examined my rectum for drugs. I felt intimidated. I wasn't used to it. I knew I had lost my freedom and I was very tearful. Why was I going through this? I couldn't believe that I had come to this country to help, and now I was going to prison, but I deserved it. They then took a photo with me holding a custody badge. I had already been suspended by the GMC but till the moment they took me downstairs I was still a doctor. Now I was nothing. I felt completely alien, a nobody. I travelled to the prison with other prisoners – we were all in a tiny individual caged cell inside a large van. Once I arrived at the prison I was put in another small room, on my own – it was very smelly, I had no blankets, I had to sleep on a rubber mattress as I was considered a suicide risk. I had had my last drink that morning before I went to court, and for the next five days I was having alcohol withdrawal. Terrible symptoms, I felt I was climbing up the walls. I was psychotic. I spoke to the officers and they said they couldn't do anything for me. My mind was all over the place and I didn't think I would survive.

This doctor did survive his first few days in prison and went on to serve 18 months of his sentence. He was discharged early due to good behaviour. When in prison he studied law and taught reading and writing to the other prisoners. He is now applying to be restored back onto the medical register. He remains abstinent. His only regret is that he did not seek help for his alcohol addiction earlier.

This is another account of a doctor who was found guilty for dishonesty at the High Court and given a suspended prison sentence. His crime related to dishonesty, which had its roots in a mental health problem:

> *I was devastated after the decision. To be labelled as a dishonest person was the worst thing that has happened in my professional life, and now to be a convicted criminal was catastrophic. I felt ashamed and guilty of letting myself, my family, my colleagues and my profession down. Sitting down with my wife and children to tell them was one of the most difficult things I have done in my life. One of the effects of this experience has been for me to reconsider what I want and wanted in life. I entered medicine because I wanted to help and treat people. As my focus shifted, I lost sight of why I loved this job and why I had committed to it. I ended up on a hamster wheel. I never took the time to stop and reflect on where I was and where I was going. I now have had that time to do so very deeply. I am, in a way, glad that this has happened as it has allowed me that space for reflection.*

DOCTORS AND UNPROFESSIONAL BEHAVIOUR

Many years ago, I undertook expert witness work involving doctors with complaints made against them. The cases would usually involve transgressions involving inappropriate prescribing (usually of controlled drugs) or prescribing to family or friends who resided overseas, or doctors who were accused of dishonesty at work. Despite my role, which was to give an impartial analysis of how I saw the facts, I nevertheless could not help but be affected by these doctors, who through a lapse in professionalism risked losing their licence to practise. I wished, more than anything else, that someone had had a conversation with them, and explained in plain language, why they shouldn't have set out to do what they did. That it would only lead to intense mental pain, grief and potentially loss of their livelihood. I stopped doing the legal work (I found it too painful to be part of the process) and instead focused on trying to understand why these doctors, who in every other aspect of their personal and professional lives were good citizens, behaved as they had. This is how this chapter came to fruition. I have looked at the determinations from the MPTS (which are available on their website) and devised a taxonomy that describes what I suspect was the 'frame of mind' the doctor was in when they crossed their professional boundary. In using these headings, I am in no way condoning the behaviour or undermining the severity of their actions, but merely trying to understand their behaviour and, in so doing, help other doctors not to follow the same path. I am not suggesting that doctors who transgress are mentally unwell at the time, though pressure of work, absence of peer support, lack of supervision or mentoring might have a role to play in pushing doctors over their 'professional' edge.

The areas are

- It was only a 'little lie' (dishonesty, fraud, probity).
- What harm can it do (dishonesty, violations)?
- I only wanted to be friendly (sexual boundary violations).
- I forgot (dishonesty).

These are only a small sample of the many determinations that are available for scrutiny.

It was only a 'little lie' (dishonesty, fraud, probity)

The majority of cases brought before a medical tribunal are to do with cases concerning probity, fraud and dishonesty, and they tend to lead to the harshest of sanctions. Acting with honesty and integrity is a fundamental tenet of the medical profession. *Good Medical Practice* states that a doctor must be *honest and open and act with integrity* and departures from this are serious transgressions. The need to be honest is a requirement for doctors since Hippocrates the world over.

This group, 'It's only a little lie' includes doctors who commit what they might consider to be small deceits, maybe in a genuinely perceived belief that what they are doing is 'almost true' and no harm will be done. They might even believe that it is justifiable, given how busy they are, to take a short cut to obtaining the necessary paperwork or doing the required training. They might also feel no one will find out and no harm will be done by their 'little lie'. It will be found out and harm will be done. The following are examples under this category.

DISHONESTY WITH RESPECT TO HAVING UNDERTAKEN PARTICULAR TRAINING

A doctor amended and uploaded an Advanced Life Support course certificate, adding it to his training portfolio. This came to light. When given the opportunity by his employer to 'come clean' he tried to cover up what he had done, blaming others, including members of his family, claiming they had access to his home computer and had inadvertently altered the certificate and added it to his training portfolio. He escaped erasure, which reading the determination was seriously considered by the panel. In the end, they were swayed by mitigating factors, glowing testimonials from colleagues and a previous unblemished record. He was instead suspended for one month.

Despite the relatively light sanction, the doctor had to still go through 18 months of investigation and shame. His name and what he did will appear on the website for years, and he will have to disclose this misdemeanour whenever he applies for a new job. For a senior doctor (which he was), this is a high price to pay for not doing half a day's training.

A similar case is of a doctor who falsely claimed he had been signed off as competent in cardiopulmonary resuscitation. The doctor received a harsher sanction as his transgression was compounded by claiming he'd attended the training and took time off as study leave (the training had in fact been cancelled), illustrating how one lie leads to another. He was suspended for four months, which resulted in his career plans being de-railed.

DISHONESTY WITH RESPECT TO REFERENCES

In reading the determinations, I am surprised how many cases involved falsifying references or aspects of one's curriculum vitae. These are not minor errors (which we are all guilty of) but major falsehoods, such as claiming to have obtained degrees. These cases tend to result in harsh sanctions.

As part of a planned move overseas, a doctor submitted two false references with his application. His actions involved the manufacturing of references from start to finish, including false letterhead, false representations, fake personalities from human resources and fake signatures. The references were designed to look different in order to avoid suspicion being aroused. The country he was emigrating to carried out the necessary checks and discovered the forgery. The doctor did not attend his tribunal, nor did he submit any statements in his defence, nor anything that could be considered remediation or contrition. He was erased from the medical register, a high price to pay for wanting to speed up an administrative process.

This doctor could easily have obtained the necessary references, there were no reasons why they would not have been provided. Instead, in his haste to emigrate, he forged them and lost his livelihood.

DISHONESTY WITH RESPECT TO CLAIMING SICK PAY WHILE WORKING

Doctors do not tend to take sick leave, rather being more likely to have 'present-eeism' (that is working when ill) than taking time off. However, if on sick leave it is important to obey the rules, including not working in another role. There are circumstances when a doctor can work in one role where they will be medically fit to do so, but be signed off sick for another (for example, a surgeon with a broken arm cannot operate but can do outpatient work). This should be made transparent to both the place one is working and the place where one is receiving sick pay. A common error is where a doctor regularly works across two sites, maybe a substantive job with the NHS but also a small amount of self-employed private work elsewhere. If signed off as unwell and receiving sick pay, it is important to stop all work, including teaching, training, academic, medico-legal, private, media and so on, **unless** agreement has formally been agreed from the employer issuing the sick pay.

DISHONESTY IN SUBMITTING TIME SHEETS

Given electronic rostering, the use of smart cards to start and end shifts, and computerised records noting our every action, it seems odd that doctors think they can get away with submitting time sheets falsifying the hours they have worked.

My advice, is don't. The risks of a few extra hours of pay can result in a lifetime of lost earnings.

What harm can it do?

This section is closely aligned to the 'it's only a little lie', except here it is not the individual doctor who sets out to benefit from their actions but instead someone close to them.

DISHONESTY AROUND PRESCRIPTIONS

There are many examples of doctors who fall foul of their professional code or even commit an overt crime by trying to help members of their families or friends. This might take the form of writing prescriptions in other patient's names or using NHS prescriptions for those who are not entitled to NHS care. It is tempting to help one's relatives; we have all been pressurised, for example, perhaps by an elderly mother residing overseas, nagging to send her medicines she can't obtain at her home, but this desire must be curtailed unless there is a proper clinical relationship and if using NHS resources, that the individual is entitled to this care (otherwise it is theft).

A doctor wrote prescriptions for patients whose names he had taken randomly from the hospital computer database and took the prescriptions to the hospital pharmacist who noticed discrepancies in the prescription. He admitted that he wrote the prescriptions for a friend who lived overseas. He was erased from the medical register.

It is unusual to get such a harsh sanction, but it shows the risk.

I only wanted to be friendly (boundary violations)

Given the changing nature of medicine, with less formal, more collaborative working and with fuzzy boundaries created by social media, it is becoming harder to maintain clear professional and personal borders between patient and doctor. I have lived and worked in the same geographical area for three decades. I often meet with patients at social events, my children attended the same school as my patients' children, I shop in the same places and use the same local restaurants. I have had to learn, as had my father 30 years before, how to navigate and maintain boundaries alongside my changing identities as parent, mother, student, citizen, friend and local doctor. This can be difficult, but vital for the practise of safe medicine. By its nature, medicine involves an intimate and personal relationship with one's patient, and this has to be predicated on trust. All of this can be undermined by doctors who do not respect professional boundaries.

Boundary issues involve departures from usual professional practice and can be thought of as being along a spectrum, from 'crossings' to 'violations'. Boundary crossings are not necessarily exploitative. I have disclosed personal information, as when I shared that my father had severe dementia as part of empathising with a patient with their struggles caring for elderly parents. Nevertheless, at other times, boundary crossings may occur as part of a 'slippery slope' of moving from outside usual practice to inappropriate practice and become boundary violations.

Violations are unethical and unprofessional because they exploit the doctor–patient relationship, undermine the trust patients and the community have in us and can cause psychological harm to patients, compromising their ongoing medical care. It also breaks a founding ethical principle of medicine, dating back to the Hippocratic Oath:

> Into whatsoever houses I enter, I will enter to help the sick, and I will abstain from all intentional wrong-doing and harm, especially from abusing the bodies of man or woman, bond or free.

Hippocratic Oath, 274 AD

The GMC GMP uses similar sentiments, advising:

> 'you must not use your professional position to pursue a sexual or improper emotional relationship with a patient or someone close to them' and 'you must make sure that your conduct justifies your patients' trust in you and the public's trust in the profession.'

The most serious of all boundary violations are those involving sexual contraventions. These cover a range of behaviours including inappropriate contact with staff, colleagues or in unequal relationships, such as with medical students and patients.[13] Doctors are powerful authoritative figures and in exploiting patients for their own gratification, transgress a position of trust, which can have a similar effect as a parent abusing a child.

It is difficult to know how many doctors have crossed a sexual boundary as they are unlikely to self-disclose and patients are reluctant to disclose this form of abuse to authorities, due to embarrassment, fear or even misplaced loyalty towards their doctor. Reviews involving doctors in different countries over a number of years suggest that between 0.2% and 10% of doctors admit to a sexual relationship with a patient and that around 1.6% doctors are sanctioned.[14,15] These doctors are more likely to work in general practice, psychiatry and obstetrics and gynaecology, reflecting the greater likelihood of physical contact and/or psychological intimacy.

A striking feature of the literature into sexual boundary violations is the absence of 'red flags', meaning that the doctors who perpetrated the violations had no features that could be identified through screening tests. Except for rape, cases occurred without obvious signs of a personality disorder in the doctor, in both single-handed and larger medical practices, and involved both patients who were particularly vulnerable as well as those who exhibited no special vulnerabilities other than being a patient.[16] However, there are some consistent factors among the cases. Almost all were male doctors, most doctors were older than 39 years (92%), were not board certified – this was an American study (70%) and 72% were not in senior consultant positions or were in non-academic medical work settings. These five variables accounted for over 70% of all cases. However, they are extremely common variables, and the vast majority of individuals with all five do not commit sexual boundary violations.

While the literature is rich in examples of doctors who commit sexual crimes against their patients, there is very little actual data with respect to understanding their motives or any predictive personality characteristics. An extremely small study, using a validated personality questionnaire, compared two male psychiatrists whose licences were revoked for sexual misconduct compared to 38 male psychiatrists without similar allegations. The questionnaire had been administered during their earlier training and before any offence had been committed. The pre-offence profiles of the two sexual offenders were character-istic of individuals with anti-social and often narcissistic personality traits, and also of individuals exhibiting high levels of defensiveness.[17] This study (albeit very small) implies that even before they committed their violation, the doctors were outliers in terms of personality profile. A study compared 19 male doctors who had sexually assaulted adult women with a matched group of well-educated non-doctors who had committed similar offences.[18] The personality profile of both groups was very similar. Another study examining the personality profiles of 88 doctors referred to a physician behavioural programme found that those who had been referred for sexual boundary violations (as opposed to behaviourally dis-ruptive or other misconduct) had personality profiles that were most indicative of a pathological character. As a group, the sexual boundary violator tended to be more self-centred, less empathetic, less likely to take responsibility for their own offences (such that they were more likely to blame others or circumstances) and less likely to be influenced by societal norms.[19]

I think it is fair to say that currently there is no actual reliable way of predicting which of the many hundreds of thousands of doctors will commit crimes of this nature, given the only reliable discriminant is being male.

It is difficult to assign motives to why doctors conduct themselves in this manner, other than the performance of the sexual act itself. Nevertheless, as with all of life, it's not always so clear cut. The daily practice of medicine is filled by opportunities to develop intense emotions between the patient and clinician. These emotions engendered might include hostility, aggression, despair or even love. Patients can evoke powerful responses in the clinician who cares for them, these responses are called counter transference. If recognised and understood, they can be a tool in gaining a better understanding of the patient. If not, as for example, where the patient evokes feelings of love in the clinician, it can have destructive and damaging sequelae. Doctors themselves, in a vulnerable position from their own life events, might find themselves in a psychological state where compromising their professionalism is possible. This might be where the doctor becomes emotionally entangled with a patient, due in part to what has been thrown up by the doctor's own life experiences during the doctor–patient interaction. This is why it is so important that we have access to supervision, especially when we are in susceptible psychological states.

EXAMPLES OF SEXUAL BOUNDARY VIOLATIONS WITH A PATIENT

> A GP treated a patient (much younger than himself) with counselling following a bereavement. While still a patient they met accidentally at a social event. Over the next few months, he invited her to other events. At their last consultation (as she was moving out of the area) he hugged her. He then contacted her once she left the practice. Over a short period of time, hugging moved to a sexual relationship.

Sexual relationships, as in this case, between doctor and patient, are often the culmination of a series of 'boundary crossings' where the first one might be perceived as entirely innocent; for example, seeing the patient for extended appointments at the end of the day or giving one's personal phone number. Other examples might be texting or offering to do home visits rather than ask the patient to attend the practice. Each has the effect of drawing the patient emotionally closer, using the therapeutic relationship essentially to entrap them in a psychological bind.

A quote from a patient illustrates the abuse of the imbalance of power:

> He put his hand on top of mine, which was on my leg. I would not pull him towards me. I'm a layman. I did not think he would contact me, and I was not going to push myself onto the doctor, a doctor to me is upper class I'm just nobody. When he first contacted me, I was over the moon.

This doctor was subsequently erased from the GMC register.

SEXUAL INAPPROPRIATE BEHAVIOUR WITH MEMBER OF STAFF OR COLLEAGUE

Sexual boundary violations also extend to doctors abusing their position with students and staff. One such doctor, undergoing marital problems at home, made sexual advances to a medical student. The Tribunal found that his conduct was sexually motivated and represented an escalating pattern of inappropriate behaviour within a professional context and one where there was a power imbalance. He was suspended for 9 months.

I forgot (dishonest)

This category includes omitting to do things that a doctor is mandated to do. For example, have up-to-date medical indemnity, renewing necessary training (such as Section 12 Approval for conducting assessments under the Mental Health Act) or forgetting to inform the GMC if one obtains a caution or conviction.

FAILING TO DISCLOSE DRINK-DRIVING OFFENCES

A surgeon forgot to inform the GMC of a drink-drive offence. Once they were made aware of this, they issued him with a warning. A few years later he received further motoring charges. He again 'forgot' to inform the GMC. It was only when he was applying for a substantive post, where a full criminal record search was done that the omissions came to light. He claimed he had genuinely forgotten. However, the Tribunal noted the repeated nature of his omissions and found his actions to be dishonest and consequently erased him from the medical register.

RISKS OF UNPROFESSIONAL BEHAVIOUR

The chances of being referred to the GMC and receiving harsh sanctions are not randomly distributed among the general medical profession. Four out of five cases involved a male doctor. Doctors aged over 49 years are over-represented in cases resulting in suspension or erasure. One-half of all cases involved a doctor of black or minority ethnic origin, though they make up just 30% of all licenced doctors on the medical register. Out of the cases where the eventual sanction applied was suspension or erasure, only around one-third qualified in the UK.

- Proportionately, male doctors are four times as likely to be erased or suspended as female doctors.
- Hospital specialists are erased or suspended at around one-half the rate of GPs and other non-specialist doctors working in hospitals or community settings.
- Doctors in all career groups are more than twice as likely to be erased or suspended in later life.
- Doctors who obtained their primary medical qualification overseas are more than twice as likely to be erased or suspended as those trained in the UK.[6]

CONCLUSION

The vast majority of doctors have an unblemished record for their entire career. Hopefully, with more accessible, confidential treatment services, doctors in whom health problems have been the underlying issue will come forward for treatment instead of risking the medical career by suffering in silence.

REFERENCES

1 WMA. Declaration of Geneva. Available from: www.wma.net/policies-post/wma-declaration-of-geneva.
2 General Medical Council. Good medical practice [Internet]. Gmc-uk.org. 2019 [cited 1 November 2019]. Available from: www.gmc-uk.org/ethical-guidance/ethical-guidance-for-doctors/good-medical-practice.
3 Davies M. Fat doctors should be struck off to help tackle obesity epidemic. [Internet]. Mail Online. 2015 [cited 18 January 2020]. Available from: www.dailymail.co.uk/health/article-3150888/Fat-doctors-struck-setting-bad-example-obese-patients-weight-loss-expert-tells-NHS-chief.html.
4 Editorial on GMC and Shipman Report. GMC: expediency before principle. *BMJ* 2004. Available from: www.bmj.com/content/suppl/2004/12/13/329.7479.DC1.
5 Wakeford R. Who gets struck off? *BMJ* 2011;**343**(2):d7842.
6 DJS Research Ltd. Analysis of cases resulting in doctors being erased or suspended from the medical register Report prepared for: General Medical Council [Internet]. 2015. Available from: www.gmc-uk.org/-/media/documents/Analysis_of_cases_resulting_in_doctors_being_suspended_or_erased_from_the_medical_register_FINAL_REPORT_Oct_2015.pdf_63534317.pdf.
7 General Medical Council. Reporting criminal and regulatory proceedings within and outside the UK [Internet]. Gmc-uk.org. 2013 [cited 18 January 2020]. Available from: www.gmc-uk.org/ethical-guidance/ethical-guidance-for-doctors/reporting-criminal-and-regulatory-proceedings-within-and-outside-the-uk.
8 Bonta J, Hanson K, Law M. The prediction of criminal and violent recidivism among mentally disordered offenders: a meta-analysis. *Psychol Bull* 1998;**123**:123–42.
9 Hanson RK, Bussiere MT. Predicting relapse: a meta-analysis of sexual offender recidivism studies. *J Consult Clin Psychol* 1998;**66**:348–62.
10 Whitley BE. Factors associated with cheating among college students. A review. *Res High Educ* 1998;**39**:235–74.
11 McMillan J, Wright B, Davidson G, Bennett J. Criminal records and studying medicine. *BMJ* 2009b2076.
12 Personal communication from confidential assessment, as verbal communication from patient about their experiences in court, NHS PHP.
13 Galletly C. Crossing professional boundaries in medicine: the slippery slope to patient sexual exploitation. *Med J Aust* 2004;**181**(7):380–3.

14 Sansone, RA, Sansone LA. Crossing the line. Sexual boundary violations by physicians. *Psychiatry* 2009;**6**(6):45–8. Available from: www.ncbi.nlm.nih.gov/pmc/articles/PMC2720840.

15 Galletly C. Crossing professional boundaries in medicine: the slippery slope to patient sexual exploitation. *Med J Aust* 2004;**181**(7):380–3.

16 DuBois JM, Walsh HA, Chibnall JT, *et al*. Sexual violation of patients by physicians: a mixed-methods, exploratory analysis of 101 cases. *Sexual Abuse* 2019;**31**(5):503–23.

17 Garfinkel P, Bagby R, Waring E, *et al*. Boundary violations and personality traits among psychiatrists. *Can J Psychiatry* 1997;**42**(7):758–63.

18 Langevin R, Glancy G, Curnoe S. Physicians who commit sexual offences: are they different from other sex offenders? *Can J Psychiatry* 1999;**44**(8):775–80.

19 Roback HB, Strassberg D, Iannelli RJ, Reid Finlayson AJ, Blanco M, Neufeld R. Problematic physicians: a comparison of personality profiles by offence type. *Can J Psychiatry* 2007;**52**(5):315–22.

26

Making Sense of the Regulatory Process

ZAID AL-NAJJAR AND CLARE GERADA

Tim ran to the front door having heard the 'thwack' of the mail on the floor after the postman had been. Today was Saturday. He knew, but didn't know why, that the letter that had just arrived was from the GMC. Two weeks ago, someone had come to his home from work, 'a welfare check' they'd called it. He had not been to work for two days and had been too unwell (suffering from the side-effects of crystal meth) to contact his boss to let them know he wouldn't be in. If only he had known they would be calling, he would have cleared up the paraphernalia. What once had been occasional recreational use, had turned into using every and all weekend. The last time he had used it, he had lost consciousness. By not showing up to work his colleagues had been so worried that someone came to check on him at home. Now, the letter marked 'confidential' was on his doorstep and his heart stopped. This was it, the end of everything he had worked so hard for. Despite himself, he ripped the envelope open and read the letter. The GMC were investigating him following concerns raised by his employer, he was asked to attend an Interim Orders Tribunal (IOT) the next week as restrictions might need to be placed on his registration. He stopped reading after the front page as he was so frightened. He collapsed on the sofa, not knowing what this meant and what to do.

Tim had no idea what receiving the letter from the General Medical Council (GMC) meant, other than something terrible was happening. He had no idea what an Interim Orders Tribunal was, how it fitted into the GMC process or how his career was now going to pan out. All he knew and saw were the words GMC.

While working with doctors in different guises over the last two decades, it is clear that most are unfamiliar with the GMC Fitness-to-Practise processes (even the more senior and experienced ones) – **what** happens, **when** and **how**. For most doctors, their only contact with the GMC is paying its annual subscription and possibly looking up the requirements for revalidation. Unless they have been unfortunate enough to have a complaint made against them, they will never have seen the need to familiarise themselves with the workings of the regulator, in particular the disciplinary processes. Given the number of referrals to the GMC, it is perhaps prudent we all understand the basics. Hopefully this and other chapters in this section will de-mystify the GMC Fitness-to-Practise procedures and give the reader a broader understanding of them. It is always better to be prepared.

This chapter is not a replacement for specialist advice from a lawyer who has a background in medical regulation or from a Medical Defence Organisation who deals with the GMC day in, day out.

While these chapters are relevant to doctors practising in the UK, many of the issues discussed will be applicable to doctors in other jurisdictions.

REFERRALS TO THE GMC

Each year, the GMC receives 8,000–9,000 complaints and around 200–300 of these ends in a Fitness-to-Practise (FtP) tribunal, resulting in between 60 and 80 doctors per year having their licence to practise removed and another 100 or so receiving a suspension. The remaining cases end without any sanction or with a warning, undertakings or letter of advice.

Anyone can make a complaint if they are concerned about a doctor's fitness to practise, and do not need to be personally or professionally involved with them (for example, a doctor might be referred by a member of the public following a newspaper story about them). Doctors may also self-refer – in some circumstances they are professionally obliged to, or before waiting for someone else to do so. In some situations, self-referral can illustrate important aspects of insight, honesty and determination. Around two-thirds of complaints are made by members of the public, and the remainder from public organisations, including employers, the police and others.

The vast majority of referrals the GMC receive every year do not progress beyond the early triage or investigation stage. Between 2018 and 2019, 73% of cases were closed at triage stage.[1] Around 5% were referred back to the employer or 'Responsible Officer' (a senior doctor within a healthcare organisation who has responsibility for overseeing the conduct, monitoring performance and evaluating the fitness to practise of doctors linked to that organisation). Another 6% were closed at Provisional Enquiry (PE) stage (see later). In total therefore, over 80% of all cases were closed at an early stage.[2] A fairly consistent percentage of cases are closed with no formal action being taken against the doctor (for example between 2010 and 2013, 82% of investigations were closed).

> Most complaints to the GMC do not progress beyond the initial triage stage.

PROVISIONAL ENQUIRIES

In 2014, the GMC introduced the ability to conduct what they call 'provisional enquiries' (PEs). A provisional enquiry involves obtaining targeted information and uses criteria to decide whether a complaint should progress to a full fitness-to-practise investigation (FTP) investigation.[3] The GMC aims to complete a PE within 63 days, compared with six months for a full investigation. In 2017 65% of cases referred for PEs were closed with no action, saving these doctors the burden of a full investigation.

> A doctor who can demonstrate insight, has undergone a period of reflection and has instituted remedial action enhances their chances of their case being closed after the Provisional Enquiry.

WHAT DOES THE GMC INVESTIGATE?

A diverse range of complaints are referred to the GMC from the seemingly trivial (for example, the doctor's garden hedge is too high) to the very serious (fraud, sexual misconduct). As mentioned, in comparison to the number of referrals received, only a relatively small number of complaints go on to formal investigation stage (18% in 2018). This might not be reassuring for those where the complaint is escalated, but even if the complaint continues, the chances are that it will be subsequently closed, unless it is deemed too serious to do so. For cases that are closed at the triage stage, doctors may not even know that the GMC has ever received a complaint against them.

As a matter of course the GMC will investigate:

- Serious repeated mistakes and failures with respect to the doctor's medical treatment of patients (poor performance or misconduct).
- Fraud or dishonesty (misconduct or criminal conviction or caution).
- Discrimination against patients or colleague (misconduct).
- Violence, sexual assault, indecency (sexual relationship) and driving offences (criminal conviction or caution).
- Breaches of patient confidentiality (misconduct).
- A determination by another regulatory body.
- Insufficient knowledge of the English language.
- Physical or mental ill- health that may impact on a doctor's ability to practise medicine (health).

The GMC does not usually investigate allegations that are more than five years old, unless they deem that it is in the public interest to do so. This might include cases such as serious sexual allegations or significant fraud.[4]

INTERIM ORDERS TRIBUNAL

The GMC can bring a case against a doctor either to an IOT, or a full FtP tribunal. These are both run by the Medical Practitioners Tribunal Service (MPTS), whose panelists are independent of the GMC to ensure fair process.

Tim went to the GMC offices in Manchester along with the lawyer his defence
organisation had instructed to represent him. His IOT was due to take place as
the third hearing of the day. He had travelled up the night before and stayed in a
hotel to make sure he was there on time, but he needn't have worried about that
as the panel was already running significantly behind. He hadn't told his family
or friends as he was so ashamed, and it would break his mother's heart to find
out that the son she was so proud of was in this mess. Lunch came and went
and finally, it was time for his case to be heard. He was advised that he wasn't
to speak at the IOT, apart from confirming his GMC registration number. The
GMC presented their case against him, and his lawyer gave his defence. It was
reassuring to the panelists that Tim had, in the short space of time since being
found at home, already sought medical help. Although the GMC had asked for his
registration to be suspended until they had had time to finish their investigation,
because of the help he had already sought, that he accepted his use and that he was
doing all he could to stop his use, the MPTS panelists instead imposed conditions
on his registration, meaning that he could still go back to work. He was however
obliged to continue engaging with his treating doctor and agree to medical super-
vision. He was relieved, although dreaded the thought of going back to work with
everyone knowing what had happened. His lawyer had also managed to present
several glowing testimonials to the panelists; his health issue aside, it was clear
that Tim was a highly thought of doctor and colleague.

IOTs decide if a doctor's practice should be restricted while an investigation takes place or following completion of an FtP tribunal.[5] They are able to put in holding arrangements (suspension or conditions) without making any judgement on the validity of the complaint or concern, only that if it were true, this would pose a risk to patient safety or seriously jeopardise the public interest in the profession, or where there is a concern that a doctor's fitness-to-practise maybe impaired by reason of ill-health, deficient performance or misconduct. Any doctor can be asked to attend an IOT at any stage, though it is usually quite early on once the GMC are first aware of the complaint.[6] Tim was asked to attend an early IOT as their might have been concerns that he used drugs at work.

If a doctor is suspended following an IOT hearing, this period of suspension will not normally be taken into account or deducted from any suspension period given as a sanction following an FtP tribunal. Suspensions or conditions imposed by the IOT are reviewed every six months and may remain in place for up to 18 months if it takes that long for the GMC to undertake a full investigation into the allegations. They may be extended by a High Court order if the GMC investigation has not concluded by then. A doctor can ask for an early review (after three months), if s(he) feels that there should be a relaxation or lifting of an Interim Order.

While the doctor cannot present 'evidence' to the IOT in defence of their case, they can provide information for the panel to consider when making their decision pending completion of the GMC investigation. This will be covered in more detail in Chapter 27, but briefly if, as with Tim, the doctor can demonstrate they are addressing any underlying health issues head on (engaging in treatment, stopping drugs and/or alcohol) this will help at this stage. Being able to demonstrate they have reflected and even started remediable action (such as attending or planning to attend relevant courses or seeking out a mentor or supervisor), can also improve the outcome.

In our experience of working with hundreds of doctors who are involved in GMC processes, it is helpful if the doctor is working when they appear at an IOT. This might not always be possible, for example, if they are unwell or suspended from work by their employer. Working provides some distraction, income and prevents de-skilling. It also allows for the doctor to demonstrate that they can be trusted to work, and this can be invaluable. In some cases, the reason a doctor is not working is self-imposed. For example, one doctor removed himself from the workplace, even though he was not unwell, 'I thought I was a "marked man" and would not get any career development anyway'.

In response to the initial letter that the GMC had sent him informing him of the investigation, Tim replied with his employer's details as the GMC would be contacting them, to make sure there were no other concerns about him at work. His lawyer wrote a very short letter to the GMC confirming he was engaged with treatment and had no further comment to make at that time, but reserved the right to, once the investigation had concluded.

INVESTIGATION STAGE

If the complaint is not closed at the triage stage or after a PE, it will be opened as an official investigation. This is where the case managers gather information from various relevant diverse sources (employers, witnesses, experts, forensic computer experts, GMC-appointed psychiatrists) and try to determine whether the complaint needs to be passed onto a FtP tribunal or can be closed with or without a sanction. If the complainant has not already told the doctor, the first indication that they are under a GMC investigation will be when they receive what is called a '**Rule 4 letter**'. This outlines the concerns and the nature of the investigation and will invite the doctor to make comments, although they are under no obligation to do so. These comments usually have to be returned within 28 days. It is important to take this letter seriously; the problem will not go away just because the doctor ignores the process. In fact, it may only get worse. In some cases, notably where health is involved, the GMC have recently introduced the ability to pause investigations to allow doctors to obtain medical treatment. As said, even at this preliminary stage, *how* a doctor responds can have a significant impact on the outcome of their case. Where there is merit to the complaint, they are best advised to demonstrate insight, reflect on their actions and the impact of these on others (the patient, profession and their employers) and to commence remedial action.

At this stage, the GMC will write to the doctor's employers to enquire about concerns. It might be wise to pre-empt the letter arriving and let employers know in advance that the GMC is conducting an investigation and will be contacted in due course. The doctor does not need to give details of any of the allegations (unless they choose to). It can feel embarrassing to know that employers will be approached. However, remember in a large Trust, a doctor being investigated by the GMC is not an uncommon occurrence. Even in a small general practice setting the doctor will not be the first to have had a complaint made about them and referred to the GMC.

The process of 'trawling' for evidence might feel unfair – and to a certain extent it is, but it is important for the GMC to make sure that the doctor does not pose a risk to patients.

> Do not try to go through this process alone, **seek professional legal advice**. Remember, you are a doctor not a lawyer.

What happens next is largely dependent on the nature of the complaint and whether other concerns come to light (for example from employers). In our experience, doctors, having received a Rule 4 letter, feel so shocked and ashamed that they just want to hide away. Some want to stop work. Others do not tell their nearest and dearest and lose out on the support (and 'wise counsel') family members can provide. Some doctors in our service, have gone through months of GMC investigations and a full FtP tribunal, only telling their loved one once erased. This is a great burden for any individual.

> Get emotional support from friends, family, colleagues or services specifically designed to help doctors.

A few weeks after attending the IOT, Tim was asked to attend two health assessments, both assessors were consultant psychiatrists. They were very much repetitions of each other (it was strange telling the same story twice in the same week). He had to tell the doctors what had happened, and they took a detailed mental health history from him, and organised blood and hair tests. These tests confirmed his prior drug use, and Tim received copies of the reports advising the GMC that he was probably fit to practise subject to restrictions on his registration, which were similar to the ones already imposed by the IOT.

Where health is suspected reports from two independent, but GMC-approved health assessors (these tend to be psychiatrists but other specialists such as occupational health doctors might carry out the assessments) will be arranged. These assessors will provide a report outlining their views on diagnosis as well as whether they believe the doctor is fit to practise, either generally or on a limited basis, and make recommendations for the management of the case. It is important to remember you have a choice whether you feel comfortable seeing the person allocated to assess you. If you have a personal or professional relationship with them (which is not uncommon) then you must let the GMC know as soon as possible. While it might seem obvious, the purpose of the consultation with the assessor is for them to furnish a report to the GMC. It is not to provide treatment, counselling or advice to the doctor. The psychiatrist might suggest you seek help if they are concerned about you, but that will be the limit of their duty of care.

The doctor's legal team may instruct their own psychiatrist at various procedural stages.

The GMC specifically asks the health assessors to provide a written opinion on a doctor's fitness to practise, by asking them to comment on whether the doctor:

- Is fit to practise without restriction.
- Is not fit to practise.
- Is not fit to practise except on a limited basis.
- Is not fit to practise except under medical supervision.
- Is not fit to practise except on a limited basis and under medical supervision.
- Suffers from a recurring or episodic condition that although in remission at the time of assessment, may be expected in future to render him/her unfit to practise, or unfit to practise except on a limited basis or under medical supervision or both.

In some cases where there are concerns about clinical practice (competence), the doctor will be invited to undergo a performance assessment.[7]

The time between receiving the Rule 4 letter and the outcome of the investigation can seem like an eternity (it is not unusual for the process to last 12–18 months, or even longer). Feelings of helplessness, hopelessness and isolation can be especially evident if the doctor is suspended from work. It is important to try and seek help – at least from someone who has been through a similar process.

The case examiners will consider all the evidence when deciding whether to progress a case to a tribunal, including the doctor's response to the Rule 4 letter and what they have done since the incident leading to the complaint. The case examiners will apply what is known as the 'realistic prospect' legal test. This means that only cases with a realistic prospect of establishing that the doctor's fitness to practise is sufficiently impaired to justify action on registration will be referred to an FtP tribunal. When the case examiners have nearly reached the end of their investigation, the GMC will send a Rule 7 letter to the doctor. This letter outlines the allegations and the evidence they have collected and the decisions that are available to the case examiners. The doctor is invited to respond in writing to the GMC, usually within 28 days (though an extension can be given in certain exceptional circumstances).

OUTCOMES OF THE CASE EXAMINERS' INVESTIGATION

A few weeks after the health assessments, Tim received a letter from the GMC inviting him to agree to undertakings. He called his lawyer, who explained that these are similar to the conditions that were placed on his registration by the IOT, but rather than be imposed he was invited to agree to them, which would conclude the investigation and halt the FtP investigation going any further. If he accepted the undertakings, then the prior conditions could be revoked, and he could continue to work. Although at first, he felt the undertakings were too onerous, he spoke to his treating doctor who explained that these safeguards may serve a helpful therapeutic purpose on his road to recovery, and that if he adhered to them, they would not be forever. They could be reviewed after a year or two, with a view to lifting them. He thought about it and agreed to accept them. He was however worried about the impact that they would have on his ability to secure a consultant post, but thought he'd cross that bridge when he came to it.

At conclusion of the investigation stage, the case examiners have a number of options open to them. These include taking no further action, issuing a warning or letter of advice. This will be a great relief to the doctor, and hopefully (s)he can resume their life where it was left off. If a warning is offered, a doctor may not wish to accept it, and can ask to be referred to the GMC's Investigation Committee. This committee can hear evidence, make a factual finding and decide if a warning is appropriate, or if the case should be concluded with no action. In exceptional circumstances, a GMC Investigation Committee can refer a case for FtP but only if new evidence has come to light during the hearing.

The GMC's case examiners can also agree **undertakings** with a doctor as an outcome of their investigation before inviting them to respond to allegations (the Rule 7 stage) if they feel any risk posed by an health condition can be safely mitigated with them in place. Undertakings are restrictions on practice (or behaviour) agreed between the doctor and the GMC. These may include restrictions to work in particular places or to no longer carry out particular procedures. In essence, they are 'promises' which, if broken, might lead to further sanctions. Undertakings can be agreed by the case examiners before a matter is referred to a tribunal; and after the tribunal has made a finding of impairment. It is not unusual for doctors with addiction issues to receive undertakings, which usually include the requirement to remain abstinent, attend treatment and, most likely, to work under supervision.

HEALTH AND FITNESS TO PRACTISE

Tim's case did not progress to an FtP tribunal as there were no other issues involved, such as dishonesty or performance issues. He had also showed insight and had begun to put in place strategies to avoid drug use happening again in the future.

18 months after accepting his undertakings, Tim remained well and abstinent from drug use. He continued to attend regular group meetings and engaged with his treating team. He was reviewed by GMC health assessors who noted his progress and his undertakings were subsequently lifted thereafter. Shortly after this, he applied for a consultant post and happily was successful. Tim continues to work as a consultant and remains well and importantly abstinent from drugs. He still attends group meetings. He was grateful for the advice and support he had received from the friends he had eventually been brave enough to tell, along with his legal and medical treating team. Looking back, he was not sure how he'd have got through the ordeal without their collective help.

As demonstrated by Tim, addiction, by **itself,** rarely results in doctors losing their job, let alone losing their licence to practise. This holds the same for other mental illnesses. For the vast majority, having an illness, physical or mental, has **no** effect on their ability to care for patients or do a job efficiently and effectively. However, it would be disingenuous to suggest that mental illness **never** interferes with work, especially if the doctor lacks insight. Cognitive impairment – due for example, to neurodegenerative diseases, alcohol or drug intoxication, or even due to severe depression – can impact on the ability to make correct and timely clinical decisions. Some mental illnesses might cause problems indirectly through diminishing the public's confidence in the medical profession, for example a doctor who shoplifts in order to fund their drug habit. The GMC states that fitness to practise might be brought into question if it appears that:

> the doctor has a serious medical condition (including an addiction to drugs or alcohol); and the doctor does not appear to be following appropriate medical advice about modifying his or her practice as necessary in order to minimise the risk to patients.[8]

They also add that:

> There is no need for GMC intervention if there is no risk to patients or to public confidence because a doctor with a health issue has insight into the extent of their condition and is seeking appropriate treatment, following the advice of their treating physicians and/or occupational health departments in relation to their work, and restricting their practice appropriately.[9]

In the most part, as long as the doctor is following professional advice, and not putting patients at risk, even serious illness does not need to be disclosed to the regulator. It is only where illness overlaps with performance and/or pro-fessional conduct that regulatory involvement might be required. This would be either as the condition requires restrictions on the doctor's practice, or that their illness is associated with other conduct or performance issues. Doctors are often surprised to discover that the GMC formally assesses only a small number of health cases per year.[10] For example, in 2016, this was 187, and 51 doctors self-referred.[2,10] These tend to be where ill health blurs into misconduct (such as drink driving) or poor performance, and as such affects the doctor's fitness to practise.

The following table gives examples of the potential impact on performance and conduct of a doctor, based on our experience at Practitioner Health.

Mental illness	Potential impact on performance	Potential impact on conduct
Psychotic illness	Lack of insight Poor concentration	Inappropriate behaviour with patient Boundary violation/disinhibited behaviour

Drug misuse	Intoxication Unreliable attendance at work	Buying illegal drugs for personal use Dealing in illegal drugs Theft to fund habit Theft of drugs from employer Prescription fraud Self-prescribing Public disorder Domestic violence Fraud Possession of drugs Drug driving
Borderline personality disorder	Unpredictable behaviour	Disruptive behaviour Boundary violations
Depression	Depressed cognition, not able to think clearly, tiredness, unreliable attendance, clinical errors, lack of empathy/interest	Poor time keeping Poor record keeping Sleeping at work Self-prescribing

If the GMC receives a complaint that involves a health issues, the chances of it progressing beyond the early stages is dependent on a number of factors. The GMC help in this regard.[11] If one or more 'positive' indicators are present it will improve the chances of the case **not** progressing further than the triage stage. Such considerations include the following:

- The type and severity of the mental illness is unlikely to affect a doctor's fitness to practise or pose a material risk to patients.
- No evidence that the mental illness has had a significant impact on performance or conduct to date.
- Evidence that the doctor has insight; the doctor is receiving appropriate support or treatment, or local employers/supervisors are aware of the issues and able to provide support.
- The doctor is in stable, long-term work or training or works only in appropriately supervised environments.
- Where necessary, the doctor has agreed to restrict their working practices in line with any advice given.
- If necessary, the doctor is not working.
- There are no relevant other fitness-to-practise issues or past history.

There are some situations, where irrespective of any underlying health problem, the case will progress to full investigation and to a FtP tribunal. These include:

- Where there is a serious performance or conduct issue.
- Where the doctor has been convicted or cautioned.
- Where the doctor is not following advice of a treating clinician or appears to lack insight.

The GMC has to investigate these incidents for reasons of public safety and confidence. Details of the doctor's health are kept confidential by the GMC, and references to ill health are heard in private session. In transcripts, issues that relate to health are redacted, as are any undertakings or conditions that refer to a health issue (for example, the requirement to undergo drug testing). Most of the health cases investigated by the GMC are due to substance misuse and the majority of these are related to alcohol misuse, such that between 2014 and 2018 of the 401 doctors investigated by the GMC for substance misuse, alcohol misuse made up 57% of the cases (most of these would have come to light following a drink drive offence). The remainder involved opioids (11%), cannabis (6%), sedatives and hypnotics (6%), cocaine and stimulants (8%), multiple (11%) and other (1%).[12] Of the doctors investigated during this five-year period, 91% did not progress to a FtP tribunal and at the end of the investigation stage, the outcomes were:

- Undertakings (57%).
- Closure (25%).
- Warning (16%).
- Advice (2%).

Overall, only 9% of referrals ended in an FtP tribunal (for the years 2014–2018 this was 34 doctors). If a doctor reaches this stage the chances of a more serious outcome increases, such that 90% had restrictions on their practice, including conditions (21%), suspension (60%) and three doctors (10%), were erased. Remember these percentages are only of those that reach an FtP tribunal. This should be reassuring to doctors, as over the five years very few doctors with referrals involving substance misuse received a serious sanction and where they did there was concomitant serious misconduct (such as theft or fraud).

In our service, over the period 2008–2018, 430 patients have been involved in FtP processes, with the number reducing each year since 2008. During the first year, 33% of all new patients had some sort of regulatory involvement. This figure dropped to just over 5% by year ten (2018) and averaged 11% over the ten years (2008–2018). We hope that the reduction over the years is a result of doctors coming for treatment earlier, before their problem has begun to cause difficulties at work.

Doctors with mental illness actually need not fear the regulator, though many do. Showing insight, seeking appropriate help and following the advice of their treating clinicians means that for the vast majority of doctors the GMC **need not be involved at all**, especially where there is no impact on patient care. Even if the GMC is involved, where there is a health issue alone, **the outcome is generally**

very good. For the vast majority of doctors with mental illness they can present for care and receive treatment with no involvement of anyone other than their treating clinicians.

FITNESS TO PRACTISE (FTP) TRIBUNAL

Tim's case did not go to a FtP tribunal. FtP tribunals are held by the MPTS. During this period, it is vital that the doctor prepares well. This can be very difficult, and many will just want to avoid any reminder that they are in this nightmare and want to hide away. Only a very small percentage of original complaints, (less than 3% in 2018) are referred for a full FtP tribunal. These cases will include the most serious allegations, where if they were to be found proven, are likely to result in action being taken on the doctor's registration. These types of cases tend to fall within five main headings:

- Sexual assault or indecency.
- Violence.
- Improper sexual or emotional relationship with a patient or someone close to the patient.
- Dishonesty.
- Knowingly practising without a licence.

Registrants are expected to attend tribunals at the MPTS though every year many do not or are not represented by lawyers. There is a significant overlap between non-attendance at a tribunal and not having legal representation. Not being represented will reduce the chances of a better outcome, though in some cases, the doctor might see the writing on the wall and wish to protect themselves from an inevitable conclusion and not attend. All else being equal, personal characteristics and first place of qualification were unrelated to the seriousness of regulatory outcomes in the UK. Instead, engagement (attendance and legal representation), nature of the allegation and referral source were importantly associated with outcomes.[13]

The level of proof applied at a tribunal is lower than for criminal cases; as such, the GMC do not have to prove their case against the doctor beyond reasonable doubt but instead on the balance of probabilities (the threshold required in civil cases). This means that the GMC have to prove that the case against a doctor is more likely than not to have occurred.

During a FtP tribunal the panel will hear evidence from both sides (from the GMC and from the doctor's side), before embarking on a three-stage process:

- **Fact finding**: The panel will hear evidence and decide whether the allegations have been proven. If the allegations are proven, they will move to the second stage.
- **Impairment**: The panel will consider if the doctor's fitness to practise is impaired. Essentially, this involves deciding whether action needs to be taken

against the doctor's registration. If the panel decides that the doctor's fitness to practise is impaired, they will move to the third stage.

- **Sanctions**: The panel will refer to the GMC's Indicative Sanction Guidance, which provides guidance about appropriate sanctions.

If fitness to practise is found to be impaired, the panel will decide on the sanction that should be applied to the doctor's registration. In doing so, they have to place protection of patients, public confidence in the medical profession and the need to uphold standards of medical practice at the forefront of their thoughts. The tribunal may take into account mitigating factors such as a demonstration of insight by the doctor and any steps that they have taken to address the problem. Evidence of this may be provided through testimonials from colleagues, patients and others. The FtP tribunal can take the following actions:

- Suspend a doctor from the medical register.
- Erase a doctor from the medical register.
- Place conditions on the doctor's registration.
- Agree undertakings with the doctor.
- Give a warning.
- Decide to take no further action.

The MPTS publishes its sanction guidance for panel members.[14] It is worth reading, not just for explanation of the different sanctions that can be applied, but also as it gives an indication of what might lead the panel to choose one over another and help the doctor steer their case to a more favourable outcome.

Outcome of medical practitioner tribunals in 2014–18:

	2014	2015	2016	2017	2018
Erasure	71	72	70	62	65*
Suspension	86	95	93	76	101
Conditions	22	24	17	13	25
Undertakings	3	1	0	0	0
No Impairment -Warning	10	6	11	13	10
Impairment – No further action	4	2	2	4	2
No Impairment	37	38	34	27	41**
Voluntary Erasure	4	1	2	0	3
Total	237	239	229	195	247

* This figure does not include an additional 14 erasures by MPT review tribunals in 2018.
** This figure includes Order Expired from New and Review tribunals.

CONDITIONS AND SUSPENSION

Suspension might be the outcome if the Tribunal feel the doctor's performance is such as to impose a risk to patients. Otherwise, conditions are usually imposed. Typical conditions require a doctor to obtain further supervised training, to have a mentor and, if health is the issue, to receive and adhere to treatment.

Conditions are meant to impose safeguards on the doctor's practice in order to protect patients and also to provide an overall rehabilitative package for the practitioner. The doctor must inform his or her employer (and prospective employers) of the conditions, which need to be in place before any future work can be undertaken, to obtain reports from the mentor and supervisor and to provide evidence at a resumed tribunal that the conditions have been met. Failure to meet the conditions could result in further sanctions being applied.

ERASURE

While the numbers are low (only between 60–80 doctors per year of the 8,000–9,000 referred to the GMC end up with their licence-to-practice being removed), erasure has shattering implications for the individual doctor concerned. International regulatory information sharing agreements means that the doctor will unable to work in many jurisdictions across the world. Some doctors we meet in our service are expecting erasure as the final outcome, for others it comes as complete surprise and shock when told the determination at the end of their tribunal.

Doctors can apply for restoration of their registration after five years. There is no automatic 'ticket of return' and the doctor will have to present their case to a Tribunal and demonstrate that they have insight and have dealt with the issues that led to erasure, have up-to-date medical knowledge and skills, and can safely return to unrestricted practice. The process of restoration onto the GMC register is explained on their website.[15] It is a long hard journey, but it can be achieved. This is a personal story of a doctor, whose name was erased and who fought hard to get himself back onto the register:

> *My instinct to live was greater than that of death and my first task was to focus on my health and get better. Ultimately, I was able to accept my alcoholism by realising that it had led to a catastrophic chain of events, including a spell in intensive care with a stroke that has left me permanently disabled. I was determined to go on living and thriving and restore myself onto the medical register. I found the restoration process itself to be an incredibly rewarding process, as I was forced to confront how and why my entire life had become so publicly and dramatically de-railed by my illness. But it also enabled me to be forced to recognise that I had turned my life around. The journey back has been hard and complicated. More so for me as my disability (I have had a stroke) meant that it was not easy for me to focus for long periods of time. However, with the help of my legal team,*

psychiatrist and intense determination, after 12 years I finally received my licence to practise again. I am deeply ashamed of the consequences of my illness, but I am quite content at my attempts of personal and professional rehabilitation in the years that followed from it.

For a doctor to have their name restored, it is not enough just to 'have served the time'. They will need to demonstrate that they have reflected on the reasons why they were erased (and accept the findings) and kept up to date, ideally undertaking unpaid clinical attachments where they are able to observe clinics/operations/services. This can be very difficult to arrange, and even more so if the doctor was not in a managed system (such as a partnership, training rotation or consultant post). Ultimately the GMC need to be reassured that you are in a fit state to be performing safely on their register of medical professionals if restored. Around 20 doctors per year apply to have their name restored, and approximately four succeed.

CONCLUSION

Doctors who receive a referral might feel that the dice are stacked against them and that a negative outcome will be inevitable. We have shown in this chapter is that this is not the case. Less than 2% of doctors who have a case opened against them end up with a serious sanction (erasure or conditions).[16] The two variables that will affect the outcome are the **nature of the complaint** and the **level of engagement** the doctor has with the whole process.

Doctors often fear that if they have made a medical error that the GMC then investigates, this signals the end of their career and they catastrophise. Again, this is not true. The GMC are well aware that medical errors occur and that the system we work in is an imperfect one. As long as the doctor deals with the medical error in an open, honest and reflective fashion, demonstrating learning for future practice then it is unlikely that the case will progress to a FtP tribunal. This is of course if the doctor isn't making repeated errors, which may indicate a real performance issue. In our experience, the cases that tend to 'have legs' at the GMC are those where the doctor's honesty and integrity are seriously called into question.

Where sole mental health and addiction issues are concerned, FtP outcomes are generally positive; it is usually the process itself that can make doctors more unwell because of the associated distress. As a result, the GMC have made huge improvements to their FtP procedures in recent times to ensure that doctors suffering with health conditions are treated with more compassion and understanding. Our service strives to work with the GMC to make sure this continues and to consider any other changes to the system that can be made to provide a kinder, fairer journey for doctors suffering with mental illness.

REFERENCES

1   General Medical Council. Fitness to practise statistics 2018. Available from: www.gmc-uk.org/-/media/documents/fitness-to-practise-statistics-report-2018_pdf-80514861.pdf.

2 General Medical Council. The state of medical education and practice in the UK [Internet]. General Medical Council, 2018. Available from: www.gmc-uk.org/about/what-we-do-and-why/data-and-research/the-state-of-medical-education-and-practice-in-the-uk.

3 General Medical Council. Guidance on conducting and deciding the outcome of single clinical incident provisional enquiries [Internet]. Available from: www.gmc-uk.org/-/media/documents/dc11439-deciding-the-outcome-of-sci-pes_pdf-75558315.pdf.

4 General Medical Council. Guidance for decision makers in applying the five-year rule [Internet]. 2020. Available from: www.gmc-uk.org/-/media/documents/dc12553--guidance-for-decision-makers-on-the-five-year-rule--external-_pdf-82134517.pdf.

5 Doctors Defence Service – UK. GMC/MPTS Interim Orders (IOT) Hearings Representation [Internet]. Doctorsdefenceservice.com. [cited 18 January 2020]. Available from: https://doctorsdefenceservice.com/gmc-interim-orders-iot-hearings-representation.

6 Medical Practitioners Tribunal Service. Taking interim orders into account: supplementary guidance to the Sanctions guidance [Internet]. Available from: www.mpts-uk.org/-/media/mpts-documents/DC10553___Taking_interim_orders_into_account.pdf_72188146.pdf.

7 Doctors Defence Service – UK. GMC Performance Assessment Law [Internet]. Doctorsdefenceservice.com. [cited 18 January 2020]. Available from: https://doctorsdefenceservice.com/gmc-performance-assessment/.

8 General Medical Council. The meaning of fitness to practise [Internet]. 2014. Available from: www.gmc-uk.org/-/media/documents/DC4591_The_meaning_of_fitness_to_practise_25416562.pdf.

9 General Medial Council. Guidance on thresholds [Internet]. 2018. Available from: www.gmc-uk.org/-/media/documents/dc4528-guidance-gmc-thresholds_pdf-48163325.pdf.

10 General Medical Council. How we work with doctors with health concerns [Internet]. Medical professionalism and regulation in the UK. 2017 [cited 8 November 2019]. Available from: gmcuk.wordpress.com/2017/09/12/how-we-work-with-doctors-with-health-concerns.

11 General Medical Council. Guidance for decision makers on assessing risk in cases involving health concerns [Internet]. 2018. Available from: www.gmc-uk.org/-/media/documents/dc4315-health-concerns---assessing-risk---guidance-for-decision-makers-48690195.pdf.

12 Freedom of Information to GMC, 2019.

13 Caballero J, Brown S. Engagement, not personal characteristics, was associated with the seriousness of regulatory adjudication decisions about physicians: a cross-sectional study. *BMC Med* 2019;**17**(1):211.

14 Medical Practitioners Tribunal Service. Sanctions guidance for members of medical practitioners tribunals and for the General Medical Council's decision makers [Internet]. 2019. Available from: www.mpts-uk.org/-/media/mpts-documents/dc4198-sanctions-guidance--november-2019_pdf-80152538.pdf.

15 General Medical Council. Restore your registration [Internet]. Available from: www.gmc-uk.org/registration-and-licensing/managing-your-registration/changing-your-status-on-the-register/restoration-to-the-register.
16 Tomkins C. Should doctors fear the regulator? [Internet]. Mdujournal.themdu.com. 2019 [cited 18 January 2020]. Available from: https://mdujournal.themdu.com/issue-archive/autumn-2019/should-doctors-fear-the-regulator.

27

Improving the Outcome of a Serious Investigation

CLARE GERADA AND ZAID AL-NAJJAR

Nothing written here should replace professional legal advice.

Where a doctor finds themselves the subject of a serious complaint, disciplinary process or investigation, this chapter aims to help them prepare them for a reasonable defence.

INTRODUCTION

Many of the doctors who come to us for help do so because they have had a serious complaint or referral to the GMC, and as a consequence feel as if the bottom has fallen out of their world. Some become depressed, others anxious and others just want to disappear. Sadly, some do kill themselves before they come to us for help. Despite being highly intelligent and, until now, competent problem solvers, they feel there is nothing they can do to influence their 'certain fate of erasure from the medical register'. There is a lot that the individual doctor **can** do, and their fate is far from sealed. As we have mentioned before, less than 2% of complaints to the GMC end in a doctor getting a serious sanction. However, being the subject of a disciplinary investigation or serious complaint is very painful for the individual concerned. It is an understatement to say that each day, as the investigation or complaint progresses slowly through its course, is anxiety laden. This is an absolutely normal reaction. It would be highly unusual not to feel anything but worried. From the moment when the envelope arrives on the doormat or the email marked 'confidential' into the in-box, to the final determination, a nerve-wracking experience unfolds, and some see their professional career unravel before their eyes. The most important issue here, is to accept that this is a normal response to an abnormal (as in out of the ordinary) experience. This chapter is as much for the individual doctor passing through the process as it is for their relatives and loved ones, who want to support them during the process. As a relative, try not to reassure (this rarely helps), instead just be there, support, love and help in practical ways, such as in drafting responses.

THE PROCESS

The vast majority of doctors want to do their best for patients and receiving notice of a complaint feels like a personal attack. Having been subject to complaints both authors of this chapter know that, no matter how trivial or unfounded they are, they always jar and are never quite forgotten, no matter how much time goes by. They are scars on our professionalism. Colleagues have described receiving notice that they are under a GMC investigation as similar to receiving a diagnosis of a serious, perhaps incurable, illness. One doctor said it was easier to receive her diagnosis of breast cancer than it was to get the letter saying she had missed tuberculosis in a patient.

A doctor's initial response is often similar to the stages of a bereavement and, as with death, can feel extremely painful and shocking. The first stage of shock is often followed by denial ('this can't be happening to me'), closely followed by feelings of anger, shame and fear. Doctors experience a sense of isolation and failure, believing they are the only ones who have ever received a complaint. You are not alone. **Many thousands of doctors receive a complaint against them, every year** and **the risk of a serious sanction is very small**.

Complaints lead to an increase in the risk of depression, anxiety, suicidal thoughts and sometimes, even suicide.[1] Ask anyone who has been subject to an official complaint, and the cognitive reaction is very often one of catastrophising, '*I am going to be struck off*'.

Being referred to the regulator can also leave the individual caught in an all-enveloping and highly confusing vortex, especially hard for individuals used to being in control. The psychiatrist Max Henderson and colleagues conducted a study of mentally ill doctors' experiences of being involved in a GMC investigation.[2] The title of their paper was *You feel you've been bad, not ill: sick doctors' experiences of interactions with the General Medical Council*, which aptly described how the doctors they interviewed felt about the process.

If the complaint is serious, be prepared for a long haul, as serious complaints can lead to 'multiple jeopardy' as different organisations, including the employer, regulator, coroner or criminal justice system, completes their own processes, and each can take many months to reach conclusion.

Be prepared to do a lot of extra work in responding to the various processes that have been triggered due to the complaint, not least meeting up with your legal team, writing responses, reading information sent to you and so on. Create dedicated time, muster the support from family, friends and colleagues. Remember, it is normal to feel anxious. This is a highly stressful, unpredictable and bewildering time.

The barrister Stephen McCaffrey has summarised his view of why a GMC referral in particular feels so personally traumatic for doctors.[3] He writes that the investigations:

- Are lengthy: the median time from the complaint arriving at the GMC to conclusion at a Fitness-to-Practise (FtP) tribunal is around 107 weeks.[4]
- Are highly public processes with determinations published online.
- Are legalistic, adversarial and inquisitional.
- Change your practice, and not necessarily for the better.
- Overly lenient decisions can be appealed to the High Court.

The GMC are aware of the problems their processes can cause and in recent years have revised them to reduce unnecessary or excess anxiety. This includes changing the tone of their letters, making sure batches are not all sent on the same day, training their staff to interact in a compassionate and sensitive manner and shortening their processes. They have also begun a process of transformation, acknowledging the need to support doctors under pressure. These changes are already making an understandably stressful process less stressful.

At all stages of a complaint, from first receiving notice that you are under investigation to attending a FtP tribunal or inquest, get professional help. A problem shared really is a problem halved. Even if you are an experienced doctor who is used to handling tricky issues at work, you are not a lawyer. This might also be the first time you have received a complaint. Medical defence organisations do this for a living every day and they know what to do. Draw on their expertise, earlier rather than later. They can help guide you through the process to ensure you get the best outcome possible. Talking it through with them will also give you a reality check as to how serious this might be for you (or not). Seeking psychological help is something doctors in this position should seriously consider given the increased risk of depression and suicide.[5]

Presented below are some of the specific outcomes that might follow a GMC investigation and how the doctor might feel or respond at these stages.

SUSPENSION

Part of the process of investigation might include being suspended from work. This is hard given how integral work is to a doctor's sense of identity and they should be prepared for (and apologies for the cliché) a roller-coaster set of emotions. In the main, there are **three** situations where a doctor can be suspended from work:

- Exclusion from the workplace, often referred to as a 'neutral-act', while an employer carries out investigations into a complaint or a serious incident. A doctor can also have restrictions on the work they can do, for example not operating while allowing the doctor to be present on-site for limited administrative duties.
- Suspended by an Interim Order Tribunal (IOT) pending completion of a GMC investigation.
- As a sanction by the GMC following an FtP tribunal.

These are all formal suspensions.

Suspension by employers can also be informal, so called 'gardening leave'. This is where the doctor is asked to work at home or from another location. The use of 'gardening leave' can lead to more confusion and a sense of being in limbo, without rights or a clear pathway of action or time scale.[6] Far from feeling like a neutral act, rather it might seem that you are being found guilty before being proven innocent, and an act of punishment.

Exclusion from the workplace can be perceived as being unfair because doctors are suspended before proof of culpability or being allowed an opportunity to respond to any allegations. It can, however, be justified as a necessary and proportionate intervention to maintain patient safety. For a clinician, exclusion often results in reduced self-esteem and disturbing emotions. Wendy Savage, an obstetrician, was suspended following complaints about her clinical practice. She described:

> The loss of my job was like a bereavement. Powerful, confusing and shifting emotions swept over me – disbelief (can this really be happening?), sadness, guilt, self-doubt and anger.[7]

If a doctor is unable to work this adds financial insecurity to an already intolerable situation as many provide the main income for their family. Writing in a British Medical Association report, an overseas qualified doctor was referred to the GMC for investigation and suspended. This doctor wrote a personal view called *Stand by me: surviving a GMC investigation*. He writes:

> I was extremely anxious, and we were short of money. Each day we were thinking about what we were going to eat. We would go to the nearest shop in the evening, just before they closed and buy the cheapest bread on reduction. We went to Tesco and checked everything on sale. My wife and I would only drink water.

During this time, his sense of shame and stigma was so intense that he felt unable to speak to anyone or confide in friends or family back home about the troubles he faced. He stopped phoning his friends because he didn't know what to tell them. He also stopped going to church as he didn't have money for petrol, and he felt too ashamed to tell anyone about what had happened.[8] This doctor exemplifies the problems with suspension: isolation, fear, shame, financial insecurity, stigma and loss of confidence.

SUPPORT FOR EXCLUDED DOCTORS

As before, if you are suspended and unable to work, get as much psychological support as you can. As well as individual support there are groups available for doctors who are suspended or have had their licence revoked.[9] They can provide psychological support and practical advice on how to prepare for hearings or seek work while suspended.

FINDING INTERIM EMPLOYMENT

Doctors might need to seek alternative work that does not require medical registration and a licence to practise. It is striking how often a doctor will assume that
because they cannot work as a doctor that they cannot work in any other capacity. But this is not true. We all have a host of transferable skills: we are able
to lead teams, make decisions under pressure, are excellent communicators, have
good written and IT skills and a host of other competencies. Voluntary work is
another option open to the suspended doctor. One of the alternative career groups
is 'Medic Footprints'.[10]

It is unlikely the income through alternative employment will be as high as
working as a doctor, so at the earliest stage, even though it is very difficult to do
so, it is important to make arrangements if the doctor has large debts or expenses
(for example, mortgage repayments, school fees). Despite being high earners,
doctors tend also to spend a lot and can have limited savings. The medical charities
can offer financial support and initial enquiries can be made via a single access
portal.[11] The lack of funds may mean needing to apply for state benefits, which can
be daunting and painfully difficult for an individual.

PRESS INTEREST

In some higher profile cases, there may be press interest and it is important that
the doctor does not navigate this tricky area alone. Defence organisations and professional bodies will have access to advice on handling media interest and may
issue statements on behalf of the doctor so again, it is important to seek help if
necessary. In the main, if approached by a journalist, do not say *'no comment'*
which often looks bad. It is better to take their details and questions that they
want answered and seek advice about a response once there has been time to consider them properly. The Press will usually only be interested on the first (and
possibly last) day of any trial or tribunal. At worst, the Press might even try to
'doorstep' you, if there is a fine line perceived within the media between genuine
justice and entertainment. On the street, try not to run pass the press or cover your
head. Instead, wearing a smart, but neutral suit, keep your head high and walk at
a normal pace, looking straight ahead into an imaginary object in the distance.

ERASURE

Erasure is a rare outcome. Even the word 'erasure' brings to mind finality and eradi-
cation. It is a horrible word to describe a very painful situation that the doctor is
now confronting. One moment they are 'a doctor' with all the status and trappings
this role brings, the next, they are a disgraced individual, removed from their professional community and shamed in front of their peers and personal community.
It is however important not to lose hope as this doctor testifies:

> A rapidly worsening alcohol dependence syndrome left the GMC with the
> only option, I had to be removed from the GMC register. 'Erasure' is a highly

emotive term. It is, in a nutshell total removal from a list of professionals who can practise medicine legally. I suppose the term itself is intended to sound bad, to engender a sense of shame or guilt. It also made me feel a sense of immense stigma, absolute 'social death', otherness and of being an 'outsider'. At worst, I associated it with hatred, which I have experienced by some previous colleagues, particularly cruel if, as I was, are suffering from a life-threatening illness such as severe substance misuse disorder. The term 'erasure' implies finality, but the thing to remember about erasure is that some doctors go on, in fact, to become restored onto the medical register, as I did after more than eight years. These doctors need support, not least in dealing with a deeply traumatic emotional situation but also in being rehabilitated into a profession they probably never fell out of love with.

HOW TO IMPROVE THE CHANCES OF A GOOD OUTCOME

This section assumes that there is substance to the complaint and provides some help for the doctor to improve their chances of a more favourable outcome.

Stop digging holes

The Law of Holes is an adage that states 'if you find yourself in a hole, stop digging'; if you keep digging you will make the hole deeper and therefore harder to get back out of, that is when in an untenable position, it is best to **stop** carrying on and exacerbating the situation.

This applies to any doctor who has found themselves the subject of a complaint or investigation. Stopping digging, put your spade down and get out of the hole. Stop doing anything that will make your case worse than it might already be. The natural temptation after receiving a complaint might be to fire off a 'knee-jerk' response, formulated in anger and frustration. Don't. Put the response in the 'draft box' and come back to it the next day or maybe even three days later, when the initial feelings of anger and frustration have settled down and you can approach it more rationally and with a clear head. In the meantime, get help.

Get the first bit right

While it is always better to engage constructively in the process, this does not mean relinquishing your rights to be kept informed or to be treated fairly by the complainant. Being fairly treated means being given the time to respond appropriately. We are aware of doctors being informed of a complaint at the end of a long shift and summoned to meetings at short notice with officials and asked to give a response there and then. Such meetings can usually wait. The doctor is often tired and emotional and should be given time to seek advice and even be accompanied to meetings. How the first stages are responded to can have a major influence on what happens later. Making hasty admissions at the end of a long shift or when you haven't thought through the facts can have serious implications further down track. The person asking the questions might be in a hurry for you to 'tell them what happened' but statements cannot be rushed or given when the doctor is not thinking clearly. Neither can any promises of confidentiality be honoured. We have experience of doctors who, following the death of a patient, have blamed themselves completely (this is a natural emotion), when in fact this was not the case. This is what happened to Hadiza Bawa-Garba, a doctor who was eventually given a suspended prison sentence having been found guilty of Gross Negligent Manslaughter following the death of a child, Jack. While she clearly played a role, by all accounts there was a series of significant system errors that contributed to his death.[12] A week after his death, while still trying to process what had happened on her watch, Bawa-Garba was told to meet her consultant in the hospital canteen. She was told to list everything that she could have done differently and to share her personal reflective process with the consultant. She later wrote:

> I was beating myself up about every single detail and obviously wishing that I had recognised sepsis, so we spoke about that and I was very open and explained everything. It contained what I felt I could've done better plus some of the things that [the consultant] also felt that I could've done better.[12]

At the meeting, the consultant took notes, which he then transferred to her training encounter form, and Bawa-Garba was asked to sign this as a true reflection of their discussion. Given that this case involved the unexpected death of a child, natural justice would dictate that the doctor should be protected in what they say at the risk of implicating themselves for something they may not be fully or partly responsible for. We see this sort of issue in less tragic cases. For example, a doctor might be caught stealing an ampoule from the anaesthetic room and when 'summoned' to explain themselves they 'over admit', in as much that in their guilt and shame they confess to haven taken more drugs than they have done.

The more serious the issue, the more important it is to be prepared, rested, supported and informed than to turn up tired, frightened and alone. Seek as much information as to what the meeting is about, and then call your defence organisation, solicitor or Trade Union to speak about next steps before attending. No one can criticise you for doing this. Depending on the seriousness of the complaint, such meetings can be very important and influence how the complaint progresses and even the final outcome for the doctor.

Saying sorry

Offering an apology, does not in itself amount to an admission of negligence or breach of statutory duty and, as soon as possible after being made aware that something has gone wrong, the doctor should seek out the patient or their family to say sorry and acknowledge what has happened. Honesty is always the best policy. In Chapter 26, we provided some examples where doctors' fate appeared to be sealed by lying, trying to cover up the initial transgression. Being open and honest and apologising if something has gone wrong, rather than covering up, is always the best approach.

Insight, reflection, remediation

In our experience, engaging in any investigatory process or responding to complaints involves **three processes**:

- Demonstrating **insight**.
- **Reflecting** on the harm or impact of the action.
- Undergoing **remediation** to prevent recurrence.

These three are all interconnected and will require time and support to be done properly. Even if there appears to be no substance to the complaint, it is important that the individual thinks about these three critical areas.

> Even where a doctor does not admit to all or some of the allegations made about them, they should still work through the process of demonstrating insight, reflecting on the allegations and putting in place any possible remedial action.

Doctors who can show insight into the impact of their actions on patients and the profession more widely, who have expressed regret and apologised, who have undergone appropriate reflective learning with an expressed commitment to do better and who (ideally) have evidence of improved practice are less likely to have sanctions taken on their registration. This is borne out by cases heard at FtP tribunals relating to conduct and performance. Of 60 cases in which the doctor apologised or had remediated since the event, 5% were erased from the GMC register. In contrast, where the panel considered that the doctor had not demonstrated insight, 59% were erased. Remediation is an effective way to demonstrate insight.[13,14]

Insight requires reflection and reflection in turn, usually leads to greater insight and so on. They are part of the same process. True reflection can be a painful process, as it means exploring all aspects of oneself, including values, personality, relationships with significant others and shortcomings.

Insight

Insight is the capacity to gain an accurate and deep understanding of someone or something. Crucially it is worth noting some misunderstandings about insight. It does not necessarily mean accepting blame or admitting to having done something, but includes why others might think this to be the case. It also does not mean not defending oneself.

A place to start in demonstrating insight is to consider the following questions:

- What happened (in detail)?
- What were the circumstances, and what were you thinking/feeling at the time?
- Who else was involved?

- What were the factors leading up to event?
- Were there any other factors involved?
- What was the duration?
- What role did I play?
- What were the outcomes?

A doctor is likely to lack insight if they: refuse to apologise or accept mistakes; do not demonstrate they are thinking about what happened; and fail to tell the truth at any stage.

Reflection

There are different models to draw upon when reflecting on an event. The GMC have published a useful document on reflective practice for all doctors, *What? So what? Now what?* Framework.[15] What is important is that the doctor thinks about the impact of events from **all** perspectives. Also think about the impact under the domains of the GMC's *Good Medical Practice*, and where one's actions might be out of kilter with what is required from a doctor. It maybe that no harm has *actually been done*, but it is still worth considering each in turn.

- Impact on patients.
- Impact on the profession.
- Harm to the public.
- Harm to my organisation.
- Harm to others.

Given how much should be included under the heading 'reflection', it is easy to see how this process takes time. Done well, it can be a powerful process at the very least and can also be helpful in preparing the case. A good reflective piece of writing will assist the doctor when they have to give evidence. Where possible, any reflective writing should be supported by evidence.

Remediation

Remediation follows on from reflection. It is the process by which a doctor aims to redress aspects of poor practice, misconduct or a health issue.

Even at an early stage of a referral to the GMC or receipt of a complaint, remediation can have a significant impact on the overall outcome, irrespective of whether this is a health case or a case involving serious misconduct. We consider that remediation involves answering the following questions:

- What have I done to address the current issue that has led me to being referred to the GMC or complaint made against me?
- What will I do to prevent the same thing happening again?

How one answers these **two** questions largely depends on *why* one has been referred to the GMC in the first place. For example, if the case is one involving addiction then remediation means engaging in treatment, attending peer support groups such as Alcoholic Anonymous or the doctors' specific equivalent, the British Doctors and Dentists Group, and explaining how future management of any on-going condition or relapse will be managed.

For doctors with sexual boundary or probity issues, attending a 'boundaries course', undertaking training in medical ethics or engaging with a mentor, counsellor or personal tutor to talk through and understand the issues that contributed to the misconduct may also help.

The doctor needs to demonstrate understanding behind their behaviour, not just make a record of it. All too often the latter is done, but not the former. The doctor also needs to think about, and record what they would do in the future if they were to get into difficulties again. For a doctor with mental illness, it might be ensuring that they are registered with a general practitioner, engaging in psychotherapy, attending self-help or therapy groups and recruiting family members or friends to help. It is not enough merely to attend courses; the doctor has to make detailed reflections on the courses undertaken and what their learning is.

Examining cases on the GMC website of doctors who have appeared in an FtP tribunal shows how much importance is put by the panel members on insight, reflection and remediation. Demonstrating **all three** can make the difference between a doctor receiving a lesser sanction or erasure. The whole process of demonstrating insight, reflecting and engaging in remediation can be very painful as it will inevitably mean examining one's sense of purpose, values and desires. True reflection takes time and psychological energy. We suggest that this is done with a mentor, supervisor, partner or counsellor, wherever possible.

We are grateful to my patient and volunteer group, many of whom have been through disciplinary processes for their advice on how to prepare themselves after a referral to the GMC (or any disciplinary action). This is what they advise:

- **Recognition/realisation**: Something has happened that poses such a risk to patients, public or profession, which has meant the GMC has had to take action. Simply denying the complaint might suggest a lack insight, which will be held against you if the facts find your fitness to practice is impaired.
- **Remorse**: Not just feeling sorry for yourself but genuine regret for the damage you may have caused to patients, partners, public confidence and the reputation of the profession.
- **Reflection**: Going over what happened, what was done and why, what you would do differently.
- **Remedy**: What can be done to repair the damage, improve performance, safeguard against recurrence and change behaviour?
- **Reassurance**: What evidence can be offered or will be collected to confirm that practice/performance/behaviour has improved, and that improvement will be maintained?

Making admissions of dishonesty

If doctors *know* that they have been dishonest (for example, stealing prescriptions, shop lifting, working when on sick leave, altering a curriculum vitae or faking a reference) then it is better to admit this. Dishonesty is the most common reason why doctors receive a harsh sanction from the GMC, as all professional regulators despise dishonesty offences. If a doctor is persistently dishonest or tries to cover up their actions, they are likely to be erased from the register. Admitting dishonesty obviously needs to be done with care, and doctors are advised to take legal advice before making admissions to any charges.

We are indebted to one of our patients for sharing with us his journey from referral to suspension. It is important to keep hopeful as you negotiate what is a complicated maze if you are subject to a GMC investigation. The GMC are only trying to fulfil their functions as specified by statute law.

A reflective journey (written by a member of my Patient and Volunteer Group)

This doctor was suspended for 12 months having already been suspended for 12 months pending the Tribunal. He had provided a dishonest medical report. The piece gives an honest description of what 'reflection' meant to this doctor and the hope it created in the process:

> When a patient reported me to the GMC for having completed a private medical report dishonestly, I felt my whole world implode. I know it sounds like a cliché but in a moment your life really does change completely. The patient was an undercover journalist. Within a few days I was in a national newspaper. A few days later, I was asked to attend a GMC and suspended with immediate effect. I remember the depressing journey back home wondering how I would break the news to my family. I sat in the dark that evening and cried for what seemed like hours and the feelings of shame, guilt and how I had disappointed everyone around me were immense. I had let down my family, patients, colleagues and the medical profession.
>
> When a doctor who previously has led a frenetic life is now rendered idle it leaves a massive gap and a void that feels vast. I did not know what to do. I felt frightened, alone and for the first time in my life I had no purpose. I began visiting my mosque every day, something I had not done for years. While there a patient approached me and said he had heard about what had happened to me and was sorry. He then told me to say, 'Alhamdulillah', which means 'All praise be to Allah (God)'. He said what had happened had brought me back to my faith. That moment was an epiphany and I began my journey of reflection and remediation.
>
> I want to share what I learnt about myself.
>
> My purpose as a doctor was to help people get better; to heal them, take away their pain, prolong their healthy lives but with my dishonest medical report, I had

betrayed these principles. A map started to unfold, and I engaged in mentorship with senior colleagues, attended courses, clinics as an observer and wrote reams of personal reflection. I studied tribunal outcomes and realised the doctors who returned to practice were the ones who showed insight, expressed remorse and regret and provided evidence to the panel of their positive changes, and this is what I set out to do, as honestly and carefully as possible. The process was hard, it was also humiliating. I sat with medical students observing clinics or with previous colleagues when attending courses. I withdrew from my social circles essentially to avoid answering that terribly common question 'what do you do? I wanted to avoid that subject. The whole process has scared me for life, I will never be the same. I discovered who my true friends were. I was lucky in that most colleagues supported me and wrote supportive testimonials but there were some who shunned me completely, which was hurtful. In all of my self-pity I began to realise that I had done this to myself and I deserved what I was going through. I attended the Tribunal and was suspended for another 12 months, (remember time spent suspended is not included in any sanction post Tribunal). I was relieved not to have been erased.

However, the next 12 months were challenging as I had to keep my mind strong and focussed to prevent slipping into depression. It is easy to lose hope with the long process. There were times I felt so isolated and thought I would not make it and just wanted to die. But I kept going. My resilience was tested to the limits. I think my faith and support from family and colleagues got me through. As time went by and my remediation folder grew with all the work I was doing, and I was approaching my review hearing I was surprised as to how much I had grown as a person. I had reflected upon my multiple roles as a doctor, husband, parent, son, brother, friend, colleague. I had let down so many people I would never be able to walk away from that responsibility. At my review hearing, I was allowed back to medicine with immediate effect. I felt so grateful and yet so exhausted. My determination had paid off and I was reminded that if I had quit or lost hope it would have been all over. I want to spread the message that doctors in a similar position are not alone. How strange, that my journey has been for a purpose – to help others get better. Yes, I wanted to help patients; but doctors are also patients and they need help too.

REFERENCES

1 Bourne T, Wynants L, Peters M, et al. The impact of complaints procedures on the welfare, health and clinical practise of 7926 doctors in the UK: a cross-sectional survey. BMJ Open 2015;5(1):e006687.
2 Brooks S, Del Busso L, Chalder T, et al. You feel you've been bad, not ill: sick doctors' experiences of interactions with the General Medical Council. BMJ Open 2014;4(7):e005537.

3 GMC Fitness to Practise Investigations: 15 things you can do today to protect your medical licence and registration – Fitness to Practise Guide [Internet]. [cited 18 January 2020]. Available from: www.fitnesstopractise.uk/gmc.

4 Professional Standards Authority. Annual review of performance 2016/17: General Medical Council [Internet]. Available from: www.professional standards.org.uk/docs/default-source/publications/performance-reviews/performance-review-gmc-2016-17.pdf.

5 BMA. Doctor support service [Internet]. Bma.org.uk. 2019 [cited 18 January 2020]. Available from: www.bma.org.uk/advice/work-life-support/your-wellbeing/doctor-support-service.

6 Empey D. Suspension of doctors. *BMJ* 2004;**328**(7433):181–2.

7 Savage W. A Savage Inquiry. London: Virago, 1986.

8 BMA. Stand by me: surviving a GMC investigation [Internet]. Bma.org.uk. 2018 [cited 18 January 2020]. Available from: www.bma.org.uk/news/2015/february/stand-by-me-surviving-a-gmc-investigation.

9 Doctors' Support Group. Suspended doctors [Internet]. Doctors' Support Group. 2006 [cited 18 January 2020]. Available from: https://doctorssupportgroup.com/suspended-doctors.

10 Medic Footprints. Alternative careers for doctors [Internet]. Medic Footprints [cited 19 January 2020]. Available from: https://medicfootprints.org.

11 Help me I'm a Doctor. Financial help for doctors and their dependents [Internet]. [cited 18 January 2020]. Available from: www.doctorshelp.org.uk.

12 www.bbc.co.uk/news/resources/idt-sh/the_struck_off_doctor.

13 DJS Research Ltd. Analysis of cases resulting in doctors being erased or suspended from the medical register Report prepared for: General Medical Council [Internet]. 2015. Available from: www.gmc-uk.org/-/media/documents/analysis-of-cases-resulting-in-doctors-being-suspended-or-erased-from-the-medical-register--63534317.pdf.

14 General Medical Council. The state of medical education and practice in the UK [Internet]. 2018. Available from: www.gmc-uk.org/about/what-we-do-and-why/data-and-research/the-state-of-medical-education-and-practice-in-the-uk.

15 General Medical Council. The reflective practitioner – guidance for doctors and medical students [Internet]. Gmc-uk.org. 2019 [cited 9 November 2019]. Available from: www.gmc-uk.org/education/standards-guidance-and-curricula/guidance/reflective-practice/the-reflective-practitioner---guidance-for-doctors-and-medical-students.

AFTERWORD

You may notice a common theme in this book, which is make sure you get help.

Although some of the outcomes of these processes and their impact can be life changing, the organisations set up to help doctors can make a real difference to the experience and the end result. Whether seeking advice because a journalist has contacted you for a news story or accessing Practitioner Health (www.practitionerhealth.nhs.uk) as it has all just got too much, it is important to know that you don't have to go it alone. There are many dedicated people out there who are ready to help. The most important message is that although this is a tremendously difficult time, others are, and have been, in the same situation, and they have, and you can, come out the other end and get back to work and normality. Make sure you are receiving as much emotional, medical and financial support as possible throughout the process, especially now as we enter the inevitable second wave of the Covid-10 pandemic. Now is not a time to hide away in shame but instead to reach out to friends and loved ones for support. After all, you would do the same for them if they found themselves in similar circumstances.

Finally, I would like to thank again all those practitioners who have crossed over the threshold from professional to patient. I thank you for your commitment to your own patients and your trust in my service. Thank you again to those who helped me write this book – to Shibley Rahman who read it in the early stages, to all those who contributed chapters, to Jo Koster from Routledge/CRC Press, to the Doctors in Distress team (especially Anne, Marie, Roma, Bertie, Amandip, Suzanne) who help me with my charitable work and to my partners and Rylla at the Hurley Group who have been with me through thick and thin.

Index

Note: Page numbers in **bold** refer to tables and those in *italic* refer to figures.

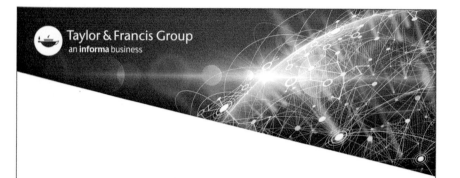